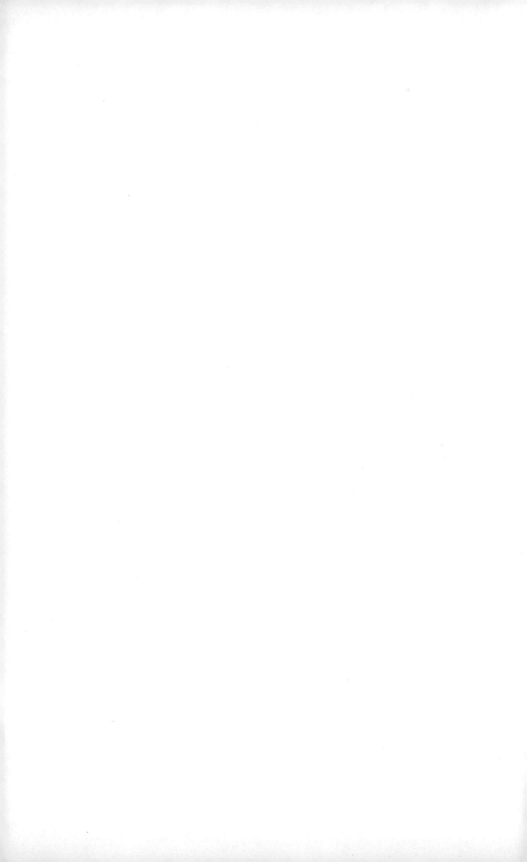

Digestive Disorders of the Abomasum and Intestines

Editors

ROBERT J. CALLAN
MEREDYTH L. JONES

VETERINARY CLINICS OF NORTH AMERICA: FOOD ANIMAL PRACTICE

www.vetfood.theclinics.com

Consulting Editor
ROBERT A. SMITH

March 2018 • Volume 34 • Number 1

ELSEVIER

1600 John F. Kennedy Boulevard ● Suite 1800 ● Philadelphia, Pennsylvania, 19103-2899

http://www.vetfood.theclinics.com

VETERINARY CLINICS OF NORTH AMERICA: FOOD ANIMAL PRACTICE Volume 34, Number 1
March 2018 ISSN 0749-0720, ISBN-13: 978-0-323-58178-3

Editor: Colleen Dietzler
Developmental Editor: Meredith Madeira

Photocopying
Single photocopies of single articles may be made for personal use as allowed by national copyright laws. Permission of the Publisher and payment of a fee is required for all other photocopying, including multiple or systematic copying, copying for advertising or promotional purposes, resale, and all forms of document delivery. Special rates are available for educational institutions that wish to make photocopies for non-profit educational classroom use. For information on how to seek permission visit www.elsevier.com/permissions or call: (+44) 1865 843830 (UK)/(+1) 215 239 3804 (USA).

Derivative Works
Subscribers may reproduce tables of contents or prepare lists of articles including abstracts for internal circulation within their institutions. Permission of the Publisher is required for resale or distribution outside the institution. Permission of the Publisher is required for all other derivative works, including compilations and translations (please consult www.elsevier.com/permissions).

Electronic Storage or Usage
Permission of the Publisher is required to store or use electronically any material contained in this periodical, including any article or part of an article (please consult www.elsevier.com/permissions). Except as outlined above, no part of this publication may be reproduced, stored in a retrieval system or transmitted in any form or by any means, electronic, mechanical, photocopying, recording or otherwise, without prior written permission of the Publisher.

Notice
No responsibility is assumed by the Publisher for any injury and/or damage to persons or property as a matter of products liability, negligence or otherwise, or from any use or operation of any methods, products, instructions or ideas contained in the material herein. Because of rapid advances in the medical sciences, in particular, independent verification of diagnoses and drug dosages should be made.

Although all advertising material is expected to conform to ethical (medical) standards, inclusion in this publication does not constitute a guarantee or endorsement of the quality or value of such product or of the claims made of it by its manufacturer.

Veterinary Clinics of North America: Food Animal Practice (ISSN 0749-0720) is published in March, July, and November by Elsevier Inc., 360 Park Avenue South, New York, NY 10010-1710. Subscription prices are $250.00 per year (domestic individuals), $413.00 per year (domestic institutions), $100.00 per year (domestic students/residents), $276.00 per year (Canadian individuals), $545.00 per year (Canadian institutions), $335.00 per year (international individuals), $545.00 per year (international institutions), and $165.00 per year (international and Canadian students/residents). To receive student/resident rate, orders must be accompanied by name of affiliated institution, date of term, and the signature of program/residency coordinator on institution letterhead. *Clinics* subscription prices. All prices are subject to change without notice. **POSTMASTER:** Send address changes to *Veterinary Clinics of North America: Food Animal Practice*, Elsevier Health Sciences Division, Subscription Customer Service, 3251 Riverport Lane, Maryland Heights, MO 63043. Customer Service (orders, claims, online, change of address): Elsevier Health Sciences Division, Subscription **Customer Service, 3251 Riverport Lane, Maryland Heights, MO 63043. Tel: 1-800-654-2452 (U.S. and Canada); 314-447-8871 (ouside U.S. and Canada). Fax: 314-447-8029. E-mail: journalscustomerservice-usa@elsevier.com (for print support); journalsonlinesupport-usa@elsevier.com (for online support).**

Reprints. For copies of 100 or more, of articles in this publication, please contact the Commercial Reprints Department, Elsevier Inc., 360 Park Avenue South, New York, NY 10010-1710. Tel.: 212-633-3874; Fax: 212-633-3820; E-mail: reprints@elsevier.com.

Veterinary Clinics of North America: Food Animal Practice is covered in *Current Contents/Agriculture, Biology and Environmental Sciences, MEDLINE/PubMed (Index Medicus), and Excerpta Medica.*

Contributors

CONSULTING EDITOR

ROBERT A. SMITH, DVM, MS
Diplomate, American Board of Veterinary Practitioners; Veterinary Research and Consulting Services, LLC, Greeley, Colorado, USA

EDITORS

ROBERT J. CALLAN, DVM, MS, PhD
Diplomate, American College of Veterinary Internal Medicine; Professor, Livestock Medicine and Surgery, Department of Clinical Sciences, College of Veterinary Medicine & Biological Sciences, Colorado State University, Fort Collins, Colorado, USA

MEREDYTH L. JONES, DVM, MS
Associate Professor, Department of Large Animal Clinical Sciences, College of Veterinary Medicine & Biomedical Sciences, Texas A&M University, College Station, Texas, USA

AUTHORS

LUCIANO S. CAIXETA, DVM, PhD
Department of Clinical Sciences, Colorado State University, Fort Collins, Colorado, USA

ROBERT J. CALLAN, DVM, MS, PhD
Diplomate, American College of Veterinary Internal Medicine; Professor, Livestock Medicine and Surgery, Department of Clinical Sciences, College of Veterinary Medicine & Biological Sciences, Colorado State University, Fort Collins, Colorado, USA

CHRISTOPHER C.L. CHASE, DVM, MS, PhD
Diplomate, American College of Veterinary Microbiologists; Professor, Department of Veterinary and Biomedical Sciences, South Dakota State University, Brookings, South Dakota, USA

MUNASHE CHIGERWE, BVSc, MPH, PhD
Diplomate, American College of Veterinary Internal Medicine; Associate Professor of Livestock Medicine and Surgery, Department of Veterinary Medicine and Epidemiology, University of California, Davis, Davis, California, USA

THOMAS M. CRAIG, DVM, PhD
Diplomate, American College of Veterinary Microbiologists; Professor Emeritus, Department of Veterinary Pathobiology, Texas A&M University, College Station, Texas, USA

ANDRÉ DESROCHERS, DMV, MSc
Diplomate, American College of Veterinary Surgeons; Clinical Sciences Department of Université de Montréal, Saint-Hyacinthe, Québec, Canada

GILLES FECTEAU, DMV
Diplomate, American College of Veterinary Internal Medicine; Professor, Department of Clinical Sciences, Faculté de Médecine Vétérinaire, Université de Montréal, Saint-Hyacinthe, Québec, Canada

MARIE-EVE FECTEAU, DVM
Diplomate, American College of Veterinary Internal Medicine; Associate Professor of Food Animal Medicine and Surgery, Department of Clinical Studies-New Bolton Center, University of Pennsylvania School of Veterinary Medicine, Kennett Square, Pennsylvania, USA

DAVID FRANCOZ, DMV, MSc
Diplomate, American College of Veterinary Internal Medicine; Clinical Sciences Department of Université de Montréal, Saint-Hyacinthe, Québec, Canada

MEERA C. HELLER, DVM, PhD
Diplomate, American College of Veterinary Internal Medicine; Assistant Professor of Clinical Livestock Medicine and Surgery, Department of Veterinary Medicine and Epidemiology, University of California, Davis, Davis, California, USA

JULIA A. HERMAN, DVM, MS
Department of Clinical Sciences, Colorado State University, Fort Collins, Colorado, USA

CHELSEA L. HOLSCHBACH, DVM
Resident, Large Animal Medicine, Department of Medical Sciences, University of Wisconsin-Madison School of Veterinary Medicine, Madison, Wisconsin, USA

ALEXANDRA HUND, Dr med vet
Diplomate, European College of Bovine Health Management; Department for Farm Animals and Veterinary Public Health, University Clinic for Ruminants, University of Veterinary Medicine Vienna, Vienna, Austria

GREG W. JOHNSON, DVM
Cows Come First, LLC, Ithaca, New York, USA

SARAH TAMMY NICOLE KEETON, PhD, MS
Assist Faculty and House Officers with Research Endeavors, Department of Veterinary Clinical Sciences, School of Veterinary Medicine, Louisiana State University, Baton Rouge, Louisiana, USA

JESSICA A.A. McART, DVM, PhD
Department of Population Medicine and Diagnostic Sciences, Cornell University, Ithaca, New York, USA

CHRISTINE B. NAVARRE, DVM, MS
Diplomate, American College of Veterinary Internal Medicine; LSU AgCenter, School of Animal Sciences, Louisiana State University, Baton Rouge, Louisiana, USA

SYLVAIN NICHOLS, DMV, MS
Diplomate, American College of Veterinary Surgeons; Associate Professor, Department of Clinical Sciences, Faculté de Médecine Vétérinaire, Université de Montréal, Saint-Hyacinthe, Québec, Canada

SIMON F. PEEK, BVSc, PhD
Diplomate, American College of Veterinary Internal Medicine; Clinical Professor of Medicine, Department of Medical Sciences, University of Wisconsin-Madison School of Veterinary Medicine, Madison, Wisconsin, USA

KATHARINE M. SIMPSON, DVM, MS
Diplomate, American College of Veterinary Internal Medicine; Livestock Clinician, Livestock Medicine and Surgery, Department of Clinical Sciences, College of Veterinary Medicine & Biological Sciences, Colorado State University, Fort Collins, Colorado, USA

DAVID C. VAN METRE, DVM
Diplomate, American College of Veterinary Internal Medicine; Professor, Livestock Medicine and Surgery, Department of Clinical Sciences, College of Veterinary Medicine & Biological Sciences, Colorado State University, Fort Collins, Colorado, USA

THOMAS WITTEK, Prof Dr med vet
Diplomate, European College of Bovine Health Management; Department for Farm Animals and Veterinary Public Health, University Clinic for Ruminants, University of Veterinary Medicine Vienna, Vienna, Austria

Contents

In this article, key concepts important for enteric immunity are discussed. The gastrointestinal tract is the largest immune organ of the body. The mucosal barrier, the tight junctions, and the "kill zone," along with the gut mucosa and maintaining an "anti-inflammatory" state, are essential for "good gut health." The microbiome, the microorganisms in the gastrointestinal tract, which has more cells than the entire animal's body, is essential for immune development, immune response, and maximizing ruminant productivity. Direct-fed microbials aid in both microbiome stability "homeostasis" and immune function.

Acute abdomen is a term used to characterize an animal presented as an emergency, in a more or less severe critical state, and for which medical and possibly surgical treatment is necessary. To succeed, the clinician should use a systematic approach, have an excellent knowledge of the bovine abdominal anatomy, and have a good understanding of the pathophysiology of abdominal pain. Good clinical judgment, critical analysis, and good client communication skills are also essential. This article presents and discusses those necessary skills in the context of field practice.

Abomasal ulcers are frequent incidental findings in necropsies of domestic ruminants and South American Camelids (SAC) or in slaughter animals and are a frequent cause of death in the most affected group of cattle, veal calves. Their true prevalence and significance is unknown owing to limitations in diagnosing the condition in live animals. This article discusses the types of ulcers, possible causes of ulceration, and clinical consequences, symptoms, and differential diagnoses, as well as further diagnostics in cattle, small ruminants, and SAC. The limited treatment options and possibilities for prevention are reviewed.

A bovine practitioner should master abdominal exploratory surgery (laparotomy). Several gastrointestinal (GI) problems require surgical correction to save the animal's life and to keep it in production. This article reviews the

dairies presents new challenges to producers and veterinarians. No current discussion of bovine salmonellosis is complete without acknowledging the increasing public health concern. Increasing antimicrobial resistance among enteric pathogens brings the use of antimicrobials by veterinarians and producers under ever stricter scrutiny. This article provides a comprehensive review of *Salmonella* etiology, prevalence, pathogenesis, diagnostics, treatment, and control.

Katharine M. Simpson, Robert J. Callan, and David C. Van Metre

Clostridial abomasitis and enteritis are important alimentary diseases observed in all domestic ruminant species. These diseases most commonly result from overgrowth of *Clostridium perfringens* types A, B, C, D, and E with the associated release of bacterial exotoxins that result in necrosis of the abomasal or intestinal mucosa. *Clostridium difficile* may also be associated with enteritis in calves but is much less common than disease caused by *C perfringens*. This article reviews the causes, pathophysiology, clinical signs, diagnosis, treatment, and prevention of clostridial gastrointestinal diseases in ruminants. Particular emphasis is given to describing the various forms of disease and treatment of individual cases.

Thomas M. Craig

Disease caused by nematodes in the gastrointestinal tract of cattle has primarily economic impacts, and the effect of treatment is that cattle grow larger faster because of increased feed intake. The disease, control measures, and drugs used must be focused on for different ages and environments. Different drugs that specifically affect the parasites should be used and administered in a manner and time that accomplishes the best sustainable control. Management needs to ensure that at-risk animals are exposed to sufficient worms to stimulate their immunologic response but not overwhelm it.

Sarah Tammy Nicole Keeton and Christine B. Navarre

Coccidiosis is an important parasitic disease of young ruminant livestock caused by the protozoan parasite of the genus *Eimeria*. Infection with *Eimeria* can lead to subclinical production losses and clinical disease. The most common clinical sign is diarrhea. Control of coccidiosis in cattle, sheep, and goats is based on sound management, the use of preventive medications, and treatment of clinical cases as necessary.

Marie-Eve Fecteau

Paratuberculosis remains one of the most important diseases of cattle worldwide. In cattle, the disease is debilitating and is characterized by weight loss and chronic diarrhea in the later stages of infection. However, cattle in the subclinical stages of the disease often show decreased milk production and are at higher risk for development of other common production diseases. Infections with *Mycobacterium avium* ssp *paratuberculosis* are difficult to control because of long incubation periods, the absence of clinical signs until advanced stages of the disease, and the lack of completely reliable diagnostic methods in the preclinical stages of the disease.

VETERINARY CLINICS OF NORTH AMERICA: FOOD ANIMAL PRACTICE

THE CLINICS ARE NOW AVAILABLE ONLINE!
Access your subscription at:
www.theclinics.com

Preface

Digestive Disorders of the Abomasum and Intestines

 CrossMark

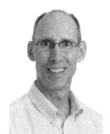 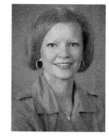

Robert J. Callan, DVM, MS, PhD   Meredyth L. Jones, DVM, MS

Editors

This issue follows the November 2017 *Veterinary Clinics of North America: Food Animal Practice* issue on Digestive Disorders of the Forestomach. Like the previous issue, it is an attempt to provide clinically relevant reviews on ruminant digestive disorders that are common, relevant, and yet still challenging to both new and seasoned veterinarians. In this issue, we continued with the theme to provide a mix of general and specific disease topics as well as both herd level and individual animal concepts. These articles also present comparative principles that exist between diseases in cattle, sheep, goats, and camelids where appropriate. This aspect of comparative medicine remains vital as we see both species and discipline specialization becoming more and more common in veterinary medicine.

Ruminants are susceptible to a wide range of infectious, parasitic, and morphologic disease of the abomasum and intestines. There are also important differences between the three major ruminant species of cattle, sheep, and goats, as well New World camelids. General clinical approaches may vary, but they all depend on thorough physical examination followed by appropriate ancillary diagnostic tests. This issue combines articles focused on general assessment of the ruminant abomasum and intestines with articles providing detailed review of the epidemiology, pathogenesis, diagnosis, and treatment of specific diseases. Given that many of the disease conditions are infectious in nature, we took this opportunity to include a review on enteric immunity. Surgical conditions of the abomasum and small intestine are also common, and a review of the most common surgical conditions is included in this issue and supports previous *Veterinary Clinics of North America: Food Animal Practice* issues on ruminant surgery. While individual animal disease identification and treatment are a cornerstone of food animal veterinary practice, they also provide the key disease observations that are the foundation of herd health management and production. Several of these intestinal disorders, including displaced abomasum, salmonellosis,

https://doi.org/10.1016/j.cvfa.2017.10.012
0749-0720/18/© 2017 Published by Elsevier Inc.
vetfood.theclinics.com

parasitism, and Johne's disease, were included because they have major herd health and public health implications.

The goal of this issue is to provide food animal practitioners with the most up-to-date information to help evaluate and treat both the individual animal and the herd health problems relevant to ruminant abomasal and intestinal disorders. We were fortunate to obtain some of the top researchers and clinicians in the field to provide these in-depth reviews of topics relevant to the practicing food animal veterinarian. It is our hope that this issue will broaden the practicing clinician's understanding of abomasal and intestinal diseases and provide useful approaches to the diagnosis, treatment, prevention, and herd management of these common and important disorders.

Robert J. Callan, DVM, MS, PhD
Department of Clinical Sciences
College of Veterinary Medicine and
Biomedical Sciences
Colorado State University
Fort Collins, CO 80523, USA

Meredyth L. Jones, DVM, MS
Department of Large Animal Clinical Sciences
College of Veterinary Medicine and
Biomedical Sciences
Texas A&M University
4475 TAMU
College Station, TX 77843, USA

E-mail addresses:
Robert.Callan@ColoState.edu (R.J. Callan)
MJones@cvm.tamu.edu (M.L. Jones)

Enteric Immunity
Happy Gut, Healthy Animal

 CrossMark

Christopher C.L. Chase, DVM, MS, PhD

KEYWORDS

- Bovine • Mucosal • Immunology • Enteric • Microbiome

KEY POINTS

- The largest organ of the immune system is the gastrointestinal (GI) mucosa, making the management of it essential for productivity and health.
- The barrier that consists of mucous, defensins, and immunoglobulin A is a "kill zone" to prevent microbial invasion of the GI epithelium.
- The enterocytes are key cells that maintain the "kill zone" and respond to metabolites and microbial components from the lumen and signals from immune cells to maintain tight junctions and prevent "leaky gut."
- Passive enteric immunity is essential for disease protection of the neonate; anti-inflammatory enteric response is essential disease protection for the growing and adult animal.
- Direct-fed microbials, including nutraceuticals, prebiotics, probiotics, and other dietary supplements, affect commensal "homeostasis" and mucosa immunity to maintain GI health.

INTRODUCTION

In the last decade, there has been an explosion of knowledge on the immune system with substantial implications for enteric health. This increase in knowledge revolves around the realization that the gastrointestinal (GI) tract is the largest immune organ of the body. It is understood that the mucosal immune system begins development in the fetus but does not become functional until epithelial cells of the mucosa in the neonate interact with microorganisms (microbiome) and/or their products in the gut lumen. The interaction between the epithelial cells and the microbiome is necessary for proper immune development, including immune system maturation, regulation, and maintenance of homeostasis. In this article, the interaction of immune system, microbiome, and the ability to maximize immunity are discussed.

Disclosure Statement: Dr C.C.L. Chase has received research funding and/or compensation for continuing education speaking events from Bayer Animal Health, Boehringer Ingelheim Vetmedica, Diamond V, Elanco Animal Health, Hipra, Merck Animal Health, Merial Animal Health, Novartis Animal Health, Zinpro, and Zoetis Animal Health.
Department of Veterinary and Biomedical Sciences, South Dakota State University, PO Box 2175, SAR Room 125, North Campus Drive, Brookings, SD 57007, USA
E-mail address: Christopher.Chase@sdstate.edu

vetfood.theclinics.com

ONTOGENY AND ORGANIZATION OF ENTERIC MUCOSAL SYSTEM

The bovine mucosal immune system prevents bacterial invasion and shapes the gut microbiota, whereas the gut microbiota influences immune system development. The fetal calf is predominately protected by the innate immune system (**Fig. 1**).[1] The innate immune response of phagocytic cells (neutrophils and macrophages) does not fully develop until late gestation and declines before gestation because of fetal cortisol levels.[2] Humoral elements such as complement are present but are at levels below that of the adult. Interferon can be induced in the fetus as early as 60 days of gestation.[3] All of the cellular components of the acquired immune response are present in the fetal calf.[4] The number of peripheral blood T cells dramatically decrease, beginning 1 month before birth of the calf, as they traffic and populate lymphoid tissues of the fetal calf before birth (decrease ~60% to 30% at birth). B cells are much lower in the developing fetus (1%–2%).[4,5] The enteric mucosal lymphoid organ system begins developing at 100 days of gestation when the mesenteric lymph nodes are present (**Fig. 2**).[6–8] The continuous ileal Peyer patch (IPP) (see **Fig. 2**) becomes quite active by day 85 of gestation.[9] The B lymphocytes present are almost exclusively immunoglobulin M (IgM)[+] cells, and if the IPP are removed, the animals remain deficient in B cells for at least 1 year because the IPP is the major source of the peripheral B-cell pool.[9] Because the IPP is the site of both proliferation and negative selection, IPP follicles can be inferred as the major site for generation of the preimmune B-cell repertoire in ruminants,[8–10] whereas the discreet Peyer patches (PPs), distributed throughout the jejunum, function as induction sites for the generation of IgA plasma cells (see **Fig. 2**).[10] The role of the rumen in mucosal immunity is unclear because there are few leukocytes in the developing rumen. The first few weeks after birth are essential for long-term enteric immunity as the expression of host microRNAs (miR), and the presence of commensal microorganisms determines long-term gut and host health.[11] By day 21 of age, there is a maximum induction of host miR by high levels of microorganisms of the microbiome.[11] These immune developments include induction of

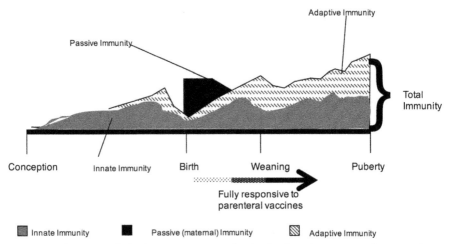

Fig. 1. Development of the immune response in the bovine: from conception to puberty. The calf's passive maternal immunity is only transferred after birth due to its unique placentation. (*Adapted from* Chase, Hurley DJ, Reber AJ, et al. Neonatal immune development in the calf and its impact on vaccine response. Vet Clin North Am Food Anim Pract 2008;24:88; with permission.)

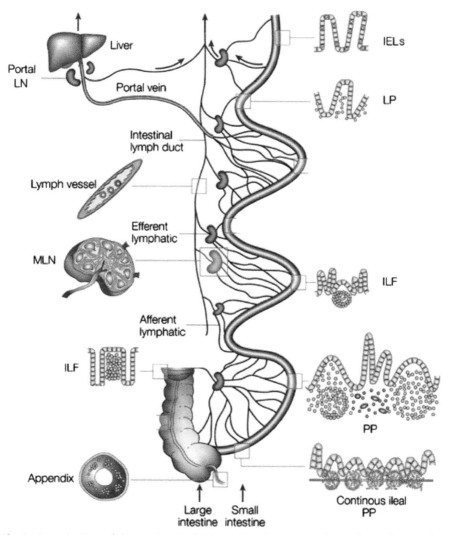

Fig. 2. Organization of the gut lymphoid tissue. Lymphocytes can leave the surface epithelium (intraepithelial lymphocytes [IEL]) or Lamina propria (LP) via draining afferent lymphatics to mesenteric lymph nodes (MLNs), or via portal blood reaching the liver where induction of tolerance occurs. The M cells in the follicle-associated epithelium of PPs transport antigen to prime B cells in the isolated lymphoid follicles (ILF) of the PPs of the jejunum, ileum, and the large intestine. The continuous IPPs are a primary lymphoid organ responsible for B-cell development. The IPP can be up to 2 m long and constitute 80% to 90% of the intestinal lymphoid tissue. LN, lymph node. (*Adapted from* Brandtzaeg P, Kiyono H, Pabst R, et al. Terminology: nomenclature of mucosa-associated lymphoid tissue. Mucosal Immunol 2008;1(1):35; with permission.)

tolerance to dietary components, reduction of mast cells that causes increased gut permeability, and decreased pathogen responses. Changes in diet in the early period of 7 to 21 days of age greatly influence microbiome and miR and therefore the level and longevity of the enteric immune response.[11,12]

COLOSTRUM AND ENTERIC IMMUNE DEVELOPMENT

Colostrum is composed of antibodies, cytokines, and cells. Antibody is the most important component of colostrum and provides an immediate source of antibody for the intestinal tract. Bovine colostrum contains ~55 mg/mL of total IgG (48 mg/mL IgG1, 3 mg/mL IgG2, and 4 mg/mL IgA).[13] Preparturient vaccination of the cow for enteric diseases, such as colibacillosis, *Clostridium perfringens*, cryptosporidiosis,[14] and rotaviruses,[15] results in production of pathogen-specific antibodies that provide protection for the neonate against severe disease. A second component of colostrum is cytokines.[16,17] These immunologic hormones help in the development of the fetal immune response. These cytokines are produced by the immune cells that traffic to the mammary gland. Interleukin 1-beta (IL-1β), IL-6, tumor necrosis factor alpha (TNF-α), and interferon-gamma are present in bovine colostrum and associated with a proinflammatory response and may help in the recruitment and development of neonatal lymphocytes into the gut to aid in normal immune development. Colostrum rapidly improves the ability of neutrophils to phagocytize bacteria, which is accomplished by absorption of proinflammatory cytokines.[18] Colostrum also contains high levels of the anti-inflammatory cytokines IL-10[19] and transforming growth factor beta (TGF-β)[20] that suppress local secretion of proinflammatory cytokines in the intestine to maintain tight junctions and also allow gut microbial colonization. The third component of colostrum is cells. Colostrum contains viable leukocytes in percentages similar to peripheral blood with more macrophages (40%–50%) and less lymphocytes (22%–25%) and neutrophils (25%–37%).[21,22] The vast majority of lymphocytes are T lymphocytes with less than 5% being B lymphocytes. Some of these maternal cells enter the circulation and reach peak levels 24 hours after birth.[23] Animals that receive colostrum containing maternal leukocytes develop gut antigen-presenting cells (APC; macrophages and dendritic cells [DC]) faster,[22] which is important because APCs are the keystone cell for the development of an acquired immune response to pathogens or vaccines. Additional pathogen-specific maternal T lymphocytes from vaccinated cows have been isolated from the neonatal calf with maximum proliferation at 1 day following birth.[24] The exact role of these cells in the long-term development of pathogen-specific mucosal-acquired immunity is not clear, because they are no longer detectable at 7 days of age.

FUNDAMENTALS OF ENTERIC IMMUNITY

The enteric mucosal immune system provides the first immune defense barrier for more than 90% of potential pathogens (**Figs. 3** and **4**). The gut mucosal immune system alone contains more than a trillion (10^{12}) lymphocytes and has a greater concentration of antibodies than other tissue in the body. It protects against harmful pathogens but also tolerize (induces tolerance) the immune system to dietary antigens and normal microbial flora. The components of the gut mucosal immune system are integrated together (see **Figs. 3** and **4**).[25] The health of the enterocytes, which are the epithelial cells that line the GI tract, is important not only for the growth and development of cattle, through secretion and absorption in the gut, but also to provide a first immune response to microorganisms (see **Fig. 4**). The goblet cells secrete mucous and mucins (the enterocytes also secrete mucins) that provide the initial mucous barrier (see **Fig. 4**).[26–29] The mucosal barrier contains defensins (also known as antimicrobial peptides [AMP] and host defense proteins [HDP]) produced by the enterocytes (see **Fig. 4**). Secretory immunoglobulin A (sIgA) is produced when dimeric IgA is secreted by the plasma cells in the lamina propria (LP) and is transported to the mucosal surface of the epithelial cell. The inner mucous layer along with the AMP

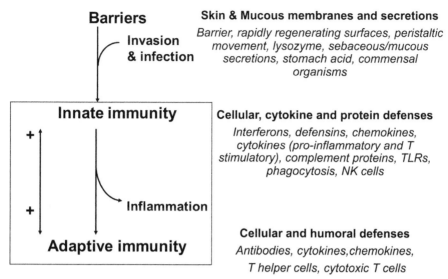

Barriers   **Skin & Mucous membranes and secretions**

Barrier, rapidly regenerating surfaces, peristaltic movement, lysozyme, sebaceous/mucous secretions, stomach acid, commensal organisms

Invasion & infection

Innate immunity   **Cellular, cytokine and protein defenses**

Interferons, defensins, chemokines, cytokines (pro-inflammatory and T stimulatory), complement proteins, TLRs, phagocytosis, NK cells

Inflammation

Adaptive immunity   **Cellular and humoral defenses**

Antibodies, cytokines, chemokines, T helper cells, cytotoxic T cells

Fig. 3. Gut immune responses: the barrier, innate, and adaptive immune components. (*Adapted with permission from* D. Topham, PhD, Rochester, NY.)

and sIgA forms a "kill zone" that few pathogens or commensals have evolved strategies to penetrate (see **Fig. 4**).[26] The "kill zone" along with the tight junctions that knit the enterocytes together forms a "barrier" against pathogens.

Once microorganisms breech the barriers, the innate immune system is the first responder to pathogen invasion. The system consists of white blood cells (macrophages, monocytes, DC, basophils, neutrophils, eosinophils, mast cells, and natural killer [NK] cells) (**Fig. 5**), complement, and the secreted immune system mediators, including chemokines and cytokines. These innate immune mediators include interferon, the proinflammatory mediators TNF-α, IL-1β, IL-6, macrophage inflammatory protein 1-alpha, and the anti-inflammatory mediator IL-10.[30] The innate response occurs in 2 waves. The first wave that occurs in the first few hours following damage or infection features the activation of macrophages, the major producer of proinflammatory cytokines that recruit other white blood cells and activate neutrophils, nonspecific killers of bacteria to increase killing of pathogens. If the proinflammatory response in the gut mucosa is excessive, "leaky gut" will occur (**Fig. 6A**).[31,32] The proinflammatory cytokines, particularly TNF-α, stimulate the myosin II regulatory light chain kinase (MLCK), which causes the tight junctions to break down so the epithelium becomes leaky (see **Fig. 6A**). Mucosa epithelium needs to be hyporesponsive under the influence of the anti-inflammatory cytokines[31] so healthy mucosa enterocytes will maintain tight junctions. A local increase of the anti-inflammatory cytokine IL-10 results in inhibition of the local proinflammatory response and increases eosinophils in the tissue. Cattle that are resistant to GI parasites like *Cooperia* and *Ostertagia* have an increase of both proinflammatory and anti-inflammatory mediators in the mucosa with a large influx of eosinophils into the tissue and lumen.[33] With only a proinflammatory response, there is little resolution of disease and enhanced collateral damage and immunopathology.[34] Immunopathology is seen in protozoal diseases like cryptosporidia, where localized neutrophilia is enhanced in young animals[34–36] and also has been hypothesized as the major contributor to the lesions of *C perfringens* alpha toxin.[37] The proinflammatory anti-inflammatory mucosal response increases with

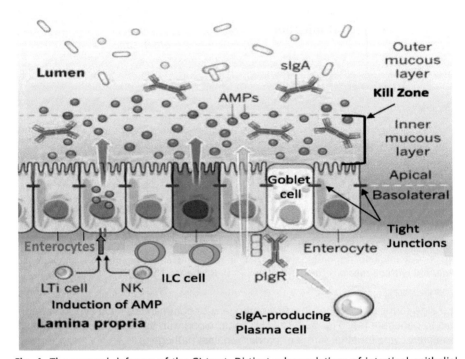

Fig. 4. The mucosal defenses of the GI tract. Distinct subpopulations of intestinal epithelial cells are integrated into a continuous, single-cell layer that is divided into apical and basolateral regions by tight junctions. Enterocytes sense the microbiota and their metabolites to induce the production of AMPs. Goblet cells produce mucin and mucous that is organized into a dense, more highly cross-linked inner proteoglycan gel that forms an adherent inner mucous layer, and a less densely cross-linked outer mucous layer. The outer layer is highly colonized by constituents of the microbiota. The inner mucous layer is largely impervious to bacterial colonization or penetration due to its high concentration of bactericidal AMPs, as well as commensals sIgA, which is moved from their basolateral surface, where it is bound by the polymeric Immunoglobulin receptor (pIgR), to the inner mucous layer. Responding to the microbiotal components, innate lymphoid cells (ILC), lymphoid tissue inducer cells (LTi), and NK produce cytokines, which stimulate AMP production and maintain the epithelial barrier. (*Adapted from* Maynard CL, Elson CO, Hatton RD, et al. Reciprocal interactions of the intestinal microbiota and immune system. Nature 2012;489:235; with permission.)

age and results in less disease. Neutrophils (see **Fig. 5**) also known as polymorphonuclear cells die after a short time at sites of inflammation. The hydrolytic enzymes are released and contribute to the inflammatory response and tissue destruction, which contributes to collateral damage and enhanced disease. Neutrophil granule proteins induce adhesion and emigration of inflammatory monocytes to the site of inflammation. Neutrophils also create extracellular defenses by the formation of neutrophil extracellular traps (NETs) (**Fig. 6B**).[38–40] The NET formation is induced by agents like bacterial aggregates and biofilms, fungal hyphae, and protozoan parasites (cryptosporidia, *Neospora*, and coccidiosis) that cannot be phagocytized.[35,36,41,42] Neutrophils use the potent oxidative metabolism system to kill bacteria. The NET reaction is one of the most potent bactericidal mechanisms of neutrophils and is

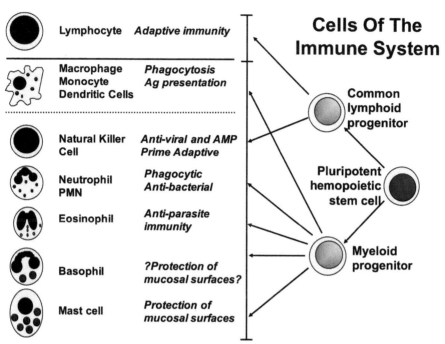

Fig. 5. The cells of the immune system. The innate and acquired immune cell lines have overlap with the macrophages and NK cells having important innate and acquired responses. Ag, antigen; PMN, polymorphonuclear cells. (*Adapted with permission from* D. Topham, PhD, Rochester, NY.)

potentially fungicidal, parasiticidal, and virucidal. The eosinophil is capable of the same phagocytic and metabolic functions as the neutrophils but focuses the host's defense against the tissue phase of parasitic infections (see **Fig. 5**). Eosinophils are more capable of exocytosis than phagocytosis; that is, rather than ingesting and killing small particles, they efficiently attach to and kill migrating parasites that are too large to be ingested. Eosinophils are also important in helping to control certain types of allergic responses. Basophils and mast cells (see **Fig. 5**) have been associated primarily with allergic reactions because of their binding of IgE. These cells have an important regulatory role. They release inflammatory mediators necessary for the activation of the acquired immune response.[43,44] Interferon, the last component of the innate response, sets up an immediate wall against virus infections. The second wave that occurs a day or 2 later is the NK cells (see **Fig. 5**) that enhance defensin production,[25,26] kill parasites,[35,36] and virally infect cells[45] but also produce cytokines to help the adaptive immune response.[45]

The adaptive phase occurs in the organized gut-associated lymphoid tissues (GALT) described above.[8] GALT is the initial induction site for mucosal immunity for antigens that are sampled from mucosal surfaces. The number and maturity of DCs and T cells in the GALT in the jejunum and ileum are very similar in the newborn and the weaned calf, indicating that the mucosal adaptive response is functional at birth.[46] The DCs are important because they are APCs that help in discriminating between dietary antigens, commensal microflora, and pathogens, and in providing a proper adaptive immune response with T cells.

These mucosal aggregates or follicles of B cells, T cells, and DCs are covered by epithelium that contains specialized epithelial cells called dome or M cells that are found

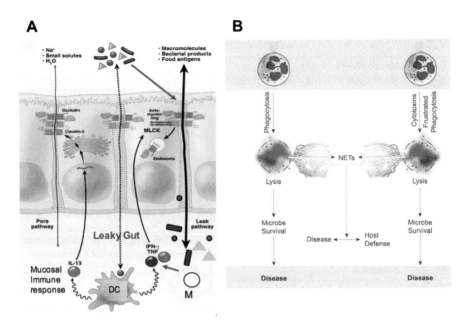

Fig. 6. Innate immunity and the mucosa. (*A*) Pathogenesis of leaky gut. The epithelial barrier normally restricts passage of luminal contents, including microbes and their products, but a small fraction of these materials do cross the tight junction. This diagram shows how DCs, and macrophages (M) react to these materials. These innate immune cells release cytokines that exert proinflammatory (TNF and interferon-gamma [IFN-γ]) and anti-inflammatory (IL-13) effects. If proinflammatory signals dominate and signal to the epithelium, MLCK can be activated to cause barrier dysfunction through the "leak pathway," allowing an increase in the amount of luminal material presented to immune cells. In the absence of appropriate immune regulation, immune activation may cause further proinflammatory immune activation, cytokine release, and barrier loss, resulting in a self-amplifying cycle that can result in disease. (*B*) Neutrophil collateral damage from NET formation. Neutrophil lysis after phagocytosis. Cytolysis can be programmed, for example, necroptosis, or caused by direct damage. Neutrophil lysis is caused by cytolytic toxins, pore-forming agents, physical injury, or frustrated phagocytosis. This can result in the formation of NETs during neutrophil lysis. Hydrolytic enzymes–DNA complexes are released in the NETs, enhancing the proinflammatory response and tissue destruction, contributing to collateral damage and disease. ([A] *Adapted from* Odenwald MA, Turner JR. Intestinal permeability defects: is it time to treat? Clin Gastroenterol Hepatol 2013;11(9):1078, with permission; and [B] Kobayashi SD, Malachowa N, DeLeo FR. Influence of microbes on neutrophil life and death. Front Cell Infect Microbiol 2017;7(4):159, with permission.)

in the GALT. These dome cells pinocytose antigen and transport it across the epithelial layer (**Fig. 7**).[47] The antigen may then be processed by APCs and presented to T and B lymphocytes; indeed, intestinal APCs play a central role in the induction and maintenance of mucosal immunity.[47] These follicles are organized like lymph nodes with T-cell areas and B-cell germinal centers.[7,46] The lymphocytes that emigrate from these organized areas into the surrounding LP are referred to as diffuse lymphocytes.[48] The hallmark of the mucosal immune system is that local stimulation will result in memory T and B cells in the nearby mucosal tissue but also in other mucosal tissues.

In the mucosal lymphoid tissues, mature T cells and B cells that have been stimulated by antigen and induced to switch to produce IgA will leave the submucosal lymphoid tissue and reenter the bloodstream.[49] These lymphocytes will exit the bloodstream through

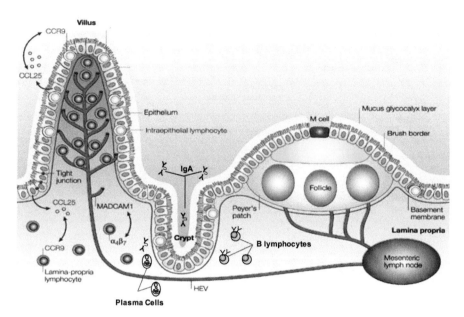

Fig. 7. Mucosal immune system of the gut epithelium. The LP contains scattered T cells and lies beneath the epithelium, which contains intraepithelial lymphocytes (IEL). B cells are scattered in the LP but are more frequent in the crypt regions along with plasma cells that produce IgA that is transported and secreted into the lumen. M cells facilitate antigen uptake and delivery to the organized lymphoid tissues. T cells activated in the PP and mesenteric lymph node express mucosa specific receptors, which interact with cell-adhesion molecules on the HEVs, assisting in homing these T cells to the mucosal LP. The chemokine CCL25 produced by epithelial cells recruits lymphocytes expressing CCR9 receptors to the LP. (*Adapted from* Cheroutre H, Madakamutil L. Acquired and natural memory T cells join forces at the mucosal front line. Nat Rev Immunol 2004;4(4):291; with permission.)

high endothelial venules (HEV) as described above and locate in the LP (see **Fig. 7**). B cells will differentiate into plasma cells that will secrete dimeric IgA. Many of these cells will return to the same mucosal surface from which they originated,[49] but others will be found at different mucosal surfaces throughout the body. The homing of lymphocytes to other mucosa-associated lymphoid tissue sites throughout the body is referred to as the "common mucosal immune system" (**Fig. 8**). Therefore, oral immunization can result in the migration of IgA precursor cells to the bronchi in the respiratory tract and subsequent secretion of IgA onto the bronchial mucosa.

MICROBIOME AND ENTERIC IMMUNITY

The microbiome is essential for immune development in the neonatal calf; then the microbiome-gut-immune-brain axis maintains the health of the calf.[50–53] As the calf develops, there is a "succession" of microbes that finally culminates in what is called a "climax" community that occurs as the gut transitions to an anaerobic environment.[50,54] Microbiome succession is influenced by nutrition, stress, and environment. This microbial community of commensals and their metabolites controls the health of the gut mucosa and the underlying immune cells in the LP (**Fig. 9**).[51,55] These

The "common mucosal immune system"

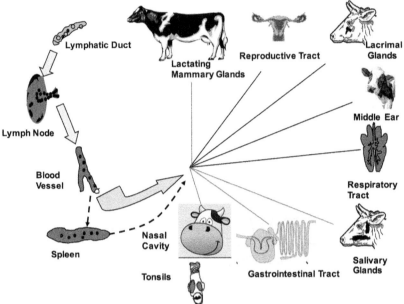

Fig. 8. Lymphocyte circulation and common mucosal immune system of the bovine. As illustrated on the left side of the figure, lymphocyte circulation with lymphocytes entering the lymph nodes by afferent lymphatics and exiting by efferent lymphatics. The common mucosal system involves the circulation of B and T cells between lymphoid tissues on mucosal surfaces.

commensal metabolites stimulate enterocytes to produce TGF-β, which is essential for the development of T-regulatory (Treg) lymphocytes that produce anti-inflammatory IL-10 (see **Fig. 9**). The microbial components in the microbiome also stimulate the enterocytes to produce serum amyloid A that stimulates DCs to activate another important mucosa regulatory T cell, T_H17 cells (see **Fig. 9**). These microbial metabolites also directly stimulate an NK-like cell, type 3 innate lymphoid cells to produce IL-22 to induce the enterocytes to produce more defensins (eg, REGIIIγ and REGIIIβ) (see **Fig. 9**). The composition of the microbiome varies by gut location with the numbers and diversity of populations being high in the rumen and increasing dramatically from the abomasum to the colon with the ileum being a key organ for microbial-immune development. These microbial communities (the microbiome) have evolved to help protect the animal by improving barrier and immune function; understanding the complexity of the gut microbial ecosystem is essential.[51,56]

The stress of weaning, co-mingling, and abrupt diet changes results in major microbial population shifts in the luminal microbial ecosystem, the microbiome. Stress lowers the defenses against pathogen entry, leading to increased risk of disease. Stress also leads to dysbiosis, the loss of good bacteria with an overgrowth of harmful organisms (**Fig. 10**).[57,58] However, dysbiosis is not just the loss of microbiome, it results in depletion of the "kill zone"(see **Fig. 4**); the mucous layer becomes thinner, and the amount of sIgA and defensins declines precipitously to allow the barrier to become weakened, allowing pathogens to interact with the mucosa and cause

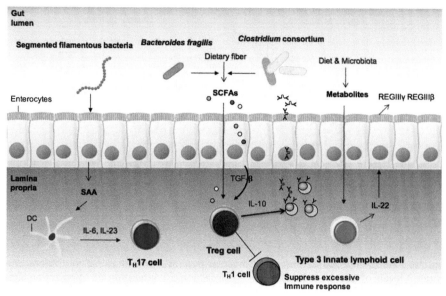

Fig. 9. Gut microbiota and their products shape the development of epithelial cells and immunity. Segmented filamentous bacteria (related to Clostridium) promote the production of serum amyloid A (SAA) protein from epithelial cells, which activates DCs to produce IL-6 and IL-23, resulting in the generation of Th17 cells that are important for T-cell development. *Clostridium consortium* and *Bacteroides fragilis* produce short chain fatty acids (SCFAs) from dietary carbohydrates that induce directly or indirectly by the production of TGF-β by the enterocytes the differentiation of Treg cells to enhance IgA production and to help minimize inflammatory response. Diet- or microbiota-derived metabolites upregulate the number of IL-22-secreting type 3 innate lymphoid cells (ILC3s) that induce the production of defensins (AMP/HDP-REGIIIβ and REGIIIγ) from epithelial cells. (*Adapted from* Kim, Yoo SA, Kim WU. Gut microbiota in autoimmunity: potential for clinical applications. Arch Pharm Res 2016;39:1568; with permission.)

disease. In addition, commensal organisms that help stimulate the mucosa to be anti-inflammatory are no longer available so tight junctions become weakened; "leaky gut" occurs, and pro-inflammatory responses occur that further weaken the gut epithelium (see **Fig. 6**A). One major factor leading to the dysbiosis and diarrhea that we can learn from pigs is low feed and water intake.[59] Dysbiosis is also associated with susceptibility to Johne disease.[60]

Homeostasis, "maintaining" a stable microbiome, is essential for good health and production. Oral antibiotics affect the microbiome homeostasis and therefore effect gut immunity and the incidence of disease. For example, the use of the antimicrobial bacitracin methylene disalicylate[61] altered the fecal microbial composition of calves by increasing the number of opportunistic pathogens such as *Escherichia*, *Enterococcus*, and *Shigella*, and decreasing beneficial bacteria. In another study, the microbiome population of *Lactobacillus* decreased with all antibiotic treatments, but the greatest reduction in *Lactobacillus* was observed with oxytetracycline, a broad-spectrum antibiotic.[61] To make things worse, the reduction of lactic acid–producing bacteria (*Lactobacillus*) during weaning raises intestinal pH, increasing disease susceptibility because low gut pH is bactericidal to *Escherichia coli*.[59] It takes weeks to months to return the microbiome populations back to normal following antibiotic treatment.

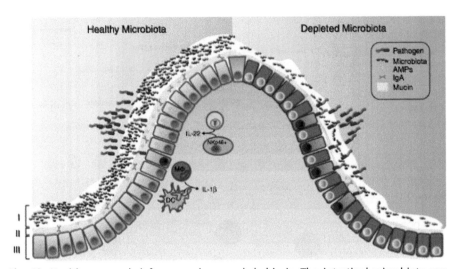

Fig. 10. Healthy mucosal defenses and mucosal dysbiosis. The intestinal microbiota promotes 3 levels of protection against enteric infection. (I) Saturation of colonization sites and competition for nutrients by the microbiota limit pathogen association with host tissue. (II) Kill zone: Commensal microbes prime barrier immunity by driving expression of mucin, IgA, and AMPs that further prevents pathogen contact with host mucosa. (III) Finally, the microbiota enhances immune responses to invading pathogens. Enhanced immune protection is achieved by promoting IL-22 expression by T cells and NK cells, which increases epithelial resistance against infection, as well as priming secretion of IL-1b by intestinal monocytes (MΦ) and DCs, which promotes recruitment of inflammatory cells into the site of infection. In conditions in which the microbiota is absent, there is reduced competition, barrier resistance, and immune defense against pathogen invasion. (*From* Khosravi A, Mazmanian SK. Disruption of the gut microbiome as a risk factor for microbial infections. Curr Opin Microbiol 2013;16(2):222; with permission.)

MAXIMIZING ENTERIC IMMUNITY: PASSIVE IMMUNITY, VACCINES, AND DIRECT-FED MICROBIALS

Passive immune therapy has been used for more than 50 years in calf enteric disease. Polyclonal antisera has been administered orally and/or subcutaneously to prevent/ treat bacterial diarrheal diseases colibacillosis and *C perfringens* type A and C with variable results.[62] One of the first successful uses of passive treatment was the oral administration of K-99 monoclonal antibody for the prevention/treatment of colibacillosis in calves.[63] Antirotavirus chicken egg yolk immunoglobulins fed in milk replacer decreased rotavirus diarrhea and enhanced rotavirus antibody-secreting cells.[64] Major success has been obtained by vaccinating cows before calving to enhance passive colostral antibodies for the protection of the calf against colibacillosis, *C perfringens* type C enterotoxemia, rotavirus, and coronavirus diarrhea.[62,65,66]

Both parenteral and mucosal vaccinations have been used to prevent enteric disease. Immune protection has been done indirectly by vaccinating the cow to obtain high levels of colostral antibodies for passive transfer to the calf against the neonatal diseases discussed above.[62,65,66] In the neonate, acquired immunity with parenteral vaccination of the neonatal calf has been used for *C perfringens* type C in herds wherein the disease occurs in calves older than 14 days of age.[62] Although oral and intranasal vaccines for rotavirus and coronavirus have the potential for active mucosal immunity in the neonatal calf (less than a week of age),[67] early onset of these diseases

(<14 days of age) along with the induction time for the immune response (7–10 days) makes efficacy poor in young calves (<14 days of age). Interestingly, oral coronavirus infections result in infection of both the enteric and the respiratory system[68] so coronavirus vaccines administered intranasal stimulated the common mucosal system and provided respiratory protection (see **Fig. 8**).[69] Several *Salmonella* vaccines: inactivated (whole cell; Rough mutants lacking oligosaccharide side chains (Re) mutant common core), MLV (genetically altered), and subunit (siderophores) vaccines have been licensed for parenteral administered but efficacy has been less then optimal.[70,71] A major problem with *Salmonella* vaccines has been adverse reactions. The off-label oral administration of MLV *Salmonella* vaccines also has variable efficacy.[70,72] There is a single *Mycobacterium avium subsp paratuberculosis* (MAP; paratuberculosis; Johne disease) vaccine available. The vaccine is efficacious and used in sheep.[73] The parenterally administered whole inactivated bacterin with Freund's adjuvant also produces cross-reactivity to both paratuberculosis and bovine tuberculosis tests.[74,75] These false positives interfere with national bovine tuberculosis eradication testing programs, which limits the use of the vaccine to approval by regulatory officials. Cross-reactivity is also a major deterrent for animal health companies to design new MAP vaccines for cattle.

Mucosal delivered vaccines have the advantage of not being affected by maternal antibody interference, being able to induce a response in neonates less than 7 days of age, and priming the common mucosal immune system (for example, oral coronavirus vaccination would provide specific coronavirus immunity to the respiratory mucosa).[67] The use of novel adjuvants with parenteral vaccines[76] that induce mucosal responses in addition to novel mucosal delivered adjuvants will also enhance enteric immunity.[77]

The area with the most opportunity that is also the least characterized is the use of direct-fed microbials to enhance enteric immunity and animal health while reducing antimicrobial usage.[78] Direct-fed microbials includes nutraceuticals, prebiotics, probiotics, and other dietary supplements. The effect of these direct-fed microbials on gut mucosal immunity and health has generated much interest.[50,51,54,56,61] Prebiotics (oligosaccharides, beta-glucan, and fiber), fiber metabolites (butyric acid and other short chain fatty acids), organic acids (ie, formic acid, citric acid), and botanicals (ie, vanilla, oregano, pepper oil) enhance the tight junctions in mucosal barrier and have an anti-inflammatory effect on mucosa (see **Fig. 9**).[79–82] Probiotics (ie, yeast, *Lactobacillus*, *Bifidobacteria*, and their metabolites) maintain microbiome homeostasis, increase secretory IgA, and decrease local inflammatory and APC responses to improve mucosal immunity (see **Fig. 9**).[83–88] This anti-inflammatory activity could have an impact on protozoal (eg, coccidia and cryptosporidia) and bacterial diseases (eg, *Salmonella* and Johne disease) where a proinflammatory response is part of the pathogenesis mechanism. Additional research needs to be done to further understand mechanisms and develop formulations that contain combinations of direct-fed microbials for different applications and age groups.

SUMMARY

The enteric mucosal immune system provides the first immune defense barrier for more than 90% of potential pathogens. The gut mucosal immune system alone contains more than a trillion (10^{12}) lymphocytes and has a greater concentration of antibodies than other tissue in the body. It protects against harmful pathogens but also induces immune system tolerance to dietary antigens and normal microbial flora. The health of the enterocytes, which are the epithelial cells that line the GI tract, is important not only for the growth and development of cattle, through secretion and absorption in the gut, but also to provide a first immune response to enteric microorganisms. The enterocytes maintain a "kill zone" barrier to keep out pathogens in concert with the commensal microorganisms (microbiome) and other cells of the immune system. The microbiome functions best when it is in a stable condition, "homeostasis." Disruptions in the microbiome's homeostasis result in dysbiosis, which decreases the "kill zone," allows "leaky gut," and increases inflammation. Increased inflammation is seen as an important part of pathogenesis of infectious diseases, including coccidia, cryptosporidia, C perfringens type A, Salmonella, and Johne disease. Maintaining microbiome homeostasis, the "kill zone," and the mucosa anti-inflammatory response are the keys to maintaining good gut and animal health and reducing antimicrobial usage.

REFERENCES

1. Chase C, Hurley DJ, Reber AJ. Neonatal immune development in the calf and its impact on vaccine response. Vet Clin North Am Food Anim Pract 2008;24(1): 87–104.
2. Barrington GM. Bovine neonatal immunology. Vet Clin North Am Food Anim Pract 2001;17:463–76.
3. Charleston B, Fray MD, Baigent S, et al. Establishment of persistent infection with non-cytopathic bovine viral diarrhoea virus in cattle is associated with a failure to induce type I interferon. J Gen Virol 2001;82:1893–7.
4. Wilson RA, Zonai A, Rudas P, et al. T-cell subsets in blood and lymphoid tissues obtained from fetal calves, maturing calves, and adult bovine. Vet Immunol Immunopath 1996;53:49–60.
5. Kampen AH, Olsen I, Tollersrud T, et al. Lymphocyte subpopulations and neutrophil function in calves during the first 6 months of life. Vet Immunol Immunopath 2006;113:53–63.
6. Schultz RD, Dunne HW, Heist CE. Ontogeny of the bovine immune response. Infect Immun 1973;7(6):981–91.
7. Brandtzaeg P, Kiyono H, Pabst R, et al. Terminology: nomenclature of mucosa-associated lymphoid tissue. Mucosal Immunol 2008;1(1):31–7.
8. Liebler-Tenorio EM, Pabst R. MALT structure and function in farm animals. Vet Res 2006;37(3):257–80.
9. Butler JE. Immunoglobulin diversity, B-cell and antibody repertoire development in large farm animals. Rev Sci Tech 1998;17(1):43–70.
10. Liang G, Malmuthuge N, Bao H, et al. Transcriptome analysis reveals regional and temporal differences in mucosal immune system development in the small intestine of neonatal calves. BMC Genomics 2016;17(1):602.
11. Liang G, Malmuthuge N, McFadden TB, et al. Potential regulatory role of microRNAs in the development of bovine gastrointestinal tract during early life. PLoS One 2014;9(3):e92592.
12. Liang G, Malmuthuge N, Guan LL, et al. Model systems to analyze the role of miRNAs and commensal microflora in bovine mucosal immune system development. Mol Immunol 2015;66(1):57–67.
13. Stelwagen K, Carpenter E, Haigh B, et al. Immune components of bovine colostrum and milk. J Anim Sci 2009;87(13 Suppl):3–9.
14. Perryman LE, Kapil SJ, Jones ML, et al. Protection of calves against cryptosporidiosis with immune bovine colostrum induced by a Cryptosporidium parvum recombinant protein. Vaccine 1999;17:2142–9.

15. Parreno V, Bejar C, Vagnozzi A, et al. Modulation by colostrum-acquired maternal antibodies of systemic and mucosal antibody responses to rotavirus in calves experimentally challenged with bovine rotavirus. Vet Immunol Immunopath 2004;100:7–24.

16. Hagiwara K, Katoka S, Yamanaka H, et al. Detection of cytokines in bovine colostrum. Vet Immunol Immunopath 2000;76:183–90.

17. Yamanaka H, Hagiwara K, Kirisawa R, et al. Proinflammatory cytokines in bovine colostrum potentiate the mitogenic response of peripheral blood mononuclear cells from newborn calves through IL-2 and CD25 expression. Microbiol Immunol 2003;47(6):461–8.

18. Menge C, Neufield B, Hirt W, et al. Compensation of preliminary blood phagocyte immaturity in the newborn calf. Vet Immunol Immunopathol 1998;62:309–21.

19. Hartogden G, Savelkoul HFJ, Schoemaker R, et al. Modulation of human immune responses by bovine interleukin-10. PLoS One 2011;6(3):e18188.

20. Chun S-K, Nam M-S, Goh J-S, et al. Kinetics and biological function of transforming growth factor-β isoforms in bovine and human colostrum. J Microbiol Biotechnol 2004;14(6):1267–74.

21. Liebler-Tenorio EM, Riedel-Caspari G, Pohlenz JF. Uptake of colostral leukocytes in the intestinal tract of newborn calves. Vet Immunol Immunopathol 2002;85: 33–40.

22. Reber AJ, Hippen AR, Hurley DJ. Effects of the ingestion of whole colostrum or cell-free colostrum on the capacity of leukocytes in newborn calves to stimulate or respond in one-way mixed leukocyte cultures. Am J Vet Res 2005;66:1854–60.

23. Reber AJ, Lockwood A, Hippen AR, et al. Colostrum induced phenotypic and trafficking changes in maternal mononuclear cells in a peripheral blood leukocyte model for study of leukocyte transfer to the neonatal calf. Vet Immunol Immunopathol 2006;109:139–50.

24. Donovan DC, Reber AJ, Gabbard JD, et al. Effect of maternal cells transferred with colostrum on cellular responses to pathogen antigens in neonatal calves. Am J Vet Res 2007;68:778–82.

25. Maynard CL, Elson CO, Hatton RD, et al. Reciprocal interactions of the intestinal microbiota and immune system. Nature 2012;489(7415):231–41.

26. Maldonado-Contreras AL, McCormick BA. Intestinal epithelial cells and their role in innate mucosal immunity. Cell Tissue Res 2011;343(1):5–12.

27. Xue Y, Zhang H, Wang H, et al. Host inflammatory response inhibits Escherichia coli O157:H7 adhesion to gut epithelium through augmentation of mucin expression. Infect Immun 2014;82(5):1921–30.

28. Pelaseyed T, Bergström JH, Gustafsson JK, et al. The mucus and mucins of the goblet cells and enterocytes provide the first defense line of the gastrointestinal tract and interact with the immune system. Immunol Rev 2014;260(1):8–20.

29. Johansson ME, Hansson GC. Microbiology. Keeping bacteria at a distance. Science 2011;334(6053):182–3.

30. Villena J, Aso H, Kitazawa H. Regulation of toll-like receptors-mediated inflammation by immunobiotics in bovine intestinal epitheliocytes: role of signaling pathways and negative regulators. Front Immunol 2014;5:421.

31. Marchiando AM, Graham WV, Turner JR. Epithelial barriers in homeostasis and disease. Annu Rev Pathol 2010;5:119–44.

32. Odenwald MA, Turner JR. Intestinal permeability defects: is it time to treat? Clin Gastroenterol Hepatol 2013;11(9):1075–83.

33. Li RW, Sonstegard TS, Van Tassell CP, et al. Local inflammation as a possible mechanism of resistance to gastrointestinal nematodes in Angus heifers. Vet Parasitol 2007;145(1–2):100–7.

34. Angus KW, Tzipori S, Gray EW. Intestinal lesions in specific-pathogen-free lambs associated with a cryptosporidium from calves with diarrhea. Vet Pathol 1982; 19(1):67–78.

35. McDonald V, Korbel DS, Barakat FM, et al. Innate immune responses against Cryptosporidium parvum infection. Parasite Immunol 2013;35(2):55–64.

36. Leitch GJ, He Q. Cryptosporidiosis-an overview. J Biomed Res 2012;25(1):1–16.

37. Goossens E, Valgaeren BR, Pardon B, et al. Rethinking the role of alpha toxin in Clostridium perfringens-associated enteric diseases: a review on bovine necro-haemorrhagic enteritis. Vet Res 2017;48(1):9.

38. Kobayashi SD, Malachowa N, Deleo FR. Influence of microbes on neutrophil life and death. Front Cell Infect Microbiol 2017;7:159.

39. de Buhr N, Reuner F, Neumann A, et al. Neutrophil extracellular trap formation in the Streptococcus suis-infected cerebrospinal fluid compartment. Cell Micro 2017;19(2):e12649.

40. Branzk N, Lubojemska A, Hardison SE, et al. Neutrophils sense microbe size and selectively release neutrophil extracellular traps in response to large pathogens. Nat Immunol 2014;15(11):1017–25.

41. Bruns S, Kniemeyer O, Hasenberg M, et al. Production of extracellular traps against Aspergillus fumigatus in vitro and in infected lung tissue is dependent on invading neutrophils and influenced by hydrophobin RodA. Plos Pathog 2010;6(4):e1000873.

42. Behrendt JH, Ruiz A, Zahner H, et al. Neutrophil extracellular trap formation as innate immune reactions against the apicomplexan parasite Eimeria bovis. Vet Immunol Immunopathol 2010;133(1):1–8.

43. Abraham SN, John AL. Mast cell-orchestrated immunity to pathogens. Nat Rev Immunol 2010;10(6):440–52.

44. Galli SJ, Tsai M. Mast cells in allergy and infection: versatile effector and regulatory cells in innate and adaptive immunity. Eur J Immunol 2010;40(7):1843–51.

45. Shekhar S, Yang X. Natural killer cells in host defense against veterinary pathogens. Vet Immunol Immunopathol 2015;168(1–2):30–4.

46. Fries PN, Popowych YI, Guan LL, et al. Age-related changes in the distribution and frequency of myeloid and T cell populations in the small intestine of calves. Cell Immunol 2011;271(2):428–37.

47. Cheroutre H, Madakamutil L. Acquired and natural memory T cells join forces at the mucosal front line. Nat Rev Immunol 2004;4(4):290–300.

48. Bailey M, Haverson K. The postnatal development of the mucosal immune system and mucosal tolerance in domestic animals. Vet Res 2006;37(3):443–53.

49. Gerdts V, Mutwiri GK, Tikoo SK, et al. Mucosal delivery of vaccines in domestic animals. Vet Res 2006;37(3):487–510.

50. Malmuthuge N, Griebel PJ, Guan LL. The gut microbiome and its potential role in the development and function of newborn calf gastrointestinal tract. Front Vet Sci 2015;2:36.

51. Taschuk R, Griebel PJ. Commensal microbiome effects on mucosal immune system development in the ruminant gastrointestinal tract. Anim Health Res Rev 2012;13(1):129–41.

52. Mayer EA, Tillisch K, Gupta A. Gut/brain axis and the microbiota. J Clin Invest 2015;125(3):926–38.

53. Sherman MP, Zaghouani H, Niklas V. Gut microbiota, the immune system, and diet influence the neonatal gut-brain axis. Pediatr Res 2015;77(1–2):127–35.
54. Malmuthuge N, Guan LL. Understanding host-microbial interactions in rumen: searching the best opportunity for microbiota manipulation. J Anim Sci Biotechnol 2017;8(1):8.
55. Kim D, Yoo SA, Kim WU. Gut microbiota in autoimmunity: potential for clinical applications. Arch Pharm Res 2016;39(11):1565–76.
56. Malmuthuge N, Guan LL. Gut microbiome and omics: a new definition to ruminant production and health. Anim Front 2016;6(2):8–12.
57. Khosravi A, Mazmanian SK. Disruption of the gut microbiome as a risk factor for microbial infections. Curr Opin Microbiol 2013;16(2):221–7.
58. Gomez DE, Arroyo LG, Costa MC, et al. Characterization of the fecal bacterial microbiota of healthy and diarrheic dairy calves. J Vet Intern Med 2017;31(3):928–39.
59. Fouhse JM, Zijlstra RT, Willing BP. The role of gut microbiota in the health and disease of pigs. Anim Front 2016;6(3):30–6.
60. Derakhshani H, De Buck J, Mortier R, et al. The features of fecal and ileal mucosa-associated microbiota in dairy calves during early infection with mycobacterium avium subspecies paratuberculosis. Front Microbiol 2016;7:426.
61. Malmuthuge N, Guan LL. Understanding the gut microbiome of dairy calves: opportunities to improve early-life gut health. J Dairy Sci 2017;100(7):5996–6005.
62. Lebrun M, Mainil JG, Linden A. Cattle enterotoxaemia and Clostridium perfringens: description, diagnosis and prophylaxis. Vet Rec 2010;167(1):13–22.
63. Sherman DM, Acres SD, Sadowski PL, et al. Protection of calves against fatal enteric colibacillosis by orally administered Escherichia coli K99-specific monoclonal antibody. Infect Imm 1983;42(2):653–8.
64. Vega C, Bok M, Chacana P, et al. Egg yolk IgY: protection against rotavirus induced diarrhea and modulatory effect on the systemic and mucosal antibody responses in newborn calves. Vet Immunol Immunopathol 2011;142(3–4):156–69.
65. Parreño V, Marcoppido G, Vega C, et al. Milk supplemented with immune colostrum: protection against rotavirus diarrhea and modulatory effect on the systemic and mucosal antibody responses in calves experimentally challenged with bovine rotavirus. Vet Immunol Immunopath 2010;136(1–2):12–27.
66. Meganck V, Hoflack G, Piepers S, et al. Evaluation of a protocol to reduce the incidence of neonatal calf diarrhoea on dairy herds. Prev Vet Med 2015;118(1):64–70.
67. Griebel PJ. Mucosal vaccination of the newborn: an unrealized opportunity. Expert Rev Vaccines 2009;8(1):1–3.
68. Merck Animal Health. 2016. Pathology and detection of bovine coronavirus in tissues from calves after challenge with virulent bovine coronavirus. Available at: http://www.merck-animal-health-usa.com/binaries/Challenge_Model_Technical_Bulletin_tcm96-210964.pdf. Accessed June 10, 2017.
69. Plummer PJ, Rohrbach BW, Daugherty RA, et al. Effect of intranasal vaccination against bovine enteric coronavirus on the occurrence of respiratory tract disease in a commercial backgrounding feedlot. J Am Vet Med Assoc 2004;225(5):726–31.
70. Smith BP. Salmonellosis in ruminants. In: Smith BP, editor. Large Animal Internal Medicine. 5th edition. St. Louis MO: Mosby; 2014. p. 832–3.
71. Fuche FJ, Sow O, Simon R, et al. Salmonella serogroup C: current status of vaccines and why they are needed. Clin Vaccine Immunol 2016;23(9):737–45.

72. Habing GG, Neuder LM, Raphael W, et al. Efficacy of oral administration of a modified-live Salmonella Dublin vaccine in calves. J Am Vet Med Assoc 2011; 238(9):1184–90.
73. Bastida F, Juste RA. Paratuberculosis control: a review with a focus on vaccination. J Immune Based Ther Vaccines 2011;9(1):8.
74. Sweeney RW. Paratuberculosis (Johne's disease). In: Smith BP, editor. Large animal internal medicine. 5th edition; 2014. p. 837.
75. Sweeney RW, Collins MT, Koets AP, et al. Paratuberculosis (Johne's disease) in cattle and other susceptible species. J Vet Intern Med 2012;26(6):1239–50.
76. Cibulski SP, Mourglia-Ettlin G, Teixeira TF, et al. Novel ISCOMs from Quillaja brasiliensis saponins induce mucosal and systemic antibody production, T-cell responses and improved antigen uptake. Vaccine 2016;34(9):1162–71.
77. Savelkoul HFJ, Ferro VA, Strioga MM, et al. Choice and design of adjuvants for parenteral and mucosal vaccines. Vaccines (Basel) 2015;3(1):148–71.
78. Kogut MH, Arsenault RJ. Editorial: gut health: the new paradigm in food animal production. Front Vet Sci 2016;3:71.
79. Sahoo A, Jena B. Organic acids as rumen modifiers. Int J Sci Res 2014;3(11): 2262–6.
80. Patra AK, Yu Z. Effects of vanillin, quillaja saponin, and essential oils on in vitro fermentation and protein-degrading microorganisms of the rumen. Appl Microbiol Biotechnol 2014;98(2):897–905.
81. Ayrle H, Mevissen M, Kaske M, et al. Medicinal plants–prophylactic and therapeutic options for gastrointestinal and respiratory diseases in calves and piglets? A systematic review. BMC Vet Res 2016;12:89.
82. Eicher SD, Patterson JA, Rostagno MH. β-Glucan plus ascorbic acid in neonatal calves modulates immune functions with and without Salmonella enterica serovar Dublin. Vet Immunol Immunopath 2011;142(3–4):258–64.
83. Sandes S, Alvim L, Silva B, et al. Selection of new lactic acid bacteria strains bearing probiotic features from mucosal microbiota of healthy calves: looking for immunobiotics through in vitro and in vivo approaches for immunoprophylaxis applications. Microbiol Res 2017;200:1–13.
84. Zhang R, Zhou M, Tu Y, et al. Effect of oral administration of probiotics on growth performance, apparent nutrient digestibility and stress-related indicators in Holstein calves. J Ani Phys An Nutr 2016;100(1):33–8.
85. Novak KN, Davis E, Wehnes CA, et al. Effect of supplementation with an electrolyte containing a Bacillus-based direct-fed microbial on immune development in dairy calves. Res Vet Sc 2012;92(3):427–34.
86. Bunešová V, Domig KJ, Killer J, et al. Characterization of bifidobacteria suitable for probiotic use in calves. Anaerobe 2012;18(1):166–8.
87. Vlasova AN, Kandasamy S, Chattha KS, et al. Comparison of probiotic lactobacilli and bifidobacteria effects, immune responses and rotavirus vaccines and infection in different host species. Vet Immunol Immunopath 2016;172:72–84.
88. Uyeno Y, Shigemori S, Shimosato T. Effect of probiotics/prebiotics on cattle health and productivity. Microbes Environ 2015;30(2):126–32.

Diagnostic Approach to the Acute Abdomen

Gilles Fecteau, DMV*, André Desrochers, DMV, MSc, David Francoz, DMV, MSc, Sylvain Nichols, DMV, MS

KEYWORDS

- Bovine • Abdomen • Colic • Pain • Ancillary tests

KEY POINTS

- Whether to cut or to wait is not an easy decision and remains a challenge for most food animal practitioners.
- Optimal management depends of multiple factors, some of which are under the direct control of the veterinarian, whereas others are totally independent.
- Complete physical examination and judicious use of ancillary tests remains the best ally.
- It is important to keep in mind that exploratory laparotomy is sometimes an economical option.

BACKGROUND INFORMATION

This description of the acute abdomen and the proposed diagnostic and therapeutic approach are the result of clinical experience and interaction between clinicians specializing in surgery and in medicine. Although the authors realize that many concepts presented apply better in a teaching hospital, we think that many hints and tips remain relevant for the bovine practitioner confronted everyday with the field reality.

One of the most challenging situations in bovine medicine, the acute abdomen may evolve into a critical situation in which the client becomes nervous, especially if a valuable animal is involved. In some species, the cost and risk associated with abdominal surgery justifies completing the medical workup to avoid surgery if possible. In the bovine, the cost and risk associated to a standing laparotomy is such that, in many situations, it seems more economical to perform a diagnostic exploratory laparotomy and institute the appropriate treatment instead of adding the cost of diagnostic tests and procedures before surgery. Is this a reasonable approach? Is it always without negative consequences?

Disclosure: The authors have nothing to disclose.
Clinical Sciences Department of Université de Montréal, 3200 rue Sicotte, Saint-Hyacinthe, Québec J2S 2M2, Canada
* Corresponding author.
E-mail address: gilles.fecteau@umontreal.ca

DEFINITION

The acute abdomen is a general term often used to characterize an animal presented as an emergency, in a more or less severe critical state, and for which medical and possibly surgical treatment will be necessary. The term is often used to describe cases in which some degree of uncertainty remains in regard to the diagnosis.

INTRODUCTION

The clinician should use a systematic approach based on adequate signalment and history, complete physical examination, and judicious choice of ancillary tests. An excellent knowledge of the bovine abdominal anatomy and a good understanding of the pathophysiology of abdominal pain are additional tools often useful in difficult cases. Good clinical judgment, critical analysis, and good client communication skills are competencies that often make a difference in the outcome of a particular case.

ABDOMINAL PAIN IN RUMINANTS

Abdominal pain may be a consequence of excess distension of a hollow viscus, spasm of intestinal smooth muscle, stretching of the mesenteric supporting structure, intestinal ischemia, or chemical irritation of the visceral or parietal peritoneum. Abdominal pain may be classified into visceral pain (hollow viscus and solid organs) and parietal pain (parietal peritoneum, abdominal muscles, rib cage). Pain sensation from the parietal peritoneum travels through the peripheral spinal nerves and usually localizes over the affected area. Because parietal pain is exacerbated by pressure and tension modification, the patient is reluctant to move and have a tonic reflex contraction of the abdominal muscles. In most cases, no active clinical signs of colic are recognized. Some pain fiber endings are located in the submucosa and muscle layers of hollow viscus (intestines, bladder), and in the capsule of solid organs (kidney, liver). Consequently, distention, forceful contraction, or traction will produce pain. Capsule stretching will also create pain. Visceral pain is most often associated with active manifestation of colic: kicking at the abdomen, treading with the rear feet, lying down or standing, and stretching out. Visceral pain is transmitted via sensory fibers in the autonomic nerves and is often diffuse and difficult to localize.

Differential diagnosis for colic in ruminants may be first categorized into abdominal or extraabdominal origin. Extraabdominal causes include thoracic pain, laminitis, and myopathy. Although not truly related to abdominal diseases, animals affected by those conditions can mimic clinical signs of colic. The abdominal causes can then be sub-categorized into digestive or nondigestive origin. The nondigestive causes include pyelonephritis and uterine torsion, whereas the classic abdominal digestive causes include abomasal volvulus, intussusception, and ileus.

RAPID EVALUATION OF THE PATIENT

Some patients need immediate medical assistance and the primary objective is to buy time to allow a better examination. Several abdominal emergencies are associated with either hypovolemic or septic shock. Hypovolemic shock is characterized by increased heart rate, pale mucous membranes, slow capillary refill time, and dehydration. Increased heart rate and dehydration are also observed in case of septic shock, but mucous membranes are hyperemic or bluish in color, and scleral vessels are engorged and dark. Intensive fluid therapy is the treatment of choice for both hypovolemic and septic shock.[1] Consequently, an intravenous (IV) catheter should be placed and fluid therapy instituted immediately. IV administration of hypertonic saline provides a rapid resuscitation in dehydrated or endotoxemic ruminants.[2] A rate of 4 to 5 mL/kg of hypertonic solution should be administered IV through the jugular vein over 4 to 5 minutes. Animals should be provided with a supply of fresh water immediately after the treatment or an IV infusion of an isotonic crystalloid solution should be instituted. Cattle not observed to drink within 5 minutes should have 20 L of water pumped into the rumen.[2] In the authors' clinics, unless the animal is unable to stand or is showing clinical signs of acute blood loss, hypertonic solutions are not used routinely in cases of acute abdomen. Most patients would already have received nonsteroidal antiinflammatory drugs (NSAIDs) before presentation; however, if not previously administered, they should be given to provide some degree of comfort and to allow the complete evaluation of the animal.

HISTORY

Age, sex, breed, and production stage are important parameters to take into consideration when elaborating the differential diagnosis. For example, abomasal volvulus develops more frequently in dairy cows than in beef cattle.[3,4] Similarly, uterine torsions are essentially observed at the time of parturition or in the last trimester.[5] Colic in a wether or a buck goat should be considered a result of urolithiasis until proven otherwise. Nutrition program and management system are important parts of the history. Previous surgery, recent calving, and obstetric manipulations are important risk factors for peritonitis. Recent estrus could be associated with hypocalcemia and results in paralytic ileus.[6] Previous treatments, especially those that can modify clinical signs or the interpretation of laboratory results, should also be noted. Description of the clinical signs observed by the owner and the chronologic sequence of events are of particular interest. Fecal output, consistency, and appearance are relevant information.

PHYSICAL EXAMINATION
Hemodynamic State

Assessment of cardiovascular status is essential and based on heart rate, mucous membranes, capillary refill time, and dehydration. Determination of rectal temperature, pulse or heart rate, and respiratory rate (TPR) should always be performed first because manipulations performed during the physical examination of an abdominal emergency can elicit pain, modifying the heart rate. The TPR and amount of pain exhibited may also be used to monitor the evolution of the condition and the response to the initiated treatment. Once vital parameters have been evaluated and the animal seems hemodynamically stable, a thorough physical examination of the body systems should be performed.

Profile, Auscultation

The abdominal profile should be observed from the rear and both sides to detect and characterize abdominal distention.[7,8] An arched back may be observed in cases of cranial abdominal pain or laminitis (sore feet). Examination of the thorax (pleuropneumonia, rib fractures) and the musculoskeletal system (laminitis, myopathy) are important in eliminating diseases that mimic abdominal pain. Abdominal examination is performed by auscultation, percussion, and succussion of the abdomen. The authors think that the rumen auscultation is of particular interest and should last at least 2 minutes. The rumen contractions should be counted and characterized. Three complete contractions per 2 minutes are normal. Incomplete and frequent (>5 per 2 minutes) are not normal. Complete absence of contraction for 2 minutes is also abnormal. The rumen auscultation should be repeated after the initial treatment is done to evaluate the improvement. Pings are tympanic resonance caused by a gas-fluid interface in a distended organ and can be detected by simultaneous auscultation and percussion.[7] Ping detection should be performed before rectal palpation because the procedure may create an area of increased resonance on the right dorsal part of the abdomen. On the right side of the abdomen, many organs may cause a ping. Location, pitch characteristics, and variability of the ping are essential to establish a differential and precise diagnosis. On the left side, pings are principally associated with left abomasal displacement, ruminal collapse, and pneumoperitoneum. Simultaneous auscultation and ballottement (succussion) of the abdomen may permit detection of fluid trapped within the intestine or in a hollow viscus, such as the rumen or abomasum. The location of the fluid splashing sounds on auscultation-succussion may help to confirm and differentiate among auscultation-percussion findings.

Pain Origin

Although the task may be challenging, localization of the origin of the pain should be attempted. Cattle with cranial abdominal pain associated with peritonitis are reluctant to move; they stand with elbows abducted and back arched. During examination, bruxism (grinding of the teeth) may be present. Pain can be elicited by pinching over the withers or applying forceful movement with the knee or upward pressure with a bar or pole over the xyphoid area or anterior abdomen. In response, the animal in pain may grunt or kick and be reluctant to dip the back.[7] Sensitivity of this test may be increased by simultaneous auscultation of the trachea. Tense abdominal muscles, secondary to parietal peritoneum inflammation, may also be detected during succussion. The visceral pain is often diffuse and virtually impossible to localize with certainty.

Transrectal Palpation

Per rectum abdominal palpation of cattle is helpful in the differential diagnosis of an acute abdomen. Cecal disorders are clearly diagnosed per rectal palpation. Moreover, cecal dilatation or volvulus can be differentiated by location of the apex. Multiple, dilated, turgid small intestine loops and a firm mass may be palpated in cases of intussusception[9,10] or hemorrhagic bowel syndrome (HBS).[11] Uterine wall integrity may be evaluated. In cases of urolithiasis in bulls or steers, rectal palpation reveals a pulsatile pelvic urethra and a distended bladder. In cases of pyelonephritis, enlargement of 1 or both ureters may be palpated. The left kidney may be painful, as well as enlarged.

Fecal Output and Appearance

Presence and macroscopic appearance of feces can be evaluated during rectal examination. A decreased volume of feces is principally associated with intestinal stasis or obstruction, which may occur secondary to mechanical obstruction (requiring surgical treatment) or to gastrointestinal ileus (requiring only medical treatment). However, feces may be present in the first few days after an intestinal obstruction.[12] Macroscopic appearance of feces is sometimes helpful in the differential diagnosis. HBS is associated with feces resembling raspberry jam. Dark feces (melena) are often associated with abomasal ulcers. Fibrin and mucus without feces is more often seen in case of complete obstruction.

MEDICAL TREATMENT

If immediate surgery is not necessary, there is time to initiate a medical treatment that will first improve the general condition of the patient and sometimes will be sufficient to obtain enough improvement and avoid surgery. If the animal is considered a potential surgical patient but not in immediate need of surgery, diagnostic procedures should be considered and performed as medical therapy is administered. The goal of supportive therapy is to correct hemodynamic and metabolic imbalances, to control pain, and to prevent or treat infection when suspected.

Fluid Therapy

Crystalloid solutions (0.9% sodium chloride, Ringer solution) are indicated initially to replenish fluid loss and improve the circulating blood volume. In the authors' clinics, we often use a volume of 20 L of isotonic saline in adult cows (20 L IV in 60–90 minutes) as an initial fluid therapy. It is not unusual for a critical adult cow to receive 60 L of IV fluid over 24 hours. Ideally, correction of electrolytes imbalance should be based on laboratory results (measured in between 20 L of fluids). Most patients with acute abdomen suffer from the metabolic alkalosis associated with hypochloremia and hypokalemia. Hypocalcemia is common in dairy cattle with gastrointestinal diseases. Calcium ions are of particular importance in gastrointestinal motility. In the authors' clinics, the IV solution used for the medical treatment of an acute abdomen is most often an isotonic saline (20 L of 0.9%) in which calcium borogluconate 23% (500 mL) is added. Response to fluid therapy helps make the diagnosis because improvement with calcium-rich fluid provides insight in the likelihood of surgical problem. If the patient continues to deteriorate while receiving rapid IV fluids, the medical approach may not be sufficient. Repeated TPR and brief gastrointestinal motility assessment (rumen contractions, gut sounds, fecal output, and ultrasound assessment of motility) often indicate the benefit of medical therapy.

Pain Control

Pain is a primary cause of gastrointestinal hypomotility. Gastrointestinal pain increases sympathic tone, causing general inhibition of the gastrointestinal tract.[13,14] Peritoneal inflammation or irritation and associated pain are initiatory factors of the ileus in several species.[13,15] Consequently, analgesic and antiinflammatory drugs are often considered in the management of the bovine acute abdomen. These drugs must be used with the complete knowledge of their possible side-effects. NSAIDs may induce abomasal ulcers particularly in an anorexic patient. Analgesics may also alter clinical signs (pain, fever) used to decision-making. No single NSAID can be recommended based on scientific evidence for the management of abdominal emergencies in cattle. The choice of NSAID becomes a matter of previous experience, comparative medicine, legislation, and cost. In the authors' experiences, both flunixin and ketoprofen are adequate for the management of acute abdomen in cattle. In equine gastrointestinal pain, a poor or short duration response to NSAIDs indicates the need for surgery.[14] This concept may or may not applied to cattle because their response to pain is less predictable. Xylazine is reported to have significant effects on the gastrointestinal tract in cattle, decreasing reticuloruminal and intestinal motility.[16] Because of the hemodynamic changes associated with the administration of α_2-agonists, these drugs must be used with caution in patients with arterial hypotension and/or shock.[17]

Antimicrobial Therapy

Bacterial translocation from the intestines may occur in cases of mechanical or functional ileus secondary to bacterial overgrowth, inflammation, and impairment of the functional barrier of the intestinal wall.[15,18] The choice of antimicrobial is variable but the IV route is always the first choice because most of these patients already have an IV catheter. The choice of antibiotic should also take into consideration legal aspects and the cost of the treatment. β-lactams, tetracyclines, and trimethoprim-sulfadoxine seem to be good choices. As a rule of thumb, trimethoprim-sulfadoxine is our first choice for enteric disease, whereas β-lactams are often used with peritonitis and presurgical antimicrobial therapy. Because a significant portion of these patients will eventually need surgery, this could also justify initiating therapy. In cattle, there is no accepted recommendation for the duration of treatment. In human medicine, prolonged broad-spectrum antibiotic therapy in case of surgical acute abdomen does not seem beneficial.[19] Prevention of infective complications was not affected by prolonging the course of antibiotic treatment.[19] In human medicine, the current recommended dosage is a single prophylactic antibiotic administration when there is no or minimal evidence of contamination, and over 5 to 7 days when pus or contamination, either localized or diffuse, is present.[19]

Prokinetic Drugs

Motility-modifying agents may be used in the management of gastrointestinal disorders. In the bovine acute abdomen, it remains a difficult decision before establishing a final diagnosis because some patients suffer from a surgical condition. Prokinetics could aggravate the situation in these cases. In the authors' clinics, we use prokinetic drugs only when a final diagnosis is made either by exploratory surgery or not. Steiner[16] reviewed the different prokinetics that can be used in ruminant medicine and their clinical implication.

USEFUL DIAGNOSTIC PROCEDURES

Ancillary diagnostic tests mainly serve 3 purposes: assessment of the patient's immediate requirements, attainment of an etiologic diagnosis and help determining prognosis. The following procedures are the ones we find most useful in the management of the acute abdomen. They are described in a relative order of importance.

Blood Lactate Concentration

Blood lactate concentration is commonly used in the authors' clinics to assess cardiovascular state; to monitor the response to treatment; and, to some extent, provide an estimate of prognosis for survival. Our routine use includes an early measurement (before any treatment) and a follow-up measure after initial therapy (IV fluids, NSAIDs, or other). We found that an increase in blood lactate or very marginal reduction in blood lactate, despite aggressive therapy, indicates that surgery is needed or the prognosis is poor.

Blood Gas Analysis, Electrolytes, and Serum Biochemistry Profile

Most gastrointestinal impairment leads to sequestration of the high-chloride abomasal contents into the upper gastrointestinal system. Some degree of systemic hypochloremic hypokalemic metabolic alkalosis eventually develops in most situations. The diagnostic value of this finding is limited because it does not bring precise information on the possible cause and has controversial value as a prognostic indicator.

However, serial measurements allow the best monitoring of the evolution of a particular case. Serum calcium concentration is of great interest because it is commonly low in anorexic periparturient dairy cattle. It is so important in gut motility that the authors' think we cannot ignore even a marginal diminution. The serum biochemistry profile will also reveal any impairment in kidney or liver function, as well as liver damage (elevation of liver enzymes).

Complete Blood Count

A white blood cell count rarely provides further information to establish the precise cause of the acute abdomen. In most cases, a minimal to moderate inflammatory process characterized by a neutrophilic leukocytosis is observed. Hematologic findings may also provide information about the severity of the associated sepsis and toxemia. Severe sepsis is associated with neutropenia, degenerative left shift, toxic changes of neutrophil morphology, and lymphopenia. An inflammatory leukogram could also reflect chronic active inflammation, such as in peritonitis. Hematology is also an important ancillary test to monitor the response to treatment. Of particular interest is the relationship between plasma protein concentration and packed cell volume (PCV). An increased PCV combined with a normal to decreased plasma protein concentration often indicates an active secretion of protein-rich fluid into the peritoneal cavity. Shock, sepsis, and toxemia cause hemoconcentration and dehydration, and are associated with an increase of PCV and total solids. If a complete blood count is not available, PCV and total solids already provide some relevant information. Fibrinogen concentration could add some insights in cases of chronic inflammation. Studies in cattle report that fibrinogen concentration may increase within 1 to 2 days after induction of inflammatory conditions.[20,21] Normal fibrinogen concentration, despite severe visceral involvement, should be observed only in peracute cases, within a few hours (eg, torsion of the root of the mesentery). Moderate to marked increased fibrinogen concentration is also the signature of an active localized inflammatory condition, such as peritonitis.

Abdominocentesis and Peritoneal Fluid Evaluation

Abdominocentesis is a simple and practical procedure helpful to manage acute abdomen. However, one should remember some bovine particularities. Absence of peritoneal fluid does not rule out the possibility of peritonitis. Fluid can be evaluated macroscopically for color, volume, odor, and turbidity. A large volume of peritoneal fluid is abnormal. Peritoneal fluid changes to cloudy yellow with peritonitis, whereas blood tinged with fibrin fluid is more often seen as bowel necrosis and extravasated red blood cells occur. Normal bovine peritoneal fluid has a specific density less than 1.016. Protein content should be less than 3 g/dL, although some investigators have reported normal values up to 6.3 g/dL (the major part being albumin). Nucleated cells count should be less than 10,000 cells per μL, with most macrophages. Lymphocytes, eosinophils, and desquamated mesothelial cells may also be present. Neutrophils are rare and more than 50% neutrophils indicate peritonitis. Periparturient cattle have significantly more peritoneal fluid with a lower protein concentration. When macroscopic examination is not diagnostic, cytologic examination of the peritoneal fluid is useful. As an example, in some cases of lymphoma, abnormal lymphocytes may be observed in the peritoneal fluid. Very little is known about the most common bacteria isolated from acute or chronic peritonitis. However, because *Trueperella pyogenes (Arcanobacterium pyogenes)* is commonly isolated from abscesses in the bovine, one could assume that it may be of importance in chronic active peritonitis. Biochemical variables may be evaluated in peritoneal fluid. Lactate, glucose, alkaline phosphatase, and pH of the peritoneal fluid concentrations have been reported to be indicators of intestinal ischemia and peritonitis in horses.[22]

Medical Imaging: Ultrasound Examination, Laparoscopic Procedures, and Cranial Abdominal Radiography

Ultrasound is used to image soft tissues of the abdominal cavity. The potential of this tool is enormous. The size and anatomic relationship of lesions may be delineated.

Knowledge of the underlying anatomy is essential. Ultrasonography is a diagnostic tool readily available in large animal medicine and surgery. To evaluate the abdomen, a 3.5 MHz curvilinear or linear probe is ideal. It allows the evaluation of the reticulum; the omasum; the abomasum; the small bowel, including the duodenum; the cecum; and spiral colon (**Fig. 1**). A 7.5 MHz transrectal probe can be used to diagnose abdominal effusion. However, in adult cattle, it is difficult to use the higher frequency probe to evaluate the gastrointestinal tract.

During investigation of the acute abdomen, the ultrasound is used to identify the structure involved in the pathologic condition and to evaluate the presence of abdominal effusion (**Fig. 2**). Following an abdominocentesis, the effusion is characterized (lactate, red blood cells, leukocytes, and proteins) to diagnose the surgical abdomen.

Reticulum

The reticulum is evaluated when reticuloperitonitis is suspected. The cranial abdomen (from left to right) is evaluated. The reticulum has a biphasic contraction.[23] Abnormal contraction or presence of abdominal effusion or even an organized abscess (**Fig. 3**) suggests hardware disease.[24] A cranial abdominal radiograph would confirm the diagnosis (**Fig. 4**).

Omasum

Pathologic complications of the omasum are uncommon. This structure is located on the visceral surface of the liver. It is best seen by scanning the 6th to 11th intercostal spaces.[25] Dilatation of this structure will be recognized ultrasonographically because the liver will be cranially displaced by a thick-walled structure. When filled with fluid from a proximal gastrointestinal obstruction, the leaves of the omasum become apparent (**Fig. 5**).[26]

Abomasum

The location of the abomasum can be followed by ultrasonography.[27–29] It can be used to confirm a displacement[30,31] or to detect a focal zone of peritonitis around a chronically displaced abomasum. The distended abomasum is easily recognized by seeing mucosal folds floating in hyperechoic fluids (**Fig. 6**).

Ultrasonography is an efficient tool for investigating vagal syndrome involving the pylorus. A presumptive diagnosis of pyloric lymphoma (**Fig. 7**) can readily be

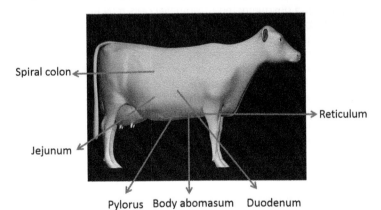

Fig. 1. Localization of abdominal structures evaluated ultrasonographically. (*Adapted from* CD on the surgery of the abomasum in cattle Faculté de Médecine Vétérinaire, Université de Montréal 2002, with permission).

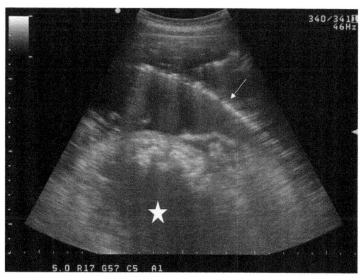

Fig. 2. Abdominal effusion. Superficial layer of the omentum (*arrow*); abomasum (*star*); effusion is present outside and inside the omental bursa. Some acoustic shadowing is present on the omentum caused by free gas within the abdomen. (*Courtesy of* Sylvain Nichols, DMV, MS.)

obtained.[32,33] The pylorus is usually located between the right mammary vein and the costochondral arch. A fine-needle aspiration performed under ultrasonographic guidance will confirm the diagnosis.

Duodenum

The cranial and the sigmoid flexure of the duodenum can be seen near the caudal edge of the liver and gallbladder in the last intercostal spaces. Its normal diameter

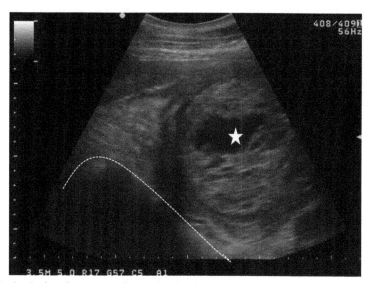

Fig. 3. Perireticular abscess. An abscess (star) is located next to the reticulum (*dotted line*). (*Courtesy of* Sylvain Nichols, DMV, MS.)

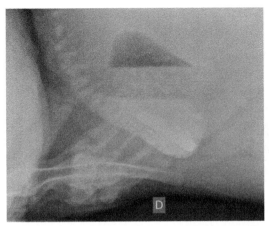

Fig. 4. Lateral radiograph of a cow with a perireticular abscess. A gas-fluid line is seen in the middle of the reticulum. A magnet with multiple foreign bodies is seen at the bottom of the reticulum. (*Courtesy of* Sylvain Nichols, DMV, MS.)

varies between 1.0 and 5.5 cm.[34] They will be distended in cases of duodenal sigmoid flexure volvulus or proximal obstruction caused by a trichophytobezoar. Their diameters will then reach 10.0 cm.[35] Peritonitis secondary to duodenal ulcers can also be seen in this area.

Jejunum

The jejunum is usually confined in the caudal lower right flank within the supraomental bursa. Normally, loops of jejunum of 2 to 4.5 cm in diameter are seen constantly moving.[34] Distended and hypomotile jejunum is frequently seen in cattle suffering from functional and mechanical ileus.[35] Presence of fluid surrounding the distended bowel suggests peritonitis.

Mechanical obstruction caused by a blood clot (HBS) or by an intussusception can sometimes be located (**Fig. 8**).[36]

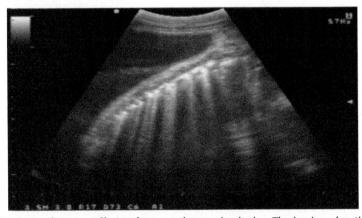

Fig. 5. Omasum of a cow suffering from an abomasal volvulus. The laminae (*vertical white line*) of the omasum are seen because of its abnormal fluid content. (*Courtesy of* Sylvain Nichols, DMV, MS.)

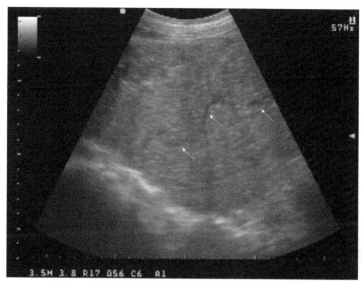

Fig. 6. Abomasum. Mucosal folds (*arrows*) can be seen floating in the normal hyperechoic content of the abomasum. (*Courtesy of* Sylvain Nichols, DMV, MS.)

Cecum and colon

The cecum and colon structures are usually filled with gas. Therefore, only their walls are seen. The spiral colon has a typical undulated shape (garland). It is located in the middle of the right paralumbar fossa just above the cecum.[37] Normally, the cecum is seen as a crescent-shaped line of 5 to 18 cm in diameter traveling from cranial to caudal. With cecal dilatation or volvulus, a large gas-filled and fluid-filled viscus (up to 25 cm), without any large mucosal folds (typical of a fluid-filled abomasum) is seen in the right paralumbar fossa.[38]

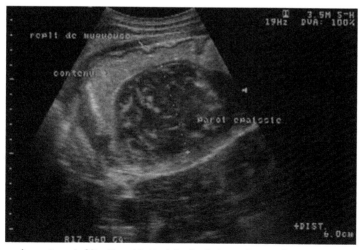

Fig. 7. Lymphomatous infiltration (*dotted line*) of the pylorus of an adult Holstein cow suffering from vagal indigestion. (*Courtesy of* Sylvain Nichols, DMV, MS.)

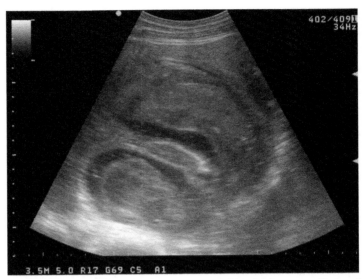

Fig. 8. Blood clot within a loop of jejunum in an adult Holstein cow suffering from HBS. (*Courtesy of* Sylvain Nichols, DMV, MS.)

Laparoscopic procedures are also import and allow visualization without the invasive procedure. This is a field in development and the future possibility seems promising.

Radiology of the cranial abdomen is a useful diagnostic aid when traumatic reticuloperitonitis is suspected. It is, however, limited to reference centers with high-quality equipment because of the difficulty to penetrate the depth and density of tissues involved.

WHEN SURGERY IS PART OF THE SOLUTION

If surgery is the only possible treatment offering a complete recovery and a long-term positive outcome, there is no reason to delay the intervention. A good example is a case of abomasal volvulus in which the definitive diagnosis is clinically achievable and in which the rate of recovery using medical treatment alone is 0%. Unfortunately, in most acute abdomens, the certainty of the clinical diagnosis is not as great as in cases of abomasal volvulus and medical treatment could seem promising at first.

Exploratory laparotomy is a valuable ancillary diagnostic procedure in ruminants. Information obtained from the physical examination and laboratory data often indicates a diagnosis but does not provide a specific cause. Moreover, the relative low cost of surgery when compared with the cost of the entire workup may justify being more aggressive toward surgical exploratory procedures. Cattle are particularly amenable to exploratory surgery because the procedure is performed standing and, with care toward asepsis, is associated with little complications. An excellent knowledge of the bovine abdominal anatomy and a good understanding of the pathophysiology of the most common abdominal conditions are additional tools often useful in difficult cases.

The criteria which the authors consider the most important in making the decision of whether to move toward a surgical approach include

- Rapidity of the evolution since the first clinical sign
- Severity of colic and its response to therapy if attempted before referral

- The severity of the abdominal distention and the absence of fecal output
- The heart rate and the rectal palpation findings
- Blood lactate, particularly if blood lactate did not return toward normal after medical therapy
- Calcium measurements, particularly if low then justifying medical therapy first.

OTHER MEDICAL AND SUPPORTIVE TREATMENTS

Several other treatments may be used before or after surgery. Only a few are described here.

The use of purgatives (magnesium hydroxide, mineral oil, liquid paraffin) in cases of suspected gastrointestinal obstruction or ileus in cattle has no therapeutic basis.[12] Moreover, these treatments may exacerbate the condition. Because the intestines are already filled with gas and fluid, purgatives only impose additional distention. Moreover, magnesium hydroxide may be responsible for detrimental effects, such as metabolic alkalosis,[39] sedation caused by hypermagnesemia,[39] increased ruminal pH,[40] and decreased ruminal microbial activity.[40] The authors strongly discourage the use of laxatives in bovine acute abdomen.

No prokinetic drug is reported to directly increase ruminal motility. In cases of prolonged anorexia or acute indigestion, ruminal flora can be disturbed and reduced. Transfaunation may help to rapidly reconstitute the ruminal flora and hasten return to normal function of the rumen and the digestive tract. The technique for and beneficial effects of transfaunation (reduction of ketonuria, increased feed intake, and higher milk yield) have been reported in the postsurgical treatment of left abomasal displacement.[41]

The Kingman tube is routinely used in the authors' clinics both before and after surgery. In fact, in several cases, as an adjunct to medical therapy, we believe that we often avoid unnecessary surgery. The procedure is performed on a standing animal. The distension must be important and the ruminal contents should be fluid. When successful, the amount of rumen fluid evacuated is spectacular. The animal is immediately relieved and time is bought for the medical therapy to become beneficial.

MONITORING

When a definitive diagnosis cannot be made, a close monitoring of the animal is indicated. Follow-up is also very important after surgery to ensure adequate response and allow possible adjustment of treatment. We think that reevaluation every 4 to 6 hours is adequate (vital parameters, rectal examination, presence and consistency of feces, and pain combined to laboratory analyses). Deterioration or persistence of clinical signs despite the initiation of supportive treatment is also an indication for surgery.

SUMMARY

Whether to cut or to wait is not an easy decision and remains a challenge for most food animal practitioners. Optimal management depends of multiple factors, some of which are under the direct control of the veterinarian, whereas others are totally independent. Complete physical examination and judicious use of ancillary tests remains the best ally. It is important to keep in mind that exploratory laparotomy is sometimes an economical option. However, it is also relevant to remember that it is not the only option to get to the final diagnosis.

REFERENCES

1. Walters PC. Approach to the acute abdomen. Clin Tech Small Anim Pract 2000; 15(2):63–9.
2. Constable PD. Hypertonic saline. Vet Clin North Am Food Anim Pract 1999;15(3): 559–85.
3. Constable PD, Miller GY, Hoffsis GF, et al. Risk factors for abomasal volvulus and left abomasal displacement in cattle. Am J Vet Res 1992;53(7):1184–92.
4. Roussel AJ, Cohen ND, Hooper RN. Abomasal displacement and volvulus in beef cattle: 19 cases (1988-1998). J Am Vet Med Assoc 2000;216(5):730–3.
5. Pearson H. Intussusception in cattle. Vet Rec 1971;89(16):426–37.
6. Goff JP. Pathophysiology of calcium and phosphorus disorders. Vet Clin North Am Food Anim Pract 2000;16(2):319–37, vii.
7. Belknap EB, Navarre CB. Differentiation of gastrointestinal diseases in adult cattlet. Vet Clin North Am Food Anim Pract 2000;16(1):59–86.
8. Navarre CB, Belknap EB, Rowe SE. Differentiation of gastrointestinal diseases of calves. Vet Clin North Am Food Anim Pract 2000;16(1):37–57.
9. Constable PD, St Jean G, Hull BL, et al. Intussusception in cattle: 336 cases (1964-1993). J Am Vet Med Assoc 1997;210(4):531–6.
10. Pearson H. Uterine torsion in cattle: a review of 168 cases. Vet Rec 1971;89(23): 597–603.
11. Dennison AC, VanMetre DC, Callan RJ, et al. Hemorrhagic bowel syndrome in dairy cattle: 22 cases (1997-2000). J Am Vet Med Assoc 2002;221(5):686–9.
12. Pearson H, Pinsent PJ. Intestinal obstruction in cattle. Vet Rec 1977;101(9): 162–6.
13. Bueno L, Fioramonti J, Delvaux M, et al. Mediators and pharmacology of visceral sensitivity: from basic to clinical investigations. Gastroenterology 1997;112(5): 1714–43.
14. Malone E, Graham L. Management of gastrointestinal pain. Vet Clin North Am Equine Pract 2002;18(1):133–58.
15. Bauer AJ, Schwarz NT, Moore BA, et al. Ileus in critical illness: mechanisms and management. Curr Opin Crit Care 2002;8(2):152–7.
16. Steiner A. Modifiers of gastrointestinal motility of cattle. Vet Clin North Am Food Anim Pract 2003;19(3):647–60.
17. Gross ME. Tranquilizers, α2-adrenergic agonists and related agents. In: Adams HR, editor. Veterinary pharmacology and therapeutics. Ames (IA): Iowa State University Press; 2001. p. 299–342.
18. Madl C, Druml W. Gastrointestinal disorders of the critically ill. Systemic consequences of ileus. Best Pract Res Clin Gastroenterol 2003;17(3):445–56.
19. Gleisner AL, Argenta R, Pimentel M, et al. Infective complications according to duration of antibiotic treatment in acute abdomen. Int J Infect Dis 2004;8(3): 155–62.
20. Conner JG, Eckersall PD, Wiseman A, et al. Bovine acute phase response following turpentine injection. Res Vet Sci 1988;44(1):82–8.
21. Earley B, Crowe MA. Effects of ketoprofen alone or in combination with local anesthesia during the castration of bull calves on plasma cortisol, immunological, and inflammatory responses. J Anim Sci 2002;80(4):1044–52.
22. Saulez MN, Cebra CK, Tornquist SJ. The diagnostic and prognostic value of alkaline phosphatase activity in serum and peritoneal fluid from horses with acute colic. J Vet Intern Med 2004;18(4):564–7.

23. Braun U, Rauch S. Ultrasonographic evaluation of reticular motility during rest, eating, rumination and stress in 30 healthy cows. Vet Rec 2008;163(19):571–4.
24. Braun U, Gotz M, Marmier O. Ultrasonographic findings in cows with traumatic reticuloperitonitis. Vet Rec 1993;133(17):416–22.
25. Braun U, Blessing S. Ultrasonographic examination of the omasum in 30 healthy cows. Vet Rec 2006;159(24):812–5.
26. Braun U, Feller B, Hässig M, et al. Ultrasonographic examination of the omasum, liver, and small and large intestines in cows with right displacement of the abomasum and abomasal volvulus. Am J Vet Res 2008;69(6):777–84.
27. Braun U, Wild K, Guscetti F. Ultrasonographic examination of the abomasum of 50 cows. Vet Rec 1997;140(4):93–8.
28. Van Winden SC, Brattinga CR, Muller KE, et al. Position of the abomasum in dairy cows during the first six weeks after calving. Vet Rec 2002;151(15):446–9.
29. Wittek T, Constable P, Morin D. Ultrasonographic assessment of change in abomasal position during the last three months of gestation and first three months of lactation in Holstein-Friesian cows. J Am Vet Med Assoc 2005;227(9):1469–75.
30. Braun U, Feller B. Ultrasonographic findings in cows with right displacement of the abomasum and abomasal volvulus. Vet Rec 2008;162(10):311–5.
31. Braun U, Pusterla N, Schonmann M. Ultrasonographic findings in cows with left displacement of the abomasum. Vet Rec 1997;141(13):331–5.
32. Braun U, Schnetzler C, Dettwiler M, et al. Ultrasonographic findings in a cow with abomasal lymphosarcoma: case report. BMC Vet Res 2011;7:20.
33. Buczinski S, Belanger AM, Francoz D. Ultrasonographic appearance of lympho-matous infiltration of the abomasum in cows with lymphoma. J Am Vet Med Assoc 2011;238(8):1044–7.
34. Braun U, Marmier O. "Ultrasonographic examination of the small intestine of cows. Vet Rec 1995;136(10):239–44.
35. Braun U, Marmier O, Pusterla N. Ultrasonographic examination of the small intes-tine of cows with ileus of the duodenum, jejunum or ileum. Vet Rec 1995;137(9): 209–15.
36. Braun U, Forster E, Steininger K, et al. Ultrasonographic findings in 63 cows with haemorrhagic bowel syndrome. Vet Rec 2010;166(3):79–81.
37. Braun U, Amrein E. Ultrasonographic examination of the caecum and the prox-imal and spiral ansa of the colon of cattle. Vet Rec 2001;149(2):45–8.
38. Braun U, Amrein E, Koller U, et al. Ultrasonographic findings in cows with dilata-tion, torsion and retroflexion of the caecum. Vet Rec 2002;150(3):75–9.
39. Kasari TR, Woodbury AH, Morcom-Kasari E. Adverse effect of orally administered magnesium hydroxide on serum magnesium concentration and systemic acid-base balance in adult cattle. J Am Vet Med Assoc 1990;196(5):735–42.
40. Smith GW, Correa MT. The effects of oral magnesium hydroxide administration on rumen fluid in cattle. J Vet Intern Med 2004;18(1):109–12.
41. Rager KD, George LW, House JK, et al. Evaluation of rumen transfaunation after surgical correction of left-sided displacement of the abomasum in cows. J Am Vet Med Assoc 2004;225(6):915–20.

Abomasal and Third Compartment Ulcers in Ruminants and South American Camelids

CrossMark

Alexandra Hund, Dr med vet*, Thomas Wittek, Prof Dr med vet

KEYWORDS

- Abomasal ulcers • South American camelids • Small ruminants • Cattle • Etiology
- Pathogenesis • Diagnosis • Treatment

KEY POINTS

- Abomasal ulcers are most frequent in veal calves and are caused by a wide array of possible factors.
- Ante mortem diagnosis of abomasal ulcers is only possible indirectly based on clinical signs, tests for fecal occult blood, and ultrasound examination, among others.
- Abomasal ulcers can be treated pharmacologically, surgically, and by alleviating concurrent disease.

INTRODUCTION: NATURE OF THE PROBLEM
Types of Ulcers and Location in Cattle

Abomasal lesions can histologically be classified as ulcers if the necrosis of the abomasal wall reaches deeper than the lamina muscularis mucosae into the submucosal layer. More superficial lesions are defined as erosions. Smith and associates[1] introduced a classification of abomasal ulcers in cattle with 4 types (modified from Fox[2] and Whitlock[3]) and Braun and colleagues[4] added 4 subtypes of type 1 abomasal ulcers (**Table 1**).

The consequences of a perforation of the abomasum differ depending on its location: If the perforation site is adjacent to a structure, like the omentum or the abdominal wall, the formation of local adhesions limiting abdominal contamination is likely (type 3 ulcers). In other cases, the ingesta contaminate the peritoneal cavity before forming adhesions and cause generalized peritonitis (type 4 ulcers). The abomasum can

Disclosure Statement: The authors have nothing to disclose.
Department for Farm Animals and Veterinary Public Health, University Clinic for Ruminants, University of Veterinary Medicine Vienna, Veterinaerplatz 1, 1210 Vienna, Austria
* Corresponding author.
E-mail address: Alexandra.Hund@vetmeduni.ac.at

Table 1
Types of abomasal ulcers with type 1 subtypes

Type	Description
1	Nonperforating ulcer with incomplete penetration of the abomasal wall
1a	Erosion with minimal mucosal defects and loss of mucosal rugae, sometimes mucosal discoloration only (often reddish-violet or green-brown)
1b	Deeper erosions with mucosal hemorrhage, sharply demarcated with a depressed center
1c	Craters with coating of detritus or fibrin, depressed center, and bulging margins
1d	Radial wrinkles with a central point, affecting gastric folds only
2	Bleeding ulcer with penetration of a major abomasal vessel and severe intraluminal hemorrhage
3	Perforating ulcer with localized peritonitis owing to adhesion to adjacent viscera
4	Perforating ulcer with diffuse peritonitis owing to spread of ingesta through the peritoneal cavity

also perforate so that ingesta leak either into the supraomental recess and cause peritonitis and adhesions of the small intestine or into the bursa omentalis with subsequent omental bursitis.[5] For this latter type of ulcer, the classification as type 5 has been used.[6]

The anatomic location of the ulcer within the abomasum may be related to differences in the pathogenesis, as discussed elsewhere in this article. There is a predisposition for calves to develop abomasal ulcers in the pyloric region (**Fig. 1**). In veal calves, 95% of nonperforating ulcers at slaughter were located mainly in the pyloric region of the abomasum.[7] In a study of feedlot cattle, both perforating and nonperforating ulcers found on necropsy were also located mainly in the pyloric region of the abomasum.[8] However, perforating ulcers in unweaned beef calves were found in the midpart of the corpus abomasi with a propensity for the greater curvature of the abomasum.[9,10] In a later study in feedlot cattle, ulcers were located mostly on mucosal folds of the corpus at the slaughterhouse.[11]

In dairy cows, erosions were found equally distributed in both parts, but bleeding ulcers occurred predominantly in the corpus of the abomasum.[12] At slaughter,

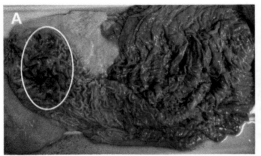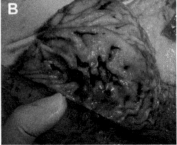

Fig. 1. Type 1 ulcer in the pyloric region of the abomasum in a slaughter veal calf. (*A*) Overview with circled ulcer in the pyloric region. (*B*) Close-up of the ulcer.

abomasal ulcers type 1a and 1c were found mostly in the pyloric region, type 1b and 1d occurred mainly in the region of the corpus abomasi.[4]

A study in slaughter calves, cows, and bulls showed that more than two-thirds of type 1 ulcers were localized in the pyloric region in all 3 groups. Type 1a ulcers were almost exclusively located in the pyloric part of the abomasum. Ulcers located in the corpus were predominantly on the tips of the abomasal folds.[13]

Specific Characteristics of the Digestive Tract of South American Camelids

South American Camelids (SAC) are ruminating animals but biologically they do not belong to the ruminants. Camelids have morphologically distinct stomachs; however, because their digestive physiology is partially similar to the ruminants, there are some similarities in anatomic structures. A number of studies describing the morphology of the gastrointestinal tract of SAC have been published.[14–18] The stomachs of camelids are also compartmentalized, but in contrast with ruminants, camels have only 3 stomach compartments. Compartment 1 (C1) is the equivalent of the rumen, where the ingesta is mixed, regurgitated, and microbially digested. A distinct anatomic structure like the reticulum in ruminants is not developed in SAC. The C1 is the largest of all compartments and contains approximately 83% of the complete volume of the stomachs, which is approximately 15 to 25 L in llamas and 8 to 12 L in alpacas. Specific for camelids are the saccular regions, which are located ventrally in the cranial and caudal sac of C1. The mucosal membrane of the saccular area secrets fluid and bicarbonate facilitating mixing and buffering of the C1 content.

Compartment 2 (C2) is the next stomach after C1 on the right side and contains about 6% of the gastric volume. C2 is a reniform organ right and cranial to C1, with thick muscular walls forming a greater and lesser curvature. C2 function is similar to the omasum in ruminants and forms the passage way to C3, where the ingesta is further mixed during the transport.

Compartment 3 (C3) is an elongated organ containing a volume of about 11% of the complete gastric volume. C3 communicates with C2 via a narrow passage and is situated ventrally and right to C1. This compartment is the true stomach; the glandular mucosal membrane is located only in the caudal third of the C3. This is where hydrochloric acid and pepsinogen are secreted into the lumen; the other parts are lined with nonglandular epithelium.

Types of Ulcers and Location in South American Camelids

Ulcers are typically seen in C3; however, from our own experience with clinical cases (necropsy) and the literature,[15] it is known that ulcers may also occur in C1 and C2. It seems that there is no specific classification for ulcers in SAC. In our opinion, it is reasonable to use the classification system (types 1–4/5), which has been developed for cattle and is described elsewhere in this article.

CAUSES OF ULCERATION

The causes of abomasal ulceration are not well-understood, and multiple contributing factors have been described. There might be similarities to the pathophysiology of gastric ulcers in monogastric animals and humans. However, the volume and pH of the abomasum is relatively constant in adult ruminants in contrast with monogastric animals; therefore, it seems reasonable to believe that there are significant differences. It can be assumed that the underlying cause is the disturbance of the equilibrium of protective and aggressive mechanisms on the gastric mucosa.[5] Stress leads to an increase in the secretion of cortisol, gastric acid, and pepsin, and to a decrease in prostaglandin secretion. This process has negative effects on the integrity of the abomasal mucosa[19] because prostaglandin E protects the abomasal wall from autodigestion by decreasing gastric acid production, increasing the secretion of protective mucus and regulating microcirculation. In combination with prolonged periods of low abomasal pH and the presence of agents like bile acids or volatile fatty acids, the mucosa becomes permeable to hydrogen ions and proteolytic enzymes, causing autodigestion.[3]

Calves and Youngstock

Feeding

In suckling calves, the most important proteolytic enzymes are pepsin and chymosin. These proteolytic enzymes are formed from their precursor enzymes pepsinogen and prochymosin in the abomasum, especially if the pH is less than 3.0.[20] If the pH remains low for a prolonged period of time, the risk for an insult of the abomasal mucosa increases. Feeding of cow's milk significantly increases abomasal pH, but the abomasal pH is higher on average over a 24-hour period and the time the pH is greater than 3.0 is longer if all milk–protein milk replacer or combined milk and soy protein milk replacer is fed.[21] Increasing the frequency of feeding increases the mean time the abomasal pH lies is greater than the critical value of 3.0 as well.[20]

In addition, feeding large volumes of milk in only 2 feedings per day in combination with strong peristalsis in the pyloric region can cause disruption of the microcirculation with ischemia and hypoxic damage of the abomasal wall and, therefore, facilitate the formation of ulcers in this area.[22]

Trauma

It is possible that trauma of the abomasal wall owing to sand and rocks or trichobezoars could be predisposing factors. However, it has been shown that it is unlikely that trichobezoars have a significant role in the development of fatal perforating ulcers in beef calves.[9,10,23,24] In contrast, coarse straw as the only roughage offered to veal calves seems to negatively affect their health and increase the incidence of ulcers.[25–28]

Management

Beside feeding, concurrent diseases or management-related events like vaccinations, dehorning, group changes,[29,30] weaning or changes in feed, and being sold at an auction and transported[31] cause stress and potentially increase the chance of developing abomasal ulcers. Feedlot cattle that experience several of these factors developed ulcers more commonly during the first 45 days of winter-initiated fattening than during other times of the year.[8]

Interestingly, studies where calves, heifers, and steers were regrouped frequently indicate that it causes stress-related behavioral changes but no detrimental health effects to the animals could be shown.[29,30,32] Diversity rather than stability of the social environment seems to be more beneficial to them.[32] Regrouped calves even had fewer ulcers than control calves. The authors assume that this may reflect feeding behavior rather than stress.[30]

Copper

In beef calves, copper deficiency has been shown to be linked with abomasal ulcers.[33] Supplementing pregnant cows and calves with copper reduced the incidence of ulcers.[34] The pathway of the interaction is speculative, but could be owing to immunoregulatory mechanisms (reduction of neutrophil function[35]) or the loss of integrity of the abomasal microvasculature owing to defective elastin and collagen as a consequence of copper deficiency.[34]

Concurrent disease

Calves that had to be euthanized owing to the severity of their disease, for example, enteritis, pneumonia, ill-thrift, or right-displaced abomasum, had abomasal ulcers as incidental finding on necropsy in about one-half of the cases (Hund, 2016, unpublished data).

Adult Cattle

Feeding

In cases of subacute or acute rumen acidosis, excessive histamine is produced. This production could either be caused by the growth of microbes that form biogenic amines from precursory amino acids (in this case histidine) owing to bacterial amino acid decarboxylases or release during bacterial lysis.[36] The increase in histamine increases abomasal acid secretion.[37] Also, excessive amounts of volatile fatty acids that cannot be absorbed in the rumen cause a decrease in abomasal motility and emptying.[38] Both factors can contribute to damaging the protective abomasal mucus layer by allowing excessive amounts of hydrochloric acid and pepsin to gravitate to and remain for a prolonged period of time in the most ventral part of the abomasum, the greater curvature, and lead to ulcer formation.[3]

Management

Recently postpartum dairy cows[3,39–41] and cows at peak production[12] are more prone to develop abomasal ulcers compared with cows in others stages of lactation. Also, in contrast with calves and youngstock, regrouping is stressful to primiparous and multiparous cows, and may increase the risk of abomasal ulcers.[42,43]

Concurrent disease

Nine of 35 cows (26%) with bleeding abomasal ulcers had at least 1 concurrent disease: ketosis, left displacement of the abomasum, stillbirth, fat mobilization syndrome, bronchopneumonia, or acute functional pyloric stenosis.[44] Smith and coworkers[1] found that concurrent disease conditions were present in 76% of cattle with abomasal ulcer disease. Displacement of the abomasum to the left or right was most frequently identified, but also mastitis, metritis, or pneumonia. Other studies found a prevalence of 90% and 100% for concurrent disease in dairy cows with perforated and bleeding ulcers, respectively. These conditions included displaced abomasum, metritis, mastitis, and ketosis.[40,41] The mucus layer can be damaged during episodes of indigestion owing to reflux of bile acids, which work as detergents, from the small intestine to the abomasum.[44,45] Additionally, abomasal lymphosarcoma can be associated with bleeding abomasal ulceration.[41]

Cattle of All Age Groups

Microorganisms

Older studies point to a possible role of bacterial and mycotic microorganisms in the pathogenesis of abomasal ulcers. Fungal hyphae could be identified in some cases in feedlot cattle[8] and in calves. However, the identification of the fungi *Absidia* spp. and *Rhizomucor pusillus* was only possible from abomasal and ruminal contents in 4 of 7 calves.[46] *Mucor* spp. and *Rhizopus* spp. were isolated from calves with abomasal ulcers, but also from healthy calves.[47] In 187 cows with type 1 ulcers, no fungal hyphae were found.[4]

Clostridium perfringens and *Campylobacter jejuni* have been described as major bacterial agents in abomasal ulcers in calves.[33,48] However, the relationship between *Campylobacter* and neonatal abomasal ulceration is undetermined.[47] More recent studies using culture-independent methods of identification of infectious agents could not show a difference between the presence of *C perfringens* in the abomasa from healthy calves as compared with ulcerations[49]; the presence of *Clostridium* spp. did not differ between healthy and ulcerated abomasal mucosa samples in calves, cows, and bulls.[50]

The bacterium *Helicobacter* spp. that plays a role in the pathogenesis of gastric ulcers in humans could not be detected in calves.[47,49] In adult cattle, *Helicobacter* spp. was the genus with the highest abundance in healthy as well as in ulcerated mucosa.[50] In type 1 ulcers, no relationship between microbiota communities associated with abomasal ulcers could be shown in cows, bulls, or calves.[50] To conclude, it can be presumed that the role of microbial agents in ulcer formation is at most limited, and potentially indirect.

Side effects of nonsteroidal antiinflammatory drugs

Steroidal and nonsteroidal antiinflammatory drugs inhibit prostaglandin synthesis by inhibiting the arachidonic acid cascade. Prostaglandin has a protective function in the abomasum owing to its ability to increase mucus production and secretion of bicarbonate, decrease gastric acid secretion, and regulate mucosal blood flow.[51] A reduction in prostaglandin synthesis in the stomach increases mucosal damage and ulceration. This change has been shown in humans, horses, and small animals,[52,53] but not in cattle to date.

The gastric side effects of nonsteroidal antiinflammatory drug administration are predominantly owing to the inhibition of the isoenzyme cyclooxygenase (COX)-1, which is constitutively expressed in the gastrointestinal tract, whereas COX-2 is mainly induced at sites of inflammation. There are preferential COX-1 inhibitors, nonspecific COX-1/COX-2 inhibitors, preferential COX-2 inhibitors, and specific COX-2 inhibitors. Truly selective COX-2 inhibitors have been shown to have no gastric side effects in humans.[54] However, this drug class is not approved for the use in food animals in the United States and the European Community. Meloxicam is the only preferential COX-2 inhibitor approved for the use in food animals. Its use could reduce the risk for gastric injury in ruminants.

Unfortunately, to date there is only one study showing that calves that received ibuprofen (a nonspecific COX-1/COX-2 inhibitor) during an infection trial had more abomasal ulcers than control calves. However, owing to the small number of animals in the study, these results were not significant[55] and the restriction to one age group prevents conclusions on older cattle.

Causes of Ulceration in Small Ruminants

The information regarding pathogenic factors for abomasal ulcers in small ruminants is limited. In a Venezuelan study examining the abomasa of goats after slaughter (no information provided if the goats had abomasal ulcers), none of the 70 goats were positive for *Helicobacter* spp. by polymerase chain reaction analysis of the DNA extracted from gastric biopsies, using genus- and species-specific primers. However, it remains unclear whether sheep harbor a gastric *Helicobacter* or not.[56] In 67 lambs with abomasal bloat, 20 also showed abomasal ulcers. *Sarcina*-like bacteria were identified in 9 of the 20 animals (45%) and *Clostridium sordellii* was more frequently encountered in cases with hemorrhage and ulcers.[57] In another study, animals with abomasal ulcers were found to have higher histamine concentrations in abomasal fluid than lambs with abomasal bloat and control animals. Isolates of *C sordellii* and *Lactobacillus* spp. from lambs with abomasal ulcers were found to be capable of producing histamine in vitro. This finding may point to a central role of bacteria and histamine synthesis in the induction of the disease. The histidine from hemoglobin associated with abomasal hemorrhage in lambs may be a precursor for bacterial histamine production.

However, it is not clear if the elevated histamine levels in the abomasa of the affected animals are solely due to bacterial production or if it is also released by damaged mast cells in the abomasal wall.[58] In lambs, there was a significant association between ulcers and the presence of bezoars.[59]

Causes of Ulceration in South American Camelids

A number of causes for ulceration have also been discussed for SAC. Similar to other animal species factors like stress, transportation, shows, concurrent diseases, treatment with nonsteroidal and steroidal antiinflammatory drugs, C1 acidosis, bacteria (*C perfringens* or *Helicobacter*), and others have been suggested.[15,60] However, most of these assumptions have been adapted from other species without clinical research. Bile acid reflux from the duodenum into the stomach has been linked with pathogenesis of gastric ulcers. A post mortem examination study performed in SAC suggests that bile acid may flow in retrograde direction into C3.[60] The role of this finding in the etiology of gastric ulcers is also unknown in SAC; it is controversially debated in other species.

Similar to cattle, little is known about the effects of nonsteroidal antiinflammatory drugs in the pathogenesis of gastric ulcers in SAC. The administration of flunixin meglumine to llamas did not result in changes of the pH value of C3 fluid.[61] Additionally, none of the five treated animals in the study developed clinical signs indicative of gastric ulcers, and no ulcers were found at necropsy. However, the results of the study do not necessarily rule out a possible effect of nonsteroidal antiinflammatory drugs on gastric ulcer pathogenesis in SAC.

PREVALENCE AND SIGNIFICANCE OF ABOMASAL AND THIRD COMPARTMENT ULCERS IN RUMINANTS AND SOUTH AMERICAN CAMELIDS
Prevalence, Mortality, and Case Fatality Rate in Cattle

The prevalence of abomasal ulcers reported in studies varies significantly owing to differences in the examined population, case definitions, and different means of diagnosis.

In a study in Austrian slaughter cattle, ulcers were found in the abomasa in 65.9% of fattening bulls, 48.5% of cows, and 59.3% of veal calves. These were all type 1 ulcers.[13] In the adult dairy cattle population admitted to a veterinary teaching hospital, 2.17% of animals were identified as having abomasal ulcers during surgery or at necropsy.[1] At slaughter, only 1% of dairy cows had abomasal ulcers, but 6.2% and 7.2% showed erosions in the fundic part and the torus pyloricus of the abomasum, respectively. Abomasal scars were found in 5.3% of cows.[12] In another study in slaughter cows, 20.5% of cows had type 1 abomasal ulcers. The subtypes 1a to 1d occurred in 29.9%, 28.9%, 32.6%, and 8.6%, respectively.[4] In feedlot cattle, perforations or hemorrhages of the abomasum were the cause of death of 1.6% of necropsied yearling cattle and a similar additional number had innocuous ulcers as incidental findings.[8] Katchuik[24] reported an incidence of 0.2% of abomasal disease in young beef calves on a herd level.

Veal calves seem to be the most severely affected group of cattle. The reported overall prevalence of nonperforating abomasal lesions in veal calves at slaughter varies from 67%[62] to 87%[28] and reaches even 95%.[7] Perforating abomasal ulcers accounted for 25% of fatal outcomes in veal calves between 3 and 16 weeks of age in Switzerland.[25] In a study in veal calves in Belgium, the digestive system accounted for 41.9% of case fatalities. The mortality risk for perforating abomasal ulceration was 0.1.[63] The case fatality rate in perforated abomasal ulcers in suckling calves was reported to exceed 50% even if treated surgically.[10] In adult cattle, case fatality rates range from 25% with type 1 ulcers to 100% with types 2 or 4 ulcers.[1]

Prevalence in Small Ruminants

In some reports of abomasal ulcers in adult sheep[64] and lambs,[57–59] prevalence information was not provided. In studies from the Middle East abomasal ulcers were found in 17.85% of sheep between 3.0 months and 3.5 years of age at slaughter[65] and in 75% of slaughtered sheep.[66] In the latter study, animals were affected by multiple ulcers: type 1a ulcers were seen in 66% of abomasa, type 1b in 38%, type 1c ulcers in 18%, and type 1d in 7%; type 2 ulcers were observed only in 1% of animals.

In another study, sheep of all ages that died suddenly were examined post mortem. The most severe gross lesions of the abomasum were observed in lambs from 4 to 10 weeks of age.[67] A study on the etiology of goat mortality in New Zealand showed that abomasal ulcers were among the least common diagnoses (no prevalence given).[68]

Prevalence, Mortality, and Case Fatality Rate in South American Camelids

It seems that no data on the prevalence of gastric ulcers in the SAC population are currently available. However, in our clinical caseload at the University Clinic for Ruminants of the University of Veterinary Medicine in Vienna, Austria, we frequently see C3 ulcers in animals that died or had to be euthanized. Typically, these animals were severely ill and gastric ulcers are likely the result of the primary disease. This finding is similar to reports from other veterinary hospitals.[15,69]

CLINICAL SYMPTOMS AND DIFFERENTIAL DIAGNOSES
Adult Cattle

In cows, type 1 ulcers seem to cause no or mild clinical signs.[4] Oftentimes, an antemortem diagnosis would not have been made without incidental identification of the ulcer during surgery. However, in 71% of cattle with types 1 to 4 ulcers at least one of the symptoms of abdominal pain, pale mucous membranes, or melena was present.[1]

A study to determine the reliability of these clinical signs showed that the presence of occult blood had a sensitivity of 0.77 and a specificity of 0.97, painful abdomen of 0.54 and 0.94, and anemia 0.31 and 0.62, respectively. Animals that met the criteria but did not have abomasal ulcers had traumatic reticuloperitonitis, displacement of the abomasum, fatty degeneration of the liver, cecal volvulus, pneumonia, or pleuritis.[70] These diseases should therefore be ruled out as differential diagnoses.

Type 2 bleeding ulcers are easier to diagnose clinically owing to the blood loss and the excretion of the digested blood via feces. In a study in 35 affected cows, their general condition was slightly, moderately, or even severely disturbed in all animals, and rumen contractions were decreased or absent. Mucous membranes were pale, the animals showed tachycardia, and some even tachypnea. The feces were dark brown to black in color (melena).[44]

The differential diagnoses for type 2 ulcers are all diseases that can cause intestinal bleeding including hemorrhagic bowel syndrome and intestinal intussusceptions. The main differential diagnosis for type 3 ulcers is traumatic reticuloperitonitis owing to a similar location of the lesions. Type 4 perforated abomasal ulcers can hardly be differentiated clinically from other causes of generalized peritonitis.

Calves

In calves, deep ulcers can be clinically inapparent until they perforate and the subsequent peritonitis causes symptoms like inappetence.[5] Further symptoms of calves with perforated abomasal ulcers are listed in **Box 1**. The differential diagnoses in

---

Box 1
Clinical symptoms in 30 calves with perforated abomasal ulcers

- No peracute progression of the disease
- No or only slight signs of colic
- Abnormal posture (arched back, head low, ears drooping)
- Dipping the mouth into water without drinking (wet chin) (**Fig. 2**)
- Painful facial expression, empty look
- Abnormal shape of the abdomen (distended)
- Increased abdominal tension
- Positive swing and percussion auscultation plus splashing
- Weak or no ruminal and intestinal motility
- Positive reaction to pain palpation over large areas of the abdomen

Data from Rademacher G, Lorch A. Verlauf und klinische Symptomatik bei Kälbern mit perforierendem Labmagengeschwür. Tierarztl Umsch. 2001;56(11):563-71.

---

calves for type 2 ulcers include bovine viral diarrhea and mucosal disease, coccidiosis, and endoparasites, especially ostertagiosis. Clinical signs of types 3 and 4 ulcers could also be caused by other septic conditions involving the abdomen, for example, omphalitis.

Small Ruminants

Like in cattle, abomasitis and abomasal ulceration often cause no apparent clinical signs in mild cases, and the most common signs are anorexia and colic.[71]

Camelids

The clinical diagnosis of gastric ulcer in SAC is difficult because, similar to cattle, the clinical signs are nonspecific. Clinical findings and necropsy results show that ulcers in

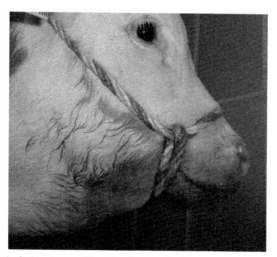

Fig. 2. Typical clinical sign in a calf with abomasal ulcer. Dipping the mouth into water without drinking (wet chin).

the third stomach compartment and the duodenum may occur in llamas and alpacas either as primary or secondary conditions.[15,72] Owing to the anatomic position of the C3 and digestive physiology, gastroscopy is not possible. Therefore, as in ruminants, only indirect diagnostic procedures are applicable. In ruminants, a number of indirect diagnostic procedures have been described and are generally feasible in SAC:

- Physical examination,
- Ultrasound examination of the ventral abdominal cavity,
- Diagnostic laparotomy,
- Fecal occult blood test,
- Hematologic parameters,
- Pepsinogen concentration in blood, and
- Gastrin concentration in blood.

Little is known about the diagnostic value of these methods and parameters in SAC, but it seems reasonable to believe that, as in other animals, a large number of animals having gastric ulcers cannot be diagnosed by clinical examination because clinical signs like decreased food intake, decreased intestinal motility, teeth grinding, and pain response to abdominal palpation likely have low sensitivity and specificity, or the animals are asymptomatic as described in cattle.[4,23]

LABORATORY DIAGNOSIS, IMAGING, AND ADDITIONAL TESTING
Blood Work

Hematology and clinical chemistry in cows with bleeding abomasal ulcers show anemia owing to blood loss: packed cell volume, hemoglobin, erythrocyte count, and mean corpuscular hemoglobin concentration are decreased. Total protein and potassium are below the reference range and urea usually above. Some cows show metabolic acidosis and some alkalosis; in some cows, rumen chloride and bile levels are slightly increased.[44]

In type 1 abomasal ulcers, hematology and clinical chemistry are of little diagnostic value. Hematocrit can be decreased and total protein increased as a sign of chronic inflammation.[4] In types 3 and 4 ulcers parameters point to the inflammatory changes owing to peritonitis.

Pepsinogen and Gastrin

Serum pepsinogen activity of greater than 5.0 U/L has been successfully used to predict abomasal ulcers in cattle.[73] Owing to increased epithelial and vascular permeability or hypersecretion by zymogenic cells, pepsinogen can leak into the blood and reflect the damage of the mucosa. However, the method is of limited value in animals with unknown or positive parasitologic status, because a higher serum pepsinogen level can also be due to other mucosal damage, for example, caused by *Ostertagia ostertagi*. This infection induces an increase in gastrin activity, which could be an additional test to diagnose abomasal ulcers in cattle.[74,75]

Fecal Occult Blood Testing

Fecal occult blood tests can be a helpful tool in determining gastrointestinal bleeding if melena is not obvious. However, they cannot differentiate whether the origin of the blood is the abomasum or other parts of the gastrointestinal tract. In nonbleeding ulcers, the sensitivity is questionable but most likely rather low. It should be noted that the orthotolidine-based test that seemed to be a good additional test even for type 1 ulcers used in the study by Smith and associates[70] is not used today owing to the high rate of false-positive results.[76] A study using 2 different fecal occult blood tests for the detection of type 1 ulcers showed a sensitivity of 0.16 and specificity of 0.94 for a guaiac test and 0.73 and 0.44 for the use of a urinary test strip, respectively. This indicated that both tests were not suitable for the detection of type 1 abomasal ulcers, likely owing to the small amounts of blood that were shed, probably intermittently, with these ulcers.[13] The limit of detection of blood using a guaiac test is 1.7 mL in 100 g feces. Testing the same animal multiple days in a row increases the sensitivity of the test.[77]

Laboratory Diagnosis in South American Camelids

As discussed, the concentration of pepsinogen and gastrin in peripheral blood can be influenced by other factors like gastrointestinal parasites in small ruminants and cattle. Because SAC have specific gastrointestinal parasites in their C3 (eg, *Camelostrongylus mentulatus*, *Graphinemia aucheniae*, *Spiculopteragia peruvianusare*) and as they are also susceptible to ruminant gastrointestinal parasites (eg, *Ostertagia* spp., *Haemonchus* spp.) it is reasonable to believe that the same interference may occur. Currently, there are no reference ranges available for gastrin and pepsinogen concentrations in healthy alpacas and llamas. The diagnostic value of fecal occult blood tests in alpacas and llamas is unknown. Based on studies in monogastric animals and ruminants, none of the indirect measurements is an objective measure that can be used as a reference method. Diagnostic laparotomy should only be considered if clinical signs indicate a perforation.[15] Currently, the definite diagnosis of gastric ulcers in ruminants and camelids can only be made after slaughter or during a post mortem examination.

Endoscopic and Ultrasound Examination and Ultrasound-Guided Abomasocentesis

The endoscopic examination of the abomasum in adult cattle via oral access is clearly impossible owing to anatomic conditions and constraints regarding the equipment. However, the attempt to examine the abomasum in calves via the reticular fold has also not been successful (Franz S, personal communication, 2017).[78]

Ultrasound examination of the abomasum has been described extensively in calves and adult cattle, and can be considered a standard diagnostic procedure.[79–84] Because of the abomasal folds and the abomasal content, the integrity of the abomasal mucosa is difficult to assess; therefore, currently ultrasound examination cannot be considered a reliable diagnostic tool for the detection of abomasal ulcers. Ultrasound-guided abomasocentesis has been established in cattle[85] and the technique has been used mainly in experimental studies.[86] It allows sampling of abomasal fluid, which can be examined for blood from bleeding ulcers. To our knowledge, the diagnostic value of the procedure has not been validated so far. Major concerns are that abomasocentesis itself may cause bleeding resulting in false-positive results, and that nonbleeding ulcers cannot be diagnosed using the method.

Although ultrasound examination is currently applied in SAC for diagnostic purposes, it seems that there is very little specific information on abdominal ultrasound examination available. Cebra and colleagues[87] described the ultrasound appearance of the abdominal organs; they were able to visualize C1 and C3. The cylindrical-shaped third compartment could be imaged in the right paramedian part of the ventral abdomen. Similar to cattle, the diagnosis of ulcers is difficult caused by the ingesta and anatomic details and as far as we know, the diagnostic value has not been evaluated.

Abdominocentesis

Abdominocentesis and peritoneal fluid analysis have been described as a diagnostic tool in ruminants[88,89] and SAC.[90] Abdominocentesis can be helpful in types 3 and 4 ulcers to diagnose the associated peritonitis. In case of localized peritonitis, the abdominocentesis could be nondiagnostic owing to the ability of cattle to effectively wall off infectious processes unless the correct location is chosen. Performing the procedure under ultrasound guidance may improve success at sampling localized lesions. Identification of a fluid exudate supports the tentative diagnosis peritonitis owing to perforated abomasal ulcer.

In 30% of calves with perforated abomasal ulcers, a direct diagnosis could be made using abdominocentesis and identifying the aspirate as abomasal content owing to pungently acid or putrid smell, low pH, and high chloride content.[5]

Exploratory Laparotomy

Another way to diagnose nonspecific abdominal symptoms is exploratory laparotomy. In rare cases in calves with a ventral midline approach, it is possible to explore the abomasum visually or by palpation and identify ulcers as a thickening of the abomasal wall or roughening of the serosal surface, both owing to inflammation at the site of ulceration. In other cases, an abomasotomy is necessary to examine the mucosa directly.

TREATMENT
Pharmacologic Treatment Options

Antacids like aluminum or magnesium hydroxide are given orally to bind hydrochloric acid, absorb pepsin, and bind bile acids[91] and, therefore, help to protect the mucosal integrity. In adult cattle, these agents have been used to treat bleeding abomasal ulcers, but their effect has not been proven to date.[41,44] On the contrary, they are most likely diluted by rumen contents and, therefore, ineffective. However, it might be possible to bypass the rumen in a higher number of adult cattle by induction of esophageal groove closure using salty or bitter solutions.[92]

In milk-fed calves, however, it has been shown that antacids administered orally transiently increase abomasal pH and could therefore play a role in the treatment of abomasal ulceration in calves. However, the clinical efficacy in calves has not been shown.[93]

Histamine type-2 receptor antagonists, for example, ranitidine and cimetidine, inhibit gastric acid secretion. Ranitidine is 3 to 13 times as potent on a molar basis as cimetidine in inhibiting gastric acid secretion.[94] It has been shown to increase abomasal pH in sheep for up to 150 minutes when given intravenously at doses of 1 to 2 mg/kg[95] and for about 60 minutes in steers when given intramuscularly at 6.6 mg/kg.[96] Given orally, ranitidine increases abomasal pH in sheep, but requires very large doses (45 mg/kg body weight by mouth).[97]

Similarly in milk-fed calves, cimetidine (50 or 100 mg/kg, by mouth, every 8 hours) and ranitidine (10 or 50 mg/kg, by mouth, every 8 hours) increased abomasal luminal pH to greater than 3.0 for greater than 75% of the 24-hour period at very high doses. The high doses that are required in calves could be due to reduced dependence on histamine-mediated stimulation of acid secretion, lower oral bioavailability of H2-antagonists, or increased volume of distribution or clearance of H2-antagonists.[98]

Omeprazole is a potent, specific, and long-acting proton pump inhibitor of basal and stimulated acid secretion. It irreversibly binds to the proton pump H^+K^+-ATPase that exchanges hydrogen ions for potassium ions at the secretory surface of the parietal cell. Thereby, it decreases gastric secretion of hydrochloric acid.[99] In milk-fed calves, the administration of omeprazole as oral formulation once daily at 4 mg/kg has been shown to significantly increase the abomasal pH over 24 hours. The effect, however, may decrease over time.[100] In adult cattle, there is no information available and orally administered omeprazole is most likely destroyed by the rumen flora and becomes ineffective. Injectable omeprazole is available as a human drug. A beneficial effect of using omeprazole to treat cattle with abomasal ulcers has not been shown.

To increase abomasal emptying and remove acidic contents, it has been suggested to use 30 mg metoclopramide at 8-hour intervals in cows.[44] However, in calves it has been shown that only erythromycin at 8.8 mg/kg but not metoclopramide and neostigmine are effective in increasing the abomasal emptying rate.[101] In adult cattle, evidence also indicates that erythromycin but not metoclopramide increases abomasal emptying. Adverse behavioral effects can occur with metoclopramide.[102] It has to be emphasized that there are no studies showing a beneficial effect of prokinetic drugs on abomasal ulcer prevention or healing.

When considering pharmacologic treatment of abomasal ulcers, national legislation and regulations regarding the extra-label use of these drugs, drug residues and withdrawal times, as well as the costs of treatment in food animals must be considered.

Pharmacologic Treatment Options in South American Camelids

The basic principles of treatment in SAC are similar to cattle. It has been shown that antiulcer agents (H2 receptor antagonists like cimetidine or ranitidine and H^+/K^+-ATPase inhibitors like omeprazole or pantoprazole), which are commonly used in monogastric species, are also effective in SAC.[61,69,103] Cimetidine (3.3 mg/kg, intramuscularly, every 12 hours) significantly increased the pH of the C3 content over a period of 30 to 60 minutes after administration.[61] A similar short reduction (<1 hour) of acid secretion into the C3 has been described by Christensen and associates[103] after intravenous application of ranitidine (1.5 mg/kg). Intravenous omeprazole (0.4 and 0.8 mg/kg) significantly reduced the C3 acid production for approximately 6 hours; the higher dosage did not have advantages.[103] Similar results were reported for pantoprazole given intravenously or subcutaneously, suggesting that pantoprazole is also suitable for ulcer treatment or prevention in SAC. Poulsen and coworkers[104] investigated the pharmacokinetics of orally administered omeprazole in adult llamas. Despite high doses, the absorption of the drug was not sufficient to yield any efficacy in camelids. These results are somehow in contrast with empirical observations of numerous clinicians suggesting that oral omeprazole treatment (4 mg/kg by mouth) has beneficial effects on gastric ulcers in SAC, including resolution of positive fecal occult blood tests, after several days of oral treatment. A possible explanation might be that esophageal groove closure results in bypassing the C1 making the drug available for absorption. Intrarectal administration of omeprazole has been studied by Marmulak and colleagues,[105] but rectal absorption was found to be poor in alpacas.

Nonpharmacologic Treatment Options

Nonpharmacologic treatment options involve treating concurrent diseases and providing supportive care, for example, blood transfusions in anemic animals.

Surgical Treatment Options

There are some reports of successfully treating ulcers by resecting the affected lesion in the abomasum. This measure has been described in a cow with a bleeding type 2 abomasal ulcer[106] as well as in 4- to 6-week old calves with perforated ulcers.[10] Four of 10 calves survived the excision of an already perforated ulcer. Abomasal contents were removed by thorough lavage of the abdomen during surgery. The remaining calves died owing to complications from peritonitis. The surgical treatment of perforated ulcers in cows is possible,[107] but the long-term survival rate of surgical treatment of concurrent abomasal displacement and perforating ulceration in cattle was only 14%.[108]

The excision of ulcers in beef calves that had not yet perforated has also been described. The calves were identified clinically owing to depression, dehydration, bloat, a distended abdomen, a fluid-filled viscus in the ventral abdomen on ballotte-ment, and subtle to severe colic. The calves underwent surgery, but ulcers were not readily detectable on palpation or visual examination of the abomasal serosa. There-fore, an abomasotomy was performed, the abomasum everted, and the entire abomasal mucosa inspected visually with a subsequent resection of all abomasal ul-cers. The overall survival of surgical cases was 74%.[24]

In the experience of these authors, however, finding nonperforated ulcers is mostly due to coincidence; in most cases, the clinical signs are too subtle to result in the consultation of a veterinarian until the ulcer has perforated and the calves are in shock. If the ulcer can be resected successfully, calves usually recover uneventfully (Flöck M, personal communication, 2016).

PREVENTION

In addition to avoiding causes of ulceration, feeding frequency and gentle contact may help to prevent abomasal ulcers in calves. Similar to monogastric animals, including humans, long periods of low abomasal pH are believed to increase the risk of injury to the abomasal mucosa and abomasal ulceration in ruminants and camelids. This finding might only apply to preruminant calves, because the pH and volume of the abomasum is relatively steady owing to a continuous flow of ingesta from the forest-omach in adult ruminants. Ahmed and coworkers[20] showed that increasing the feeding frequency in calves to 3 to 8 times per day increased the proportion of time where the abomasal pH was greater than 3 and increased the mean 24-hour abomasal luminal pH. This feeding strategy resembles the inherent suckling frequency in range calves, which is on average 5 times in 24 hours.[109]

Veal calves that received human contact for 90 seconds each day (stroking, talking to calves, and letting them suck on fingers directly after milk feeding) had significantly fewer abomasal ulcers and scars compared with control animals.[110] The authors hy-pothesized that the additional human contact decreased stress during handling and transport to the slaughterhouse or that sucking the fingers induced better digestion after the meals, resulting in fewer ulcers. In addition, gentle contact reduces the adverse response to transport shown by differences in glycolytic potential (estimator of resting glycogen level in muscle).

SUMMARY

Abomasal ulcers are an obscure, but likely underdiagnosed, problem in cattle. When they become clinically apparent, treatment is usually not economically promising or even clinically possible. Measures for prevention are not well-defined, and the general recommendation of avoiding stress is not feasible in cattle production systems. There-fore, abomasal ulcers pose a reason for frustration to producers and veterinarians, but also an opportunity for further research.

REFERENCES

1. Smith DF, Munson L, Erb HN. Abomasal ulcer disease in adult dairy cattle. Cor-nell Vet 1983;73(3):213–24.

2. Fox FH. The esophagus, stomach, intestines and peritoneum. In: Amstutz HE, editor. Bovine medicine and surgery, vol. 2, 2nd edition. Santa Barbara (CA): American Veterinary Publications; 1980. p. 667–8.
3. Whitlock RH. Bovine stomach diseases. In: Anderson NV, editor. Veterinary gastroenterology. Philadelphia: Lea and Febinger; 1980. p. 425–8.
4. Braun U, Eicher R, Ehrensperger F. Type 1 abomasal ulcers in dairy cattle. Zentralbl Veterinarmed A 1991;38(5):357–66.
5. Dirksen GU. Ulceration, dilatation and incarceration of the abomasum in calves: clinical investigations and experiences. Bovine Pract 1994;28:127–35.
6. Constable PD. Abomasal ulcers. 2014. Available at: http://www.merckvetmanual.com/mvm/digestive_system/diseases_of_the_abomasum/abomasal_ulcers.html?qt=abomasal_ulcers&alt=sh. Accessed October 6, 2016.
7. Groth W, Berner H. Untersuchungen über das Labmagengeschwür des Kalbes bei Milchaustauschermast und bei Frühentwöhnung. Zentralbl Veterinarmed A 1971;18(6):481–8.
8. Jensen R, Pierson RE, Braddy PM, et al. Fatal abomasal ulcers in yearling feedlot cattle. J Am Vet Med Assoc 1976;169(5):524–6.
9. Jelinski MD, Ribble CS, Campbell JR, et al. Investigating the relationship between abomasal hairballs and perforating abomasal ulcers in unweaned beef calves. Can Vet J 1996;37(1):23–6.
10. Tulleners EP, Hamilton GF. Surgical resection of perforated abomasal ulcers in calves. Can Vet J 1980;21(9):262–4.
11. Jensen R, Spraker TR, Glock RD, et al. Abomasal erosions in feedlot cattle. Am J Vet Res 1992;53(1):110–5.
12. Aukema JJ, Breukink HJ. Abomasal ulcer in adult cattle with fatal haemorrhage. Cornell Vet 1974;64(2):303–17.
13. Hund A, Beer T, Wittek T. Abomasal ulcers in slaughtered cattle in Austria. Tierarztl Prax Ausg G Grosstiere Nutztiere 2016;44(5):279–85.
14. Pérez W, König HE, Jerbi H, et al. Macroanatomical aspects of the gastrointestinal tract of the alpaca (Vicugna pacos Linnaeus, 1758) and dromedary (Camelus dromedarius Linnaeus, 1758). Vertebr Zool 2016;66(3):419–25.
15. Smith BB, Pearson EG, Timm KI. Third compartment ulcers in the Llama. Vet Clin North Am Food Anim Pract 1994;10(2):319–30.
16. Vallenas A, Cummings JF, Munnell JF. A gross study of the compartmentalized stomach of two new-world camelids, the llama and guanaco. J Morphol 1971;134(4):399–423.
17. Vallenas AP, Stevens CE. Motility of the llama and guanaco stomach. Am J Physiol 1971;220(1):275–82.
18. Von Engelhardt W, Höller H. Salivary and gastric physiology of camelids. Verhandlungen der Deutschen Zoologischen Gesellschaft 1982;195–204.
19. Rademacher G, Lorch A. Verlauf und klinische Symptomatik bei Kälbern mit perforierendem Labmagengeschwür. Tierarztl Umsch 2001;56(11):563–71.
20. Ahmed AF, Constable PD, Misk NA. Effect of feeding frequency and route of administration on abomasal luminal pH in dairy calves fed milk replacer. J Dairy Sci 2002;85(6):1502–8.
21. Constable PD, Ahmed AF, Misk NA. Effect of suckling cow's milk or milk replacer on abomasal luminal pH in dairy calves. J Vet Intern Med 2005;19(1):97–102.
22. Krauser K. Untersuchungen zur Pathogenese der Pylorusulzera beim Mastkalb. Berl Münch Tierärztl Wschr 1987;100:156–61.
23. Ide PR, Henry JH. Abomasal abnormalities in dairy cattle: a review of 90 clinical cases. Can Vet J 1964;5(3):46–55.

24. Katchuik R. Abomasal disease in young beef calves: surgical findings and management factors. Can Vet J 1992;33(7):459–61.

25. Bähler C, Regula G, Stoffel MH, et al. Effects of the two production programs 'Naturafarm' and 'conventional' on the prevalence of non-perforating abomasal lesions in Swiss veal calves at slaughter. Res Vet Sci 2010;88(2):352–60.

26. Mattiello S, Canali E, Ferrante V, et al. The provision of solid feeds to veal calves: II. Behavior, physiology, and abomasal damage. J Anim Sci 2002;80(2):367–75.

27. Van Putten G. Welfare in veal calf units. Vet Rec 1982;111(19):437–40.

28. Welchman DD, Baust GN. A survey of abomasal ulceration in veal calves. Vet Rec 1987;121(25–26):586–90.

29. Gupta S, Earley B, Nolan M, et al. Effect of repeated regrouping and relocation on behaviour of steers. Appl Anim Behav Sci 2008;110(3–4):229–43.

30. Veissier I, Boissy A, dePassillé AM, et al. Calves' responses to repeated social regrouping and relocation. J Anim Sci 2001;79(10):2580–93.

31. Gregory NG. Animal welfare at markets and during transport and slaughter. Meat Sci 2008;80(1):2–11.

32. Raussi S, Boissy A, Andanson S, et al. Repeated regrouping of pair-housed heifers around puberty affects their behavioural and HPA axis reactivities. Anim Res 2006;55(2):131–44.

33. Mills KW, Johnson JL, Jensen RL, et al. Laboratory findings associated with abomasal ulcers/tympany in range calves. J Vet Diagn Invest 1990;2(3):208–12.

34. Lilley C, Hamar D, Gerlach M, et al. Linking copper and bacteria with abomasal ulcers in beef calves. Vet Med 1985;80:85–8.

35. Minatel L, Carfagnini JC. Copper deficiency and immune response in ruminants. Nutr Res 2000;20(10):1519–29.

36. Straub BW, Kicherer M, Schilcher SM, et al. The formation of biogenic amines by fermentation organisms. Z Lebensm Unters Forsch 1995;201(1):79–82.

37. Plaizier JC, Krause DO, Gozho GN, et al. Subacute ruminal acidosis in dairy cows: the physiological causes, incidence and consequences. Vet J 2008; 176(1):21–31.

38. Shaver RD. Nutritional risk factors in the etiology of left displaced abomasum in dairy cows: a review. J Dairy Sci 1997;80(10):2449–53.

39. Hemmingsen I. Ulcus perforans abomasi bovis. Nord Vet Med 1967;19:17–30.

40. Palmer J, Whitlock R. Perforated abomasal ulcers in adult dairy cows. J Am Vet Med Assoc 1984;184(2):171–4.

41. Palmer JE, Whitlock RH. Bleeding abomasal ulcers in adult dairy cattle. J Am Vet Med Assoc 1983;183(4):448–51.

42. Hasegawa N, Nishiwaki A, Sugawara K, et al. The effects of social exchange between two groups of lactating primiparous heifers on milk production, dominance order, behavior and adrenocortical response. Appl Anim Behav Sci 1997;51(1):15–27.

43. Phillips CJC, Rind MI. The effects on production and behavior of mixing uniparous and multiparous cows. J Dairy Sci 2001;84(11):2424–9.

44. Braun U, Bretscher R, Gerber D. Bleeding abomasal ulcers in dairy cows. Vet Rec 1991;129(13):279–84.

45. Braun U, Hausammann K, Forrer R. Reflux of bile acids from the duodenum into the rumen of cows with a reduced intestinal passage. Vet Rec 1989;124(14): 373–6.

46. Gitter M, Austwick PKC. The presence of fungi in abomasal ulcers of young calves; a report of seven cases. Vet Rec 1957;69:924–8.

47. Jelinski MD, Ribble CS, Chirino-Trejo M, et al. The relationship between the presence of Helicobacter pylori, Clostridium perfringens type A, Campylobacter spp, or fungi and fatal abomasal ulcers in unweaned beef calves. Can Vet J 1995;36(6):379-82.
48. Roeder BL, Chengappa MM, Nagaraja TG, et al. Isolation of Clostridium perfringens from neonatal calves with ruminal and abomasal tympany, abomasitis, and abomasal ulceration. J Am Vet Med Assoc 1987;190(12):1550-5.
49. Valgaeren BR, Pardon B, Flahou B, et al. Prevalence and bacterial colonisation of fundic ulcerations in veal calves. Vet Rec 2013;172(10):269.
50. Hund A, Dzieciol M, Schmitz-Esser S, et al. Characterization of mucosa-associated bacterial communities in abomasal ulcers by pyrosequencing. Vet Microbiol 2015;177(1-2):132-41.
51. Wallace JL. Prostaglandins, NSAIDs, and gastric mucosal protection: why doesn't the stomach digest itself? Physiol Rev 2008;88(4):1547-65.
52. Schoen RT, Vender RJ. Mechanisms of nonsteroidal anti-inflammatory drug-induced gastric damage. Am J Med 1989;86(4):449-58.
53. Lees P, Higgins AJ. Clinical pharmacology and therapeutic uses of non-steroidal anti-inflammatory drugs in the horse. Equine Vet J 1985;17(2):83-96.
54. Hawkey CJ. COX-1 and COX-2 inhibitors. Best Pract Res Clin Gastroenterol 2001;15(5):801-20.
55. Walsh P, Carvallo Chaigneau FR, Anderson M, et al. Adverse effects of a 10-day course of ibuprofen in Holstein calves. J Vet Pharmacol Ther 2016;39(5):518-21.
56. Gueneau P, Fuenmayor J, Aristimuno OC, et al. Are goats naturally resistant to gastric Helicobacter infection? Vet Microbiol 2002;84(1-2):115-21.
57. Vatn S, Tranulis MA, Hofshagen M. Sarcina -like bacteria, clostridium fallax and Clostridium sordellii in lambs with abomasal bloat, haemorrhage and ulcers. J Comp Pathol 2000;122(2):193-200.
58. Vatn S, Sjaastad OV, Ulvund MJ. Histamine in lambs with abomasal bloat, haemorrhage and ulcers. J Vet Med A Physiol Pathol Clin Med 2000;47(4):251-5.
59. Vatn S, Ulvund MJ. Abomasal bloat, haemorrhage and ulcers in young Norwegian lambs. Vet Rec 2000;146(2):35-9.
60. Cebra CK, Tornquist SJ, Bildfell RJ, et al. Bile acids in gastric fluids from llamas and alpacas with and without ulcers. J Vet Intern Med 2003;17(4):567-70.
61. Drew ML, Ramsay E, Fowler ME, et al. Effect of flunixin meglumine and cimetidine hydrochloride on the pH in the third compartment of the stomach of llamas. J Am Vet Med Assoc 1992;201(10):1559-63.
62. Wiepkema PR, Van Hellemond KK, Roessingh P, et al. Behaviour and abomasal damage in individual veal calves. Appl Anim Behav Sci 1987;18(3-4):257-68.
63. Pardon B, De Bleecker K, Hostens M, et al. Longitudinal study on morbidity and mortality in white veal calves in Belgium. BMC Vet Res 2012;8(1):26.
64. Angus K, Bannatyne C. Abomasal ulceration in adult sheep: a report of two contrasting cases. Vet Rec 1970;86(18):531-3.
65. Jassim A, Yousif AAR, Kshash QH. Study on abomasal ulcer in sheep in Iraq. Int J Adv Res (Indore) 2014;2(1):342-9.
66. Khodakaram-Tafti A, Hajimohammadi A, Amiri F. Prevalence and pathology of abomasal abnormalities in sheep in southern Iran. Bulgarian Journal of Veterinary Medicine 2015;18(3):270-6.
67. Lewis CJ, Naylor RD. Sudden death in sheep associated with Clostridium sordellii. Vet Rec 1998;142(16):417-21.
68. Buddle BM, Herceg M, Ralston MJ, et al. A goat mortality study in the southern North Island. N Z Vet J 1988;36(4):167-70.

69. Smith GW, Davis JL, Smith SM, et al. Efficacy and pharmacokinetics of panto-prazole in alpacas. J Vet Intern Med 2010;24(4):949–55.

70. Smith DF, Munson L, Erb HN. Predictive values for clinical signs of abomasal ul-cer disease in adult dairy cattle. Prev Vet Med 1986;3(6):573–80.

71. Pugh DG. Sheep & goat medicine. Philadelphia: Saunders; 2002.

72. Cebra CK, Cebra ML, Garry FB, et al. Acute gastrointestinal disease in 27 New World Camelids: clinical and surgical findings. Vet Surg 1998;27(2):112–21.

73. Mesaric M. Role of serum pepsinogen in detecting cows with abomasal ulcer. Vet Arh 2005;75(2):111–8.

74. Fox MT, Carroll AP, Hughes SA, et al. Gastrin and gastrin-related responses to infection with Ostertagia ostertagi in the calf. Res Vet Sci 1993;54(3):384–91.

75. Ok M, Sen I, Turgut K, et al. Plasma gastrin activity and the diagnosis of bleeding abomasal ulcers in cattle. J Vet Med A Physiol Pathol Clin Med 2001;48(9):563–8.

76. Ostrow J. Tests for fecal occult blood. In: Walker HK, Hall WD, Hurst JW, editors. Clinical methods: the history, physical, and laboratory examinations. 3rd edition. Boston: Butterworths; 1990. Available at: https://www.ncbi.nlm.nih.gov/books/NBK445/.

77. Fischer W. Untersuchungen zum Nachweis von okkultem Blut im Kot von Rin-dern und Kälbern. Tierarztl Umsch 1985;40:931–4.

78. Franz S, Gentile A, Baumgartner W. Comparison of two ruminoscopy techniques in calves. Vet J 2006;172(2):308–14.

79. Braun U, Wild K, Guscetti F. Ultrasonographic examination of the abomasum of 50 cows. Vet Rec 1997;140(4):93–8.

80. Van Winden SC, Brattinga CR, Muller KE, et al. Position of the abomasum in dairy cows during the first six weeks after calving. Vet Rec 2002;151(15):446–9.

81. Wittek T, Constable PD, Marshall TS, et al. Ultrasonographic measurement of abomasal volume, location, and emptying rate in calves. Am J Vet Res 2005; 66(3):537–44.

82. Wittek T, Constable PD, Morin DE. Ultrasonographic assessment of change in abomasal position during the last three months of gestation and first three months of lactation in Holstein-Friesian cows. J Am Vet Med Assoc 2005; 227(9):1469–75.

83. Wittek T, Ernstberger M, Muckenhuber M, et al. Effects of wheat protein in milk replacers on abomasal emptying rate in calves. J Anim Physiol Anim Nutr (Berl) 2016;100(2):264–70.

84. Wittek T, Sen I, Constable PD. Changes in abdominal dimensions during late gestation and early lactation in Holstein-Friesian heifers and cows and their rela-tionship to left displaced abomasum. Vet Rec 2007;161(5):155–61.

85. Braun U, Wild K, Merz M, et al. Percutaneous ultrasound-guided abomasocent-esis in cows. Vet Rec 1997;140(23):599–602.

86. Wittek T, Schreiber K, Fürll M, et al. Use of the d-Xylose absorption test to mea-sure abomasal emptying rate in healthy lactating Holstein-Friesian cows and in cows with left displaced abomasum or abomasal volvulus. J Vet Intern Med 2005;19(6):905–13.

87. Cebra CK, Watrous BJ, Cebra ML. Transabdominal ultrasonographic appear-ance of the gastrointestinal viscera of healthy llamas and alpacas. Vet Radiol Ul-trasound 2002;43(4):359–66.

88. Wittek T, Grosche A, Locher L, et al. Biochemical constituents of peritoneal fluid in cows. Vet Rec 2010;166(1):15–9.

89. Wittek T, Grosche A, Locher LF, et al. Diagnostic accuracy of D-Dimer and other peritoneal fluid analysis measurements in dairy cows with peritonitis. J Vet Intern Med 2010;24(5):1211-7.

90. Cebra CK, Tornquist SJ, Reed SK. Collection and analysis of peritoneal fluid from healthy llamas and alpacas. J Am Vet Med Assoc 2008;232(9):1357-61.

91. Maton PN, Burton ME. Antacids revisited. A review of their clinical pharmacology and recommended therapeutic use. Drugs 1999;57(6):855-70.

92. Scholz H. Nutzung der Schlundrinnenkontraktion bei erwachsenen Rind - eine therapeutische Alternative für den praktischen Tierarzt? Prakt Tierarzt 1987; 18:88-91.

93. Ahmed AF, Constable PD, Misk NA. Effect of an orally administered antacid agent containing aluminum hydroxide and magnesium hydroxide on abomasal luminal pH in clinically normal milk-fed calves. J Am Vet Med Assoc 2002; 220(1):74-9.

94. Dowling PM. Therapy of gastrointestinal ulcers. Can Vet J 1995;36(5):276-7.

95. Morgado AA, Nunes GR, Martins AS, et al. Metabolic profile and ruminal and abomasal pH in sheep subjected to intravenous ranitidine. Pesqu Vet Bras 2014;34:17-22.

96. Wallace LLM, Reecy J, Williams JE. The effect of ranitidine hydrochloride on abomasal fluid pH in young steers. Agri-Practice (USA) 1994;15(6):36-8.

97. Duran S, Lin H, Tyler J, et al. PH changes in abomasal fluid of sheep treated with intravenous and oral ranitidine. Paper presented at: 11th annual ACVIM Forum. Washington, DC, May 20, 1993.

98. Ahmed AF, Constable PD, Misk NA. Effect of orally administered cimetidine and ranitidine on abomasal luminal pH in clinically normal milk-fed calves. Am J Vet Res 2001;62(10):1531-8.

99. Clissold SP, Campoli-Richards DM. Omeprazole. A preliminary review of its pharmacodynamic and pharmacokinetic properties, and therapeutic potential in peptic ulcer disease and Zollinger-Ellison syndrome. Drugs 1986;32(1): 15-47.

100. Ahmed AF, Constable PD, Misk NA. Effect of orally administered omeprazole on abomasal luminal pH in dairy calves fed milk replacer. J Vet Med A Physiol Pathol Clin Med 2005;52(5):238-43.

101. Wittek T, Constable PD. Assessment of the effects of erythromycin, neostigmine, and metoclopramide on abomasal motility and emptying rate in calves. Am J Vet Res 2005;66(3):545-52.

102. Constable PD, Nouri M, Sen I, et al. Evidence-based use of prokinetic drugs for abomasal disorders in cattle. Vet Clin North Am Food Anim Pract 2012;28(1): 51-70.

103. Christensen JM, Limsakun T, Smith BB, et al. Pharmacokinetics and pharmacodynamics of antiulcer agents in llama. J Vet Pharmacol Ther 2001;24(1):23-33.

104. Poulsen KP, Smith GW, Davis JL, et al. Pharmacokinetics of oral omeprazole in llamas. J Vet Pharmacol Ther 2005;28(6):539-43.

105. Marmulak T, Stanley S, Kass PH, et al. Pharmacokinetics of intrarectal omeprazole in alpacas. J Vet Pharmacol Ther 2010;33(4):371-5.

106. Tasker JB, Roberts SJ, Fox FH, et al. Abomasal ulcers in cattle; recovery of one cow after surgery. J Am Vet Med Assoc 1958;133(7):365-8.

107. Nuss K, Wehbrink D, Schweizer G. Operative Behandlung von Labmagenulzera Typ 3 bei einer Kuh*. Tierarztl Prax Ausg G Grosstiere Nutztiere 2005;33(6): 427-30.

108. Cable CS, Rebhun WC, Fubini SL, et al. Concurrent abomasal displacement and perforating ulceration in cattle: 21 cases (1985-1996). J Am Vet Med Assoc 1998;212(9):1442–5.
109. Odde KG, Kiracofe GH, Schalles RR. Suckling behavior in range beef calves. J Anim Sci 1985;61(2):307–9.
110. Lensink BJ, Fernandez X, Boivin X, et al. The impact of gentle contacts on ease of handling, welfare, and growth of calves and on quality of veal meat. J Anim Sci 2000;78(5):1219–26.

Surgical Management of Abomasal and Small Intestinal Disease

Sylvain Nichols, DMV, MS*, Gilles Fecteau, DMV

KEYWORDS

- Bovine • Surgery • Abomasum • Duodenum • Jejunum • Ileum • Caecum • Colon

KEY POINTS

- The right para-lumbar fossa is not always the ideal surgical approach to treat abomasal problems, such as ulcer and impaction.
- Minimally invasive procedures have the advantage of decreasing the need for perioperative antibiotics.
- The sigmoid flexure of the duodenum should be systematically evaluated in case of proximal intestinal obstruction.
- Hemorrhagic bowel syndrome remains a difficult condition to treat.
- Partial cecal amputation should be considered in cases of recurrent dislocation/dilatation.

INTRODUCTION

A bovine practitioner should master abdominal exploratory surgery (laparotomy). Several gastrointestinal (GI) problems require surgical correction to save the animal's life and to keep it in production. Time, from the onset of the clinical signs to the surgery, is a key factor in the success of the procedure. Clients need to be educated to rapidly recognize clinical signs of GI obstruction anorexia, colic, decreased fecal output, change in color of feces (melena, fresh blood, mucus). The veterinarian should evaluate cows presenting such signs as early as possible. At the farm, the tools described in Gilles Fecteau and colleagues' article, "Diagnostic Approach to the Acute Abdomen," in this issue, should be used to determine if surgery is needed (surgical abdomen). Depending on the most probable diagnosis, the attending veterinarian should then quickly decide whether or not the surgery can be performed at the farm, if he or she needs to call for help (assistant or a more experienced surgeon), or if the cow has to be euthanized because of the poor prognosis.

Disclosure Statement: The authors have nothing to disclose.
Department of Clinical Sciences, Faculté de Médecine Vétérinaire, Université de Montréal, 3200 Sicotte Street, Saint-Hyacinthe, Québec J2S 2M2, Canada
* Corresponding author.
E-mail address: sylvain.nichols@umontreal.ca

This article first reviews the surgical preparation of the abdomen and the preoperative treatments. The following part is divided in 2 sections: abomasal and intestinal surgery. For the abomasal surgery, the different surgical approaches according to suspected problems will be presented. Finally, postoperative care, including management of postoperative ileus, is presented.

PREOPERATIVE TREATMENTS

Cattle in shock should be stabilized before the surgery (fluids and blood transfusion). Preoperative antibiotics (beta-lactam) are needed when the abdomen is manually explored in a field setting. When the GI tract is open, a broad-spectrum antibiotic effective against gram-negative bacteria should be given. A nonsteroidal antiinflammatory drug (NSAID) (flunixin meglumine or meloxicam), if not already given by the owner, should be given before the surgery with the exception of when an abomasal ulcer is suspected.

Depending on the procedure, the cattle remains standing (most procedures) or is placed in dorsal, lateral, or sternal recumbency. The authors have come to prefer sternal recumbency when it is highly probable that the animal will go down during the procedure (pain or weakness). A key element when choosing this position is to provide enough padding for the down leg to avoid peroneal paresis (seen even more frequently in hypotensive animals). The upper leg should be pulled back and secured to clear the para-lumbar fossa (**Fig. 1**). Compared with the left lateral recumbency position, sternal recumbency allows better exteriorization of the jejunum and the exploratory seems easier to perform.

If a recumbent position is required, the animal will most likely need to be sedated. A ketamine stun given intravenously (IV) (butorphanol 0.025 mg/kg, xylazine 0.05 mg/kg, ketamine 0.5 mg/kg) combined with casting ropes (**Fig. 2**) is usually sufficient to get the cow to lay down safely without significantly compromising the cardiovascular system.[1,2] For the more frantic cattle, the dose of ketamine can be increased to 1.1 to 2.2 mg/kg.

PRINCIPLES OF SURGICAL PREPARATION AND ANESTHESIA
Patient (Cattle)

After identifying a clean area with appropriate lighting to perform the surgery, the animal should be brushed to remove dirt and hairs from the back and flank. Then, the

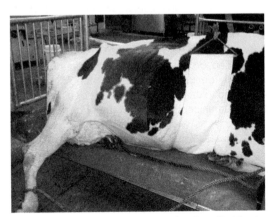

Fig. 1. Adult cow in sternal recumbency. The upper leg is pulled backward to expose the para-lumbar fossa. (*Courtesy of* Sylvain Nichols, Université de Montréal, Saint-Hyacinthe, Québec, Canada.)

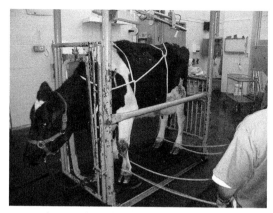

Fig. 2. Casting rope passed around the neck, the thorax, and the abdomen. By pulling on the rope, the abdomen and the thorax are squeezed. The leg ropes help to flip and secure the cow in dorsal recumbency. (*Courtesy of* Sylvain Nichols, DMV, MS, DACVS, Université de Montréal, Saint-Hyacinthe, Québec, Canada.)

surgical site is clipped using a clipper with a No. 40 blade. Using a cordless clipper removes the hassle of finding a power outlet. The razor blade has no advantages over the clipper blade and causes more skin irritation.[3] The clipped area should be a least twice the length of the incision vertically and horizontally.

The second step of the surgical preparation is cleaning. An antiseptic soap with a detergent is needed to remove all organic material from the surgery site. At least 3 rounds of cleaning and aggressive brushing should be done before anesthesia and the aseptic scrub.

Local anesthesia
Local anesthesia of the surgical field within the para-lumbar fossa may be obtained through multiple techniques. For ventral surgery, local anesthesia can only be obtained through a line block using 2% lidocaine.

The proximal and the distal paravertebral blocks have the advantage of completely anesthetizing the para-lumbar fossa. They are somewhat more challenging to perform than the line block and the inverted L. They have the negative reputation of not being efficacious 100% of the time. The percentage of failure lowers over the years of experience.

Proximal paravertebral block The nerves anesthetized are T13, L1, and L2. They are located respectively behind the same numbered vertebrae. The site is at the junction of the axial third and the middle third of the length of the vertebra's transverse process. The closer the block is performed to the spine, the more efficient it is. At this location, 30 to 60 mL of 2% lidocaine is infiltrated in 3 sites (1 cm below, at the level, and 1 cm above the transverse process) with an 18-G, 3.5-in (9 cm) spinal needle. The depth of the transverse process is evaluated by walking off the process with the needle. Before injection, aspiration is performed to check for air (needle in the peritoneum) or blood. The last transverse process to be palpated before the ilium wing is L5. Knowing this, L2 is located to start the block.

Distal paravertebral The nerves anesthetized are T13, L1, and L2. They are located above and below the tip of the vertebral transverse process of L1, L2, and L4.

At this location, 20 to 40 mL of 2% lidocaine is infiltrated in 2 sites (above and below the distal end of the transverse process) with an 18-G, 1.5-in (3.8 cm) needle. Before injection, the site is checked for air (needle in the peritoneum with the ventral injection) or blood (do not inject IV). The last transverse process to be palpated before the ilium wing is L5. Knowing this, L4 is located to start the block. The authors find that the distal paravertebral block does not have the same reliability as the proximal block. However, it is easier to perform and does not create the scoliosis caused by the proximal block.

Segmental epidural block This block is more challenging to perform. It is done at the level of L1-L2 or T13-L1. A 16-G, 12-cm in length Tuohy needle is used. After aseptic preparation, the needle is inserted in the epidural space. A hanging drop technique is used to confirm the proper placement of the needle. Air is allowed to enter the space for 1 minute before the needle is inserted 0.5 cm deeper to avoid injection in the epidural fat. A fixed volume of 4 mL of 2% lidocaine or 1 mL of xylazine (20 mg/mL) and 3 mL of 2% lidocaine is injected. The xylazine speeds up the onset of anesthesia and provides a mild sedative effect. When successfully performed, the abdominal wall is anesthetized bilaterally.[4,5]

The aseptic scrub is performed using an antiseptic soap and detergent. The shaved area is divided in 3 sections: central, mid, and external sections. The central section is located precisely where the incision line will be performed. The aseptic scrub is initiated in this area. It is scrubbed for 90 seconds before moving to the midsection. At this point, the brush should not come in contact with the central section. Another 90 seconds of scrubbing is performed at this location before moving to the external section. At this point, the brush should not come in contact with the mid and central sections. The external section is the junction between the clipped and unclipped part of the animal.

The final step of the surgical preparation is the alternating swipes of alcohol and antiseptic in a circular motion from the anticipated incision line to the outside of the prepared area. This step should be performed just before cleaning and scrubbing the surgeon's hands. Three swipes of each product are performed. The last swipes should be done with the antiseptic. The gauze is inspected to evaluate the cleanliness of the surgical field.

Commonly, iodine- (povidone-iodine) or chlorhexidine-based (4% chlorhexidine gluconate or 2% chlorhexidine diacetate) products are used for surgical preparation. It is important to use the same product throughout the preparation. Chlorhexidine is superior to iodine in the face of organic material. It also has a residual effect that iodine products are lacking. However, studies were not able to demonstrate a difference between the 2 products in regard to surgical site infection.[3-6]

Surgeon

Practitioners doing on-farm surgery are often multitasking to get the animal ready in a timely fashion. They are the anesthesiologist, technician, and surgeon at the same time. After the aseptic scrub, just before the aseptic swipes, the surgery table is set. Visualizing the procedure while opening the instrument packets is a useful review of the material that might be needed. Then, the final aseptic swipes are done just before the surgeon's preparation. The hands and forearms are thoroughly cleaned with an antiseptic and detergent soap, which is followed by a 5-minute scrub.

An impermeable surgical gown (sterile or not) and sterile gloves should be worn for all abdominal procedures.

Drapes

Sterile drapes can be used for standing or recumbent surgery. Ideally, they should be impervious. They extend the aseptic surgical field and help keep the suture material and the surgeon's hands sterile. They are held in place with towel clamps. Those clamps are essential to avoid sliding of the drapes, which will bring dirt in the surgical field. Care must be taken not to contaminate the scrubbed area when setting the drapes. Remember that the back of the drape is in contact with the unclean area so if it moves toward the prepared and aseptic site, contamination occurs.

ABOMASAL PROBLEMS/DISEASES

The most frequent problem involving the abomasum is the displacement. Two displacements have been described: the left (left displaced abomasum [LDA]) and the right side (right displaced abomasum [RDA]) displacement. The RDA is less frequent. However, this displacement can lead to a more serious condition: abomasal volvulus.

LDAs are frequently seen after calving. The cause is multifactorial. Small rumen after calving, electrolyte calcium imbalances, and any other concomitant diseases (retained membranes, mastitis, metritis) causing a decrease in food intake and reduce abomasal motility may predispose to LDA.[7–9]

The RDA can be seen at any time during the life of the animal. When an RDA progresses to a volvulus, the animal rapidly goes into cardiovascular shock (increased heart rate, severe dehydration, pale mucous membrane, slow capillary refill time).[10–12] In this case, surgery is needed as soon as possible to correct the condition and obtain a better outcome.

Other conditions affecting the abomasum are ulcers,[13,14] motility dysfunction leading to impaction,[15] and pyloric outflow obstruction caused by an intraluminal (bezoar) or an extraluminal/intramural (lymphoma, abscess) mass.

ABOMASAL SURGERIES

Multiple surgical approaches to the abomasum have been described. Some are minimally invasive (laparoscopically), and others are performed through an abdominal incision. Each technique has its pros and cons. It is important to realize that not all surgical approaches are suitable for all abomasal problems. Other factors that influence the choice of a procedure over another are surgeon experience, client budget, the value of the cow, and the environment where the animal is kept.

The blind techniques (toggle and blind stitch) are not discussed in this article.

Surgical Techniques Performed Through Laparotomy

The main advantages of laparotomy over laparoscopy are the possibility to explore the abdomen more thoroughly and to palpate the structures. However, having the abdomen open in a farm setting increases the risk of surgical wound infection and peritonitis compared with the noninvasive technique. Therefore, perioperative antibiotics are more often needed and justified with laparotomy.

Right or left paramedian (abomasopexy)

This technique became less popular when the standing right flank omentopexy was developed. It creates a strong adhesion between the abomasum and the body wall.[16] With this technique, the abomasum is secured in its normal anatomic location.

This technique is the ideal surgical technique when ventral adhesion or abomasal ulcers are suspected because it is the only technique that allows exteriorization of the greater curvature of the abomasum through the incision (**Fig. 3**). All the

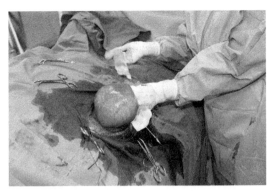

Fig. 3. Greater curvature exposed through a right paramedian incision. (*Courtesy of* André Desrochers, DMV, MS, DACVS, Université de Montréal, Saint-Hyacinthe, Québec, Canada.)

displacements can be corrected through this approach. The main disadvantages of this technique are the need for dorsal recumbency and the risk of postoperative abdominal/abomasal herniation.[17] The latter is reduced by performing a left paramedian approach with a right paramedian pexy next to the incision instead of directly in it. This technique does not allow a thorough abdominal exploration.

Abdominal surgical approach A 15- to 20-cm skin incision is performed 5 to 8 cm caudal to the sternum and lateral (right or left) to the midline. The incision is made through the skin, subcutaneous tissue, caudal deep pectoral muscle (cranially), the external sheet, the rectus abdominis, the internal sheet, and the peritoneum.

Abdominal exploration and abomasopexy The abomasum should be located right below the incision. If the abomasum is not in its place, it is located and brought back to the right side. If it cannot be replaced, adhesions should be suspected. Fibrinous adhesions can be broken down manually. Fibrous adhesions need to be sharply dissected. When the abomasum is freed, it is brought out of the incision. Any perforations or ulcers are sutured. The greater curvature and its omental attachment are identified. Caudally, the pylorus and cranially the reticulo-abomasal ligament are palpated. The abomasopexy is performed midway between those two landmarks, 2 to 4 cm lateral to the omental attachment.

Two techniques have been described:

1. The first technique incorporates the abomasal wall into the abdominal wall closure. The serosa and the muscular layer of the abomasum are attached to the peritoneum and the internal sheet of the rectus abdominis muscle with a simple continuous pattern using nonabsorbable suture material. Care should be taken not to penetrate the lumen of the abomasum by slipping the mucosa away at each bite.
2. The second technique secures the abomasum away from the incision. It reduces the risk of postoperative abomasal herniation. Three pieces of absorbable or nonabsorbable suture material are preplaced through the peritoneum, internal sheet, and rectus abdominis muscle lateral to the incision (**Fig. 4**). Then they are placed within the abomasum wall (same location as in the previous technique) making sure not to penetrate the lumen. The sutures are tightened before abdominal wall closure.

Abdominal surgical closure The abdominal incision is closed in 3 layers. The peritoneum and the internal sheet are closed in a simple continuous pattern (already done if the abomasopexy is located in the abdominal incision). An interrupted suture pattern

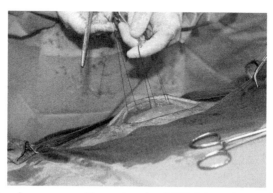

Fig. 4. Paramedian abomasopexy. Three strands of PDS 2 have been placed through the peritoneum, internal sheet, and rectus abdominis muscle before being placed within the abomasal wall. (*Courtesy of* André Desrochers, DMV, MS, DACVS, Université de Montréal, Saint-Hyacinthe, Québec, Canada.)

(cruciate or simple interrupted) is then used for the rectus abdominis and the external sheet (holding layer). Finally, cruciate sutures are used for the skin.

Left para-lumbar fossa (abomasopexy)

This technique can only be used with an LDA. It is commonly performed on cattle with displacement while in late gestation. It is also used when adhesions and ulcers are suspected up high in the flank.

Surgical approach The flank approach closer to the last rib (3–5 cm) and more ventrally on large cattle is used.

Abdominal exploration and abomasopexy The left para-lumbar approach allows the surgeon to palpate the reticulum, the rumen, the spleen, the displaced abomasum, the uterus, and the left kidney. Fibrinous adhesions should be carefully dissected. With fibrous adhesions, it is safer to dissect the parietal peritoneum with the adhesions to avoid rupturing the abomasum. The parietal defect left by this technique will heal quickly.

The omental attachment is identified, and the greater curvature of the abomasum is pulled out of the incision (**Fig. 5**). A continuous pattern (Ford interlocking) is placed 2 to 3 cm lateral to the omental attachment, midway between the reticulo-abomasal ligament and the pylorus. A long strand (2 m) of nonabsorbable suture material of US Pharmacopeia (USP) 4 is used. The length of the suture line, on the abomasum, is 5 to 6 cm. The cranial and caudal ends of the suture are kept long.

The abomasum is partially deflated. Using a 3-in straight needle or a straightened S-curve needle, the cranial end of the suture is pulled toward the pexy site making sure not to grab the omentum on the way down. An assistant can identify the pexy site by pushing on the abdominal wall with hemostatic forceps (15-20 cm caudal to xyphoid and 5-10 cm on the right side of midline). The pexy site can be identified by palpating the xyphoid intra-abdominally. The needle is pushed through the abdominal wall and grabbed by an assistant. The same process is performed with the caudal end of the suture. It is important that the length of the suture line on the abomasum is the same as the distance between the exit points on the abdominal wall. The abomasum is fully deflated (not always necessary) and pushed down into normal position (not pulled down by the assistant otherwise tearing will occur). The

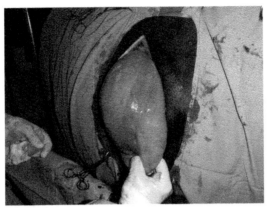

Fig. 5. Greater curvature of the abomasum exteriorized through a left para-lumbar fossa incision. (*Courtesy of* Marie Babkine, DMV, MSc, DECBHM, Université de Montréal, Québec, Canada.)

abomasum is held down while an assistant attaches the suture ends together through a roll of gauze.

Abdominal surgical closure and specific postoperative care The abdominal incision is closed in 3 layers (peritoneum and transverse muscle, external and internal oblique muscles, and skin). The ventral stitch is removed 14 to 21 days after the procedure. If the cow is not doing right early in the postoperative period with clinical signs of proximal GI obstruction, it is recommended to cut the ventral suture and perform another type of abomasal fixation. The authors have seen omental/intestinal incarceration and kink of the abomasum at the pexy site causing total outflow obstruction.

Right para-lumbar fossa (omentopexy/pyloropexy)

This technique can be used for all types of displacement. It is the ideal surgical approach for abomasal volvulus.

Abdominal surgical approach The standard right flank approach is used (8–10 cm below the transverse process and 8–10 cm caudal to the last rib).

Abdominal exploration and omentopexy The right flank approach allows for the most thorough abdominal exploration.

The abomasum is deflated and brought back to its anatomic location. The omentum and pylorus (not to be confused with the cranial duodenum) are pulled out of the incision (**Figs. 6** and **7**). The fixation site is located 10 cm caudal to the pylorus. The sow's ear (an omental fold) is rarely at this location. This should not be used as a landmark for the pexy. However, when identified, you know you are close. Allis forceps are used to mark the site.

Retention sutures are placed at the cranial and caudal aspect of the incision to enlarge the size of the adhesion. Absorbable suture material of USP 2 is used. The cranial suture is passed from outside in through all the muscle layers and peritoneum at the lower end of the incision. Then 2 to 3 large bites of omentum are taken from the bottom to the top in regard to the Allis forceps. The suture is passed through the body wall from the inside out at the top of the incision. The same manipulations are repeated on the caudal aspect of the incision. The suture ends are held together with hemostatic forceps. They will be tied before skin closure.

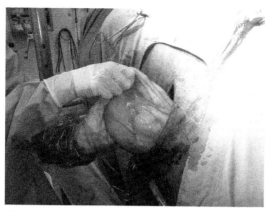

Fig. 6. Pylorus exteriorized through a right para-lumbar fossa incision. (*Courtesy of* Sylvain Nichols, DMV, MS, DACVS, Université de Montréal, Saint-Hyacinthe, Québec, Canada.)

The omentopexy is performed with absorbable suture material of USP 2 in a simple continuous pattern. The suture line includes the peritoneum, the transverse muscle, and the omentum (large bits). It starts at the bottom of the incision. Care should be taken not to incorporate the descending duodenum while closing blindly the top of the incision. The internal and external oblique muscles are then closed together with a simple continuous pattern. The retention sutures are tied before skin closure with a Ford interlocking suture pattern.

Pyloropexy A *pyloropexy* is performed when the omentum is friable, overly fat, or torn (**Fig. 8**). Several techniques have been described. The antrum can be incorporated in the suture of the ventral aspect of the flank incision when an omentopexy cannot be performed. If the omentum is still usable, a single horizontal mattress suture can be placed through all of the muscle layer of the flank and the serosal and muscular layer of the pyloric antrum at the ventral and cranial aspect of the incision. It is important to avoid the lumen of the abomasum to avoid postoperative complications (leakage

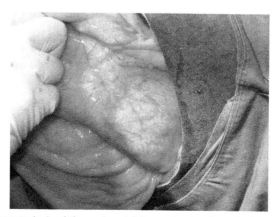

Fig. 7. Duodenum exteriorized through a right para-lumbar fossa incision. It is important to note the difference with the structure shown in **Fig. 6**. (*Courtesy of* Sylvain Nichols, DMV, MS, DACVS, Université de Montréal, Saint-Hyacinthe, Québec, Canada.)

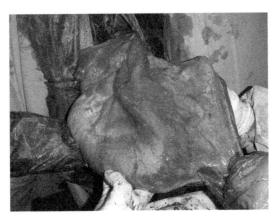

Fig. 8. Pylorus, pyloric antrum, and part of the body of the abomasum exteriorized through a right para-lumbar fossa incision. The omental attachment has been torn from the greater curvature during an abomasal volvulus. (*Courtesy of* Sylvain Nichols, DMV, MS, DACVS, Université de Montréal, Saint-Hyacinthe, Québec, Canada.)

causing peritonitis or outflow obstruction). Slowly, absorbable suture material can be used. Although somewhat infrequent, in the authors' opinion, the complications are maybe more serious with this technique if they occur.

Abomasal volvulus A large fluid-filled abomasum in volvulus can be difficult to replace. By lifting up and forward the body of the abomasum, it loosens the knot at the pylorus allowing the fluid to drain into the duodenum. This movement is repeated until the volvulus can be corrected by pushing back and down the pylorus and the greater curvature. However, if no progress is noted after several attempts at lifting the heavy abomasum, drainage is indicated. A purse string suture with an internal diameter of 5 cm is placed on the greater curvature before the incision and insertion of a gastric tube. It is not uncommon to remove more than 5 gal of abomasal fluid with this technique. When the drainage stops, the purse string is closed before being buried with an inverting suture pattern. The empty abomasum is then easily replaced in a normal anatomic position before being pexied.

Para-costal flank approach (abomasopexy or abomasotomy)
This approach is performed with the animal in lateral recumbency. From the left side, it allows the safe release of a chronically displaced abomasum adhered to the body wall. In a referral center, on anesthetized cattle, the rib cage can be lifted up to expose the adhesions (**Fig. 9**).

From the right side, it allows exteriorization of the pyloric antrum and part of the body of the abomasum to perform an abomasotomy to empty an impacted abomasum or to safely remove an abomasal foreign body.

From both sides, an abomasopexy using the transfixation technique described through the left flank approach can be used to secure the abomasum in place.

Surgical Techniques Performed Through Laparoscopy

The main advantage of laparoscopy over laparotomy is the minimal invasive approach needed to perform the procedure, thereby decreasing postoperative morbidity. However, the technique requires specific equipment and training and can only be used to correct LDA.

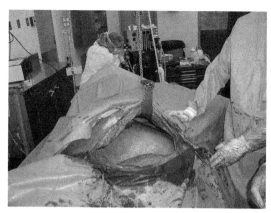

Fig. 9. Right para-costal approach to release a dilated abomasum from its abdominal adhesions. The rib cage has been lifted to improve exposure. (*Courtesy of* Marie Babkine, DMV, MSc, DECBHM, Université de Montréal, Québec, Canada.)

Two-step laparoscopic toggle pin placement (Janowitz)

The procedure starts by placing a double-strand toggle pin within the abomasum through a standing left flank laparoscopy.[18,19] Two 10 cm × 10-cm squares are shaved and prepared for the introduction of the laparoscope and instruments. The laparoscope is introduced just behind the last rib and ventral to the transverse process of the lumbar vertebras. Room air is allowed to enter the abdomen. The instrument portal is located at the 11th or 12th intercostal space at the same level or slightly ventral compared with the laparoscope portal. A long trocar and its cannula are introduced through the instrument portal into the abomasum. The trocar is removed, and the toggle pin is introduced within the abomasum. The abomasum is deflated, and the toggle ends are left in the abdomen.

The second step requires that the cow is placed in dorsal recumbency. Two 10 cm × 10-cm squares are shaved and prepared for the introduction of the laparoscope and instruments. The laparoscope is introduced 10 cm lateral (right) to midline and 30 cm cranial to the umbilicus. The instrument portal is introduced 10 cm lateral (right) to midline and 10 cm cranial to the umbilicus. The toggle ends are brought out of the instrument portal with laparoscopic forceps introduced through the instrument portal. The instruments are removed, and the cow is placed in right lateral recumbency. The sutures are tied over a roll of gauze until the markers are visualized (5 cm from the pin).

One-step laparoscopic toggle pin placement standing procedure (Christiansen)

This procedure requires a special instrument named a spieker to push the toggle ends through the ventral abdomen from a standing left flank approach.[20] Two 10 cm × 10-cm squares are shaved and prepared for the introduction of the laparoscope and instruments. The laparoscope is introduced just behind the last rib and ventrally to the transverse process of the lumbar vertebras. Room air is allowed to enter the abdomen. The instrument portal is located at the 11th or 12th intercostal space at the same level or slightly ventral compared with the laparoscope portal. A long trocar and its cannula are introduced through the instrument portal into the abomasum. The trocar is removed, and the toggle pin is introduced within the abomasum. The abomasum is deflated, and the toggle ends are kept outside the abdomen. They are passed through the push rod within the spieker. This unit is then introduced in the abdomen through the instrument portal and directed in the cranial right paramedian part of the abdomen. The tip of the spieker is felt or seen before pushing the rods through the abdominal wall. Finally, the toggle ends are tied over a roll of gauze until the markers are visualized (5 cm from the pin).

With this technique, it is possible to damage abdominal structures when the rod is pushed blindly outside the abdomen and cause GI obstruction or septic peritonitis. Therefore, if the cow is not doing right after the surgery, it is recommended to cut the ventral suture, do a complete physical examination, and modify the treatments according to the findings.

One-step laparoscopic toggle pin placement dorsal procedure (Newman)

This procedure is performed with the cow in dorsal recumbency. The ventral abdomen is prepared aseptically. The first portal is created near the umbilicus to avoid penetrating the abomasum. Because no pneumoperitoneum is created, it is more challenging to insert the cannula. Insufflation through the left para-lumbar fossa before placing the cow in dorsal recumbency can be useful to avoid inappropriate placement of the cannula. The abomasum is visualized (**Fig. 10**) and the trocar and its cannula are introduced into the abomasum in the right paramedian area (same location as the previous technique). The trocar is removed, and the toggle pin is introduced in the abomasum. The toggle ends are kept outside the animal. The abomasum is deflated. The remainder of the procedure is like the 2-step technique. With this technique, no laparoscopic forceps are necessary.[21]

Ventral laparoscopic abomasopexy (Babkine)

This technique is a minimally invasive way to perform a right paramedian abomasopexy.[22,23] The cow is positioned in dorsal recumbency. A laparoscope, grasping laparoscopic forceps, and a laparoscopic needle holder are introduced into the abdomen. The abomasum is deflated before being grasped with the laparoscopic forceps. A needle of USP 2 (polydioxanone [PDS II, Ethicon, Somerville, NJ] or polyglactin 910 [Vicryl, Ethicon, Somerville, NJ]) is straightened and introduced in the abdomen through a stab incision in the skin at the pexy site. The needle is grasped with the needle holder, and the suture is introduced in the abomasum wall. The needle is then stabbed back out where it is retrieved by an assistant through the stab skin incision. The manipulations are repeated 2 to 3 times to create the abomasopexy (**Fig. 11**). The sutures are tightened subcutaneously only when they are all in position.

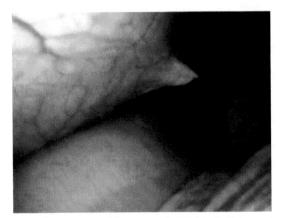

Fig. 10. Abomasum seen from a ventral laparoscopic approach. A trocar to insert the toggle within the abomasum is inserted in the abdomen (*top center of the picture*). The greater curvature with the omental attachment are seen on the right side of the abomasum. (*Courtesy of* Sylvain Nichols, DMV, MS, DACVS, Université de Montréal, Saint-Hyacinthe, Québec, Canada.)

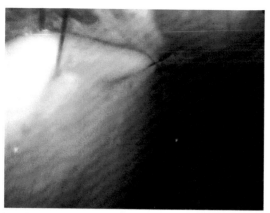

Fig. 11. Four stitches have been placed laparoscopically to perform the abomasopexy. (*Courtesy of* Sylvain Nichols, DMV, MS, DACVS, Université de Montréal, Saint-Hyacinthe, Québec, Canada.)

This technique is more challenging than the other laparoscopic procedures described previously. An assistant is needed to assist the surgeon technically.

In all the minimally invasive techniques, the skin incisions are closed with cruciate sutures. The toggle stitches are cut 14 to 21 days after the procedure.

Laparotomy Versus Laparoscopy

The 2-step laparoscopic abomasopexy seemed to improve abomasum motility when compared with the right flank omentopexy.[24] However, when the peritoneal fluid was analyzed, the laparoscopic technique seemed to create more inflammation than the right flank omentopexy.[25] It is thought that inflammation was caused by puncture of the abomasum with the toggle. The overall success rate (milk production and culling rate) are not different between techniques.[26] The main advantages of the laparoscopic technique are the rapidity of the surgery and the decreased use of antibiotics.[27]

INTESTINAL SURGERIES

Intestinal surgery can be challenging in cattle. The short mesenteric attachment of the intestinal tract (with the exception of the cecum) makes exteriorization of the devitalized segment difficult. Because most procedures are performed with the animal standing, the pain elicited increases the probability that the animal will go down, usually at the least desirable moment. Frequently, by the time the animal is evaluated, the condition has progressed to a point where the lesion has become friable and necrotic. Therefore, many cattle with intestinal problems will be euthanized before or during exploratory laparotomy.

This section is divided according to the localization of the lesion: the small intestine versus the cecum and colon. For the preoperative treatments and the surgical preparation, the reader is referred to the beginning of this article.

Small Intestines

Duodenum
Duodenum sigmoid flexure volvulus This condition is caused by a dorsal displacement followed by a counterclockwise volvulus (as seen from the top of the cow) of the duodenal sigmoid flexure (**Figs. 12–14**).[28] The cause of this condition remains unknown. Prior omentopexy seems to be a risk factor.

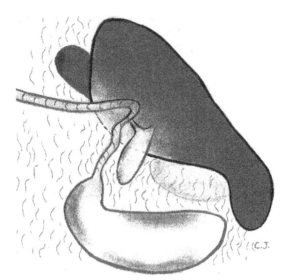

Fig. 12. The normal anatomy of the abomasum and duodenum. (*Courtesy of* Sylvain Nichols, DMV, MS, DACVS, Université de Montréal, Saint-Hyacinthe, Québec, Canada.)

This condition is diagnosed mainly on dairy cattle of any age and at any stage of lactation. The clinical signs are similar to those of an abomasal volvulus. However, the ping location and diameter are different. A high-intensity ping associated with a positive succussion will be located at the 11th and 12th ICS. Classic hypochloremia, metabolic alkalosis, and hypokalemia are present but much worse than with an abomasal volvulus. Ultrasound evaluation of the right ventral and dorsal abdomen shows a large fluid-filled abomasum and cranial duodenum. During surgery, similarly, a fluid-filled abomasum and cranial duodenum and a gas-distended duodenal sigmoid flexure are palpated. The sigmoid flexure is located cranially, just under the caudate

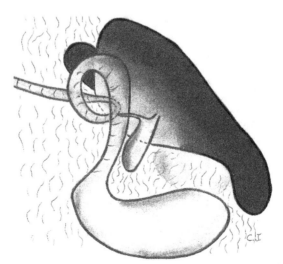

Fig. 13. The dorsal displacement of the duodenal sigmoid flexure before the volvulus. (*Courtesy of* Sylvain Nichols, DMV, MS, DACVS, Université de Montréal, Saint-Hyacinthe, Québec, Canada.)

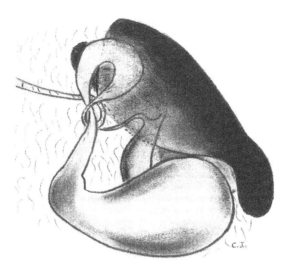

Fig. 14. Duodenal sigmoid flexure volvulus. (*Courtesy of* Sylvain Nichols, DMV, MS, DACVS, Université de Montréal, Saint-Hyacinthe, Québec, Canada.)

lobe of the liver. This area is often neglected during abdominal exploratory. A twist is often palpated at the sigmoid flexure. An empty descending duodenum is a constant finding. The volvulus is resolved by flipping the gas distended duodenum ventrally and caudally. On correction of the volvulus, the descending duodenum starts to fill with ingesta. No pexy of the duodenum is performed.

In chronic cases, peritonitis surrounding the duodenum may be present, complicating replacement of the sigmoid flexure. In this situation, a side-to-side anastomosis of the cranial duodenum to the descending duodenum is necessary.[29] This technique is not described in this section.

The abdomen is routinely closed without performing an omentopexy. It is thought that it could be a risk factor for duodenum sigmoid flexure volvulus (DSFV), because most cases had an omentopexy before presentation. In addition, the pexy creates pain because the large fluid-filled abomasum is pulling on it.

Intensive fluid therapy, systemic antibiotics, and NSAID are needed in the postoperative period. The prognosis is good with the exception of the cows with extensive peritonitis at the time of surgery.[28]

Gallbladder malposition Duodenal obstruction caused by malposition of the gallbladder shows clinical signs of proximal gastro-intestinal obstruction similar to those seen with duodenal sigmoid flexure volvulus. The obstruction is caused by a displacement of the gallbladder above the cranial duodenum. The condition is resolved by returning the distended gallbladder to its normal anatomic position.[30]

Jejunum
Hemorrhagic bowel syndrome Hemorrhagic bowel syndrome (HBS) has been recognized in veterinary medicine for more than 2 decades. It affects mostly dairy cattle in lactation consuming a high-energy diet.[31] The cause remains unclear. Clostridium perfringens type A containing the beta2 toxin is thought to be involved in the disease.[32]

The cattle are usually in shock. A blood clot in the lumen or in the intestinal submucosa creates a GI obstruction. Moderate to severe abdominal distension will be present. Bloody feces and distended loops of bowel are a frequent finding on transrectal examination. Ultrasound evaluation reveals distended jejunum. In some cases, blood clots within the intestinal lumen can be seen, as in Gilles Fecteau and colleagues' article, "Diagnostic Approach to the Acute Abdomen," in this issue.

Treating cattle with HBS is always challenging. The first reports of HBS showed that the prognosis after either surgical or medical treatment was poor.[33,34] Better understanding of the disease seems to improve the prognosis. However, after the encouraging report by Peek and colleagues,[35] it seems that the prognosis remains guarded at best (authors' clinical impression). The treatments have not changed drastically over the year with the exception that pain is better control nowadays. However, the authors think that the current cases are more challenging than they were. The single-clot obstruction is rare. Enormous clots, multifocal clots, and ruptured bowel (**Fig. 15**) at surgery are seen more frequently.

When the animal is still passing feces, medical therapy is indicated. Broad-spectrum antibiotics, including a beta-lactam, NSAID, or other analgesic, such as lidocaine, and aggressive fluid therapy, including blood transfusion, are appropriate. It is the authors' opinion that mineral oil (1 gal orally) is extremely useful to move the clot aborally. If fecal output or if the general status of the animal does not improve or worsens during medical therapy, a right flank laparotomy is warranted. Massaging (**Fig. 16**) the clot, when possible, has been shown to carry a better prognosis than resection and anastomosis.[35] Relapses have been reported with this disease after clot massaging or resection and anastomosis.

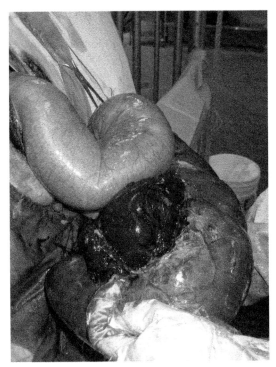

Fig. 15. Loop of jejunum suffering from hemorrhagic bowel syndrome exteriorized through a right para-lumbar fossa incision. The massive blood clot had ruptured the jejunum before the surgery. (*Courtesy of* Sylvain Nichols, DMV, MS, DACVS, Université de Montréal, Saint-Hyacinthe, Québec, Canada.)

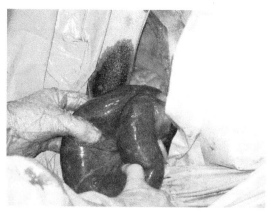

Fig. 16. Loop of jejunum suffering from hemorrhagic bowel syndrome exteriorized through a right para-lumbar fossa incision. The clot is carefully broken down and pushed in the empty jejunum. (*Courtesy of* Sylvain Nichols, DMV, MS, DACVS, Université de Montréal, Saint-Hyacinthe, Québec, Canada.)

Volvulus A volvulus is defined as a rotation of the viscera around its mesenteric attachment. Two types of intestinal volvulus are recognized in cattle: mesenteric root and jejunal flange volvulus. The flange refers to the distal portion of the jejunum, including the ileum. It has a longer mesenteric attachment that can rotate on itself and create a volvulus. Both types of volvulus are uncommon and may be present in cattle of all ages.

The mesenteric root volvulus causes a rapid obstruction of the mesenteric vein and artery of the small intestine, cecum and ascending colon with the exception of the duodenum and descending colon. The cattle show acute and severe signs of abdominal pain. They become rapidly in shock and may die suddenly. The transrectal examination reveals distended bowel with tension bands.

Cattle with jejunal flange volvulus also have acute signs of abdominal pain. However, their general status deteriorates progressively when compared with mesenteric root volvulus, which is rapid and sudden.

With both conditions, the abdomen is explored through a right flank approach. When a mesenteric root volvulus is present, discolored jejunum segments are seen in the abdomen. The mesenteric root is palpated by sliding the hand cranially to the left kidney within the supraomental recess. The volvulus is located, and the direction of the twist is determined. The jejunum is then carefully untwisted to prevent spontaneous rupture of a fragile devitalized segment. Because the jejunum cannot be completely resected, the animal should be euthanized if the jejunum is determined to be nonviable.

When a jejunal flange volvulus is diagnosed, the affected segment of bowel is gently exteriorized while reducing the volvulus. The bowel is inspected for viability. Resection and anastomosis of the devitalized segment is possible (**Fig. 17**).

The prognosis for both types of volvulus is guarded to poor. Dairy cattle seem to have a better outcome because the farm staff recognize the condition earlier.[36]

Intussusception An intussusception is a segment of bowel (intussusceptum) penetrating another segment (intussuscipiens). Several predisposing factors have been identified (diarrhea, intraluminal mass [granuloma, abscess, tumors], drugs affecting GI motility) (**Fig. 18**). It can affect cattle of all ages, but it seems more frequent in calves

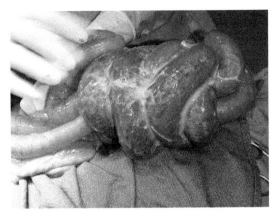

Fig. 17. Jejunal flange volvulus in a 1-year-old heifer. The affected segment has to be re-sected. An end-to-end anastomosis will be performed. (*Courtesy of* Sylvain Nichols, DMV, MS, DACVS, Université de Montréal, Saint-Hyacinthe, Québec, Canada.)

less than 2 months of age.[37] The segment most frequently affected is the jejunum. Seldom, it can affect the ileocecal junction and the spiral colon. Compared with other types of intestinal obstruction, the clinical signs appear slowly and will evolve over several days. Colics are mild and present only in the early stage. The production of feces decreases until it stops, and only fibrin and mucus are expulsed. Distended loops of the bowel are palpated during a transrectal examination, and fluid-filled jejunum is seen on ultrasound. Rarely, the supposed typical bull's eye sign is observed during ultrasound evaluation.

Through a right flank approach, the abdomen is evaluated quadrant by quadrant un-til the intussusception is localized. Frequently, fibrinous adhesions are present around the obstruction site. It is gently exteriorized to perform a resection and anastomosis. The authors have never been able to reduce the intussusception without a resection. It is, however, described in other species.

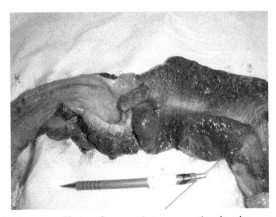

Fig. 18. A loop of jejunum suffering from an intussusception has been resected. The intus-susception has been reduced to expose a granuloma of unknown origin within the lumen of the jejunum. (*Courtesy of* Sylvain Nichols, DMV, MS, DACVS, Université de Montréal, Saint-Hyacinthe, Québec, Canada.)

The prognosis remains guarded because the long-term outcome was estimated at 35%.[37]

RESECTION AND END-TO-END JEJUNAL ANASTOMOSIS

Challenge of the procedure
1. Exteriorization (short mesentery)
2. Pain control during the procedure (difficult to anesthetize the mesentery)
3. Hemostasis (localization of vessels difficult because of the abundant fat within the mesentery)

When the affected segment is localized, it is carefully pulled out of the abdomen. Wet towels are used to isolate the bowel and protect the abdomen from any leakage during the procedure. The site of resection is determined (healthy jejunum). The mesenteric vessels are ligated (blindly) or transected using a sealing device (eg, Liga-Sure, Medtronic, Minneapolis, MN). The mesentery is cut parallel to the bowel to be resected.

The lumen is occluded with Penrose drains on the healthy section to anastomose. On the section to be resected, any type of obstructive clamps or forceps can be used (Doyen, Rochester forceps).

The aboral section is cut with a 60° angle to increase the lumen diameter. The oral portion is cut at 90°. Each side of the jejunum should be held by an assistant. The anastomosis is started at the mesenteric side. It is more difficult to obtain a tight seal at this location. Two or 3 simple continuous or Lembert sutures are made to complete the anastomosis. Absorbable suture material (Vicryl, PDS) of USP 2.0 or 3.0 is used. The Penrose drains are removed allowing the ingesta to progress through the anastomosis. The site is evaluated for leakage. The mesentery is closed with a simple continuous pattern. Absorbable suture material of USP 0 is used. The surgery site is thoroughly rinsed before being carefully replaced in the abdomen.

Internal herniation Internal herniation is diagnosed sporadically in cattle. The clinical signs are similar to other types of intestinal obstruction (abdominal distension, colic, distended loops of bowel on transrectal examination and ultrasound evaluation) and ileus. Nonresponse to medical therapy (NSAID and fluids) justifies right flank laparotomy. The abdomen is carefully evaluated quadrant by quadrant. Finding empty loops of bowel helps to localize the site of obstruction. The jejunum can be trapped through a rent in the broad ligament, the omentum, the mesojejunum, or the mesoduodenum. When the hernia ring is located, it is determined if the bowel can be pulled out safely. In most cases, the ring has to be enlarged manually. The entrapped segment is then exteriorized to evaluate their viability. If necessary, a resection and anastomosis are performed. If accessible, the rent is closed after being refreshed. If not accessible, it is enlarged to avoid further entrapment. The prognosis is good if the jejunum is viable at the time of surgery.[38]

Ileum
Impaction Ileal impaction seems to be uncommon in North America. However, it is a more frequent cause of intestinal obstruction in other parts of the world.[39] No predisposing factors have been identified other than the condition occurs more frequently during winter time. The clinical signs are more subtle than other types of obstruction (eg, intestinal volvulus). Distended loops of bowel and in some cases a firm mass (the impaction) can be palpated during a transrectal examination. A right flank laparotomy allows the localization of the obstruction, which can be broken down and massaged within the cecum. The long-term outcome following surgery is good.[39]

Cecum

Cecum dislocation After abomasal displacements, cecal dislocation is the most frequent condition affecting the GI tract. It has been associated with hypocalcemia and a diet rich in rumen-resistant starch causing an increase in carbohydrate fermentation in the cecum and large colon.[40] It is usually diagnosed in dairy cattle during their lactation.

The cecum can be dilated, retroflexed (ventral or dorsal volvulus), or twisted. The dilation will be recognized on transrectal examination. The apex of the cecum is found in the pelvic canal. With a 180° retroflexion, the apex is typically located cranially in the abdomen. This flexion can evolve to a 360° volvulus. Then, only the body of the cecum is palpated transrectally. The cecal torsion is a twist within the long axis of the organ. This presentation is less common.

Usually, with cecal dislocation, a distended structure is seen in the para-lumbar fossa. A positive percussion and succussion is present. Depending on the type of dislocation, the vital parameters will be affected with more or less severity.

Cattle with cecal dilatation without significant systemic repercussion and still passing feces are treated medically with IV fluids and NSAID. The fluids are complemented in calcium because hypocalcemia has been shown to be a predisposing factor to cecal problems.[41]

Cattle with cecal dilatation with systemic repercussion, cecal retroflexion or cecal torsion has to be treated surgically. A right para-lumbar fossa approach allows to safely mobilize and exteriorize the cecum (**Fig. 19**). A typhlotomy is performed to empty the cecum and the proximal loop of the ascending colon. If the cecum has necrotic patches or in recurrent cases, partial resection is indicated (**Fig. 20**).

The prognosis following cecal surgery is good. It is important to note that the recurrence rate of cecal dilatation is relatively high.[41–43]

TYPHLOTOMY AND PARTIAL TYPHLECTOMY

1. Typhlotomy

   The apex of the cecum is easily exteriorized after correction of the retroflexion or torsion. A typhlotomy is performed to empty the contents. An assistant holds the cecum exteriorized. The abdomen is protected with a wet sterile towel. At the apex of the caecum, a 5-cm stab incision is made (**Fig. 21**). The ingesta within the cecum and proximal loop of the ascending colon is massaged out. The typhlotomy is closed with 2 inverting layers (Cushing) with absorbable

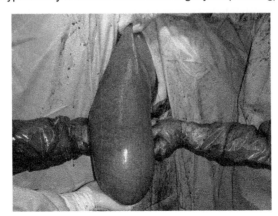

Fig. 19. Dilated cecum exteriorized through a right para-lumbar incision. (*Courtesy of* Sylvain Nichols, DMV, MS, DACVS, Université de Montréal, Saint-Hyacinthe, Québec, Canada.)

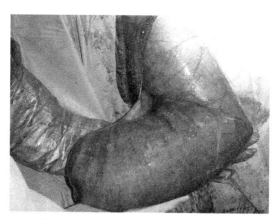

Fig. 20. Dilated cecum with necrotic patch following a volvulus exteriorized through a right para-lumbar incision. The apex of the cecum will have to be amputated. (*Courtesy of* Sylvain Nichols, DMV, MS, DACVS, Université de Montréal, Saint-Hyacinthe, Québec, Canada.)

(Vicryl, Braided Lactomer [Polysorb, Covidien, Mansfield, MA]) suture material of USP 0. The possibly contaminated part of the cecum is rinsed thoroughly before being returned in the abdomen at its normal anatomic location (apex pointing back in the right dorsal quadrant of the abdomen).

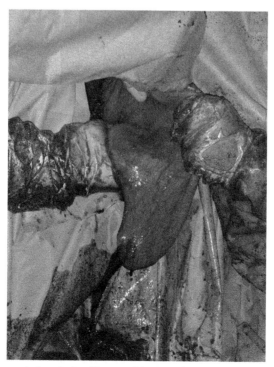

Fig. 21. Dilated cecum being drained by a typhlotomy through a right para-lumbar incision. The fluid within the proximal loop of the ascending colon has been massage back to the cecum and out by the typhlotomy incision. (*Courtesy of* Sylvain Nichols, DMV, MS, DACVS, Université de Montréal, Saint-Hyacinthe, Québec, Canada.)

2. Partial typhlectomy

This surgery is performed when the cecum is devitalized or in recurrent cases. The cecum is exteriorized and isolated from the abdomen with wet sterile towels. A typhlotomy is performed to empty the cecum and ascending colon. The ileocecal ligament is dissected toward the ileocecal junction, and the blood vessels are ligated along the way. Two Doyen forceps are placed across the cecum (**Fig. 22**). The cecum is amputated at least 3 cm away from the forceps. The cecum edges are rinsed before being closed with 2 inverting layers (Cushing) with absorbable suture material (Vicryl, Polysorb) of USP 0. The cecum is rinsed thoroughly before being returned in the abdomen.

Colon

Mechanical obstruction of the colon is uncommon in adult cattle. Adhesions, volvulus, intussusception, and phytobezoars have been described. Abdominal distension with moderate signs of colic are a common feature. No feces and distension of the cecum and part of the jejunum are present on transrectal examination.

Medication given through the peritoneal route is a risk factor to colonic adhesion.[44] Through a right para-lumbar fossa laparotomy, the obstruction is located. Most of the time, the bowels are distorted and difficult to recognize. A side-to-side anastomosis would have to be performed to bypass to obstruction.

Intussusception of the spiral colon is more frequent in calves (**Fig. 23**).[37,45] The fat surrounding the loops of colon are thought to protect against this condition in older cattle. Dissection of the intussusception within the spiral colon is difficult. The authors have come to think that the diseased segment should be left in place and a side-to-side anastomosis should be performed. Some cases can spontaneously heal and slough the intussusceptum.

A phytobezoar can be found within the spiral colon. It is usually a single mass causing a complete obstruction. The obstructed colon is pulled out of the abdomen to perform an enterotomy (**Figs. 24** and **25**). An assistant is needed to hold the spiral colon exteriorized. The incision is closed with a single inverting layer (Cushing) with absorbable suture material (Vicryl, Polysorb) of USP 0.

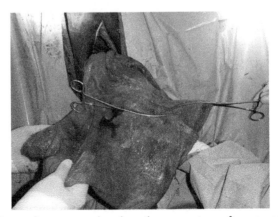

Fig. 22. Curved Doyen forceps are placed on the cecum to perform a partial typhlectomy. (*Courtesy of* Sylvain Nichols, DMV, MS, DACVS, Université de Montréal, Saint-Hyacinthe, Québec, Canada.)

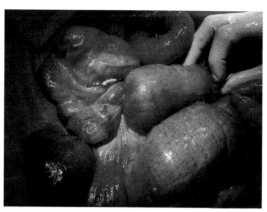

Fig. 23. Intussusception within the spiral colon of a 3-month-old calf. (*Courtesy of* Sylvain Nichols, DMV, MS, DACVS, Université de Montréal, Saint-Hyacinthe, Québec, Canada.)

POSTOPERATIVE TREATMENTS

The postoperative period can be as challenging as the surgery itself. Fluids and systemic antibiotics are frequently needed for an extended period of time. Serum electrolytes are followed to avoid functional ileus from hypocalcemia or hypokalemia.

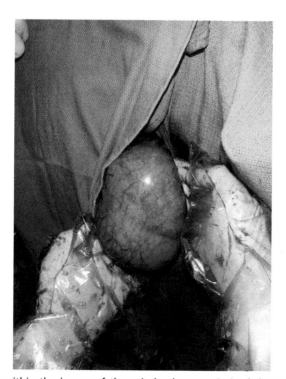

Fig. 24. Fecalith within the lumen of the spiral colon exteriorized through a right para-lumbar fossa incision. Wet sterile towels have been placed around the lesion to avoid abdominal contamination during enterotomy. (*Courtesy of* Sylvain Nichols, DMV, MS, DACVS, Université de Montréal, Saint-Hyacinthe, Québec, Canada.)

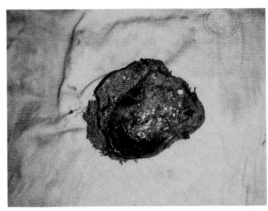

Fig. 25. Fecalith removed from the spiral colon in **Fig. 23.** (*Courtesy of* Sylvain Nichols, DMV, MS, DACVS, Université de Montréal, Saint-Hyacinthe, Québec, Canada.)

To allow the GI tract to regain its motility, pain control is essential. NSAIDs are used judiciously to avoid abomasal ulceration. Opioids should also be used carefully because they may decrease GI motility.[46] Butorphanol, a κ agonist and a μ antagonist, seems to affect GI motility to a lesser extent than other morphinics.[46] It may be used during the early postoperative period as repeated injections (0.025–0.05 mg/kg IV, intramuscularly [IM], subcutaneously) or as a continuous drip (0.01–0.02 mg/kg/h).

If a functional ileus remains despite adequate therapy, prokinetic drugs are used. Erythromycin (8.8 mg/kg IM) has the best prokinetic effect on the abomasum[47,48] and the jejunum. Neostigmine and bethanechol have been used for cecal atony.[49] Neostigmine should be used carefully because it causes anarchic contractions. Erythromycin has been shown to increase the myoelectric activity of the spiral colon.[50]

Lidocaine drips have been used in cattle based on studies performed in horses.[51] The prokinetic effect is uncertain. It is thought that the analgesic effect might explain the positive clinical result perceived during lidocaine infusion. It is important to note that cattle may be more sensitive than horses to lidocaine. Therefore, the initial bolus is not routinely given in the authors' institution to avoid the possible neurologic side effect.

REFERENCES

1. Abrahamsen EJ. Chemical restraint and injectable anesthesia of ruminants. Vet Clin North Am Food Anim Pract 2013;29:209–27.
2. Abrahamsen EJ. Ruminant field anesthesia. Vet Clin North Am Food Anim Pract 2008;24:429–41.
3. Bedard S, Desrochers A, Fecteau G, et al. Comparaison de quatre protocoles de préparation préopératoire chez le bovin. Can Vet J 2001;42:199–203.
4. Hiraoka M, Miyagawa T, Kobayashi H, et al. Successful introduction of modified dorsolumbar epidural anesthesia in a bovine referral center. J Vet Sci 2007;8: 181–4.
5. Lee I, Yamagishi N, Oboshi K, et al. Practical tips for modified dorsolumbar epidural anesthesia in cattle. J Vet Sci 2006;7:69–72.
6. Desrochers A, St-Jean G, Anderson DE, et al. Comparative evaluation of two surgical scrub preparations in cattle. Vet Surg 1996;25:336–41.

7. Rohrbach BW, Cabbedy AL, Freeman K, et al. Risk factors for abomasal displacement in dairy cows. J Am Vet Med Assoc 1999;214:1660–3.

8. Van Winden SCL, Kuiper R. Left displacement of the abomasum in dairy cattle: recent developments in epidemiological and etiological aspects. Vet Res 2003; 34:47–56.

9. Doll K, Sickinger M, Seeger T. New aspects in the pathogenesis of abomasal displacement. Vet J 2009;181:90–6.

10. Fubini SL, Gröhn YT, Smith DF. Right displacement of the abomasum and abomasal volvulus in dairy cows: 458 cases (1980-1987). J Am Vet Med Assoc 1991;198:460–4.

11. Constable PD, St-Jean G, Hull B, et al. Preoperative prognostic indicators in cattle with abomasal volvulus. J Am Vet Med Assoc 1991;198:2077–85.

12. Constable PD, St-Jean G, Hull BL, et al. Prognostic value of surgical and postoperative findings in cattle with abomasal volvulus. J Am Vet Med Assoc 1991;199: 892–8.

13. Smith DF, Munson L, Erb HN. Abomasal ulcer in adult dairy cattle. Cornell Vet 1983;73:213–4.

14. Cable CS, Rebhun WC, Fubini SL, et al. Concurrent abomasal displacement and perforating ulcerations in cattle: 21 cases (1985-1996). J Am Vet Med Assoc 1998;212:1442–5.

15. Wittek T, Constable PD, Morin DE. Abomasal impaction in Holstein-Friesian cows: 80 cases (1980-2003). J Am Vet Med Assoc 2005;227:287–91.

16. Thomas KL, Wilson DG, Bracamonte JL, et al. Quality of adhesions after sutured paramedian vs. laparoscopic toggle abomasopexy in an ovine model. Vet Surg 2016;45:488–93.

17. Sams AE, Fubini SL. Primary repair of abomasal fistulae resulting from right paramedian abomasopexy in eight adult dairy cattle. Vet Surg 1993;22:190–3.

18. Janowitz H. Laparoscopic reposition and fixation of the left displaced abomasum in cattle. Tierarztl Prax Ausg G Grosstiere Nutztiere 1998;26:308–13 [in German].

19. van Leeuwen E, Janowitz H, Willemen MA. Laparoscopic positioning and attachment of stomach displacement to the left in the cow. Tijdschr Diergeneeskd 2000; 125:391–2 [in Dutch].

20. Christiansen K. Laparoschopisch kontrollierte operation des nach links verlagerten Labmagens (Janowitz-operation) ohn Ablegen des Patienten. Tierärztl Praxis 2004;32:118–21.

21. Newman KD, Anderson DE, Silveira F. One step laparoscopic abomasopexy for correction of left-sided displacement of the abomasum in dairy cows. J Am Vet Med Assoc 2005;227:1142–7.

22. Babkine M, Desrochers A, Bouré L, et al. Ventral laparoscopic abomasopexy on adult cows. Can Vet J 2006;47:343–8.

23. Mulon PY, Babkine M, Desrochers A. Ventral laparoscopic abomasopexy in 18 cattle with displaced abomasum. Vet Surg 2006;35:347–55.

24. Wittek T, Locher L, Alkaassem A, et al. Effect of surgical correction of left displaced abomasum by means of omentopexy via right flank laparotomy or two-step laparoscopy-guided abomasopexy on postoperative abomasal emptying rate in lactating dairy cows. J Am Vet Med Assoc 2009;234:652–7.

25. Wittek T, Fürll M, Grosche A. Peritoneal inflammatory response to surgical correction of left displaced abomasum using different techniques. Vet Rec 2012;171: 594.

26. Seeger T, Kümper H, Failing K, et al. Comparison of laparoscopic-guided aboma-sopexy versus omentopexy via a right flank laparotomy for treatment of left abomasal displacement in dairy cows. J Am Vet Med Assoc 2006;67:472–8.

27. Roy JP, Harvey D, Bélanger AM, et al. Comparison of 2-step laparoscopy-guided abomasopexy versus omentopexy via a right flank laparotomy for the treatment of dairy cows with left displacement of the abomasum in on-farm settings. J Am Vet Med Assoc 2008;232:1700–6.

28. Vogel SR, Nichols S, Buczinski S, et al. Duodenal obstruction caused by a duodenal sigmoid flexure volvulus in dairy cattle: 29 cases (2006-2010). J Am Vet Med Assoc 2012;241:621–5.

29. Van der Valden MA. Functional stenosis of the sigmoid curve of the duodenum in cattle. Vet Rec 1983;112:452–3.

30. Boerboom D, Mulon PY, Desrochers A. Duodenal obstruction caused by malpo-sition of the gallbladder in a heifer. J Am Vet Med Assoc 2003;223:1475–7.

31. Berghaus RD, McCluskey BJ, Callan RJ. Risk factors associated with hemorrhag-ic bowel syndrome in dairy cattle. J Am Vet Med Assoc 2005;226:1700–6.

32. Adaska JM, Aly SS, Moeller RB, et al. Jejunal hematoma in cattle: a retrospective case analysis. J Vet Diagn Invest 2014;26:96–103.

33. Abutarbush SM, Radostits OM. Jejunal hemorrhage syndrome in dairy and beef cattle: 11 cases (2001-2003). Can Vet J 2005;46:711–5.

34. Dennison AC, VanMeter DC, Callan RJ, et al. Hemorrhagic bowel syndrome in dairy cattle: 22 cases (1997-2000). J Am Vet Med Assoc 2002;221:686–9.

35. Peek SF, Santschi EM, Liversey MA, et al. Surgical finding and outcome for dairy cattle with jejunal hemorrhage syndrome: 31 cases (2000-2007). J Am Vet Med Assoc 2009;234:1308–12.

36. Anderson DE, Constable PD, St-Jean G, et al. Small intestinal volvulus in cattle: 35 cases (1967-1992). J Am Vet Med Assoc 1993;203:1178–83.

37. Constable PD, St-Jean G, Hull BL, et al. Intussusception in cattle: 336 cases (1964-1993). J Am Vet Med Assoc 1997;210:531–6.

38. Ruf-Ritz J, Braun U, Hilbe M, et al. Internal herniation of the small and large intes-tines in 18 cattle. Vet J 2013;197:374–7.

39. Nuss K, Lejeune B, Lischer C, et al. Ileal impaction in 22 cows. Vet J 2006;171:456–61.

40. Abegg R, Eicher R, Lis J, et al. Concentration of volatile fatty acids in digesta samples obtained from healthy cows and cows with cecal dilatation or disloca-tion. Am J Vet Res 1999;60:1540–5.

41. Braun U, Beckmann C, Gerspach C, et al. Clinical findings and treatment in cattle with caecal dilatation. BMC Vet Res 2012;8:75.

42. Fubini SL, Erb HN, Rebhun WC, et al. Cecal dilatation and volvulus in dairy cows: 84 cases (1977-1983). J Am Vet Med Assoc 1986;189:96–9.

43. Braun U, Steiner A, Bearth G. Therapy and clinical progress of cattle with dilata-tion and torsion of the caecum. Vet Rec 1989;125:430–3.

44. Smith DF, Donawick WJ. Obstruction of the ascending colon in cattle: I. Clinical presentation and surgical management. Vet Surg 1979;8:93–7.

45. Strand E, Welker B, Modransky P. Spiral colon intussusception in a three year old bull. J Am Vet Med Assoc 1993;202:971–2.

46. Stock ML, Coetzee JF. Clinical pharmacology of analgesic drugs in cattle. Vet Clin North Am Food Anim Pract 2015;31:113–38.

47. Wittek T, Tischer K, Gieseler T, et al. Effect of preoperative administration of eryth-romycin or flunixin meglumine on postoperative abomasal emptying rate in dairy

cows undergoing surgical correction of left displacement of the abomasum. J Am Vet Med Assoc 2008;232:418–23.

48. Wittek T, Tischer K, Körner I, et al. Effect of preoperative erythromycin of dexamethasone/vitamin C on postoperative abomasal emptying rate in dairy cows undergoing surgical correction of abomasal volvulus. Vet Surg 2008;37:537–44.

49. Steiner A, Roussel AJ, Martig J. Effect of bethanechol, neostigmine, metoclopramide, and propranolol on myoelectic activity of the ileocecocolic area in cows. Am J Vet Res 1995;56:1081–6.

50. Zanolari P, Steiner A, Meylan M. Effects of erythromycin on myoelectric activity of the spiral colon of dairy cows. J Vet Med A Physiol Pathol Clin Med 2004;51: 456–61.

51. Malone E, Esink J, Turner T, et al. Intravenous continuous infusion of lidocaine for treatment of equine ileus. Vet Surg 2006;35:60–6.

Herd-Level Monitoring and Prevention of Displaced Abomasum in Dairy Cattle

Luciano S. Caixeta, DVM, PhD[a],*, Julia A. Herman, DVM, MS[a],
Greg W. Johnson, DVM[b], Jessica A.A. McArt, DVM, PhD[c]

KEYWORDS

- Displaced abomasum • Herd health • Dairy cows • Transition period

KEY POINTS

- Displaced abomasum is a multifactorial disorder; for this reason, veterinarians should not monitor displace abomasum alone but in association with other diseases that can lead to its development.
- Monitoring, prevention, and treatment of infectious and metabolic disorders characteristic of early lactation (eg, ketosis, retained placenta, metritis, mastitis, hypocalcemia) decreases the incidence of displaced abomasa on dairy farms.
- When formulating diets to prevent displaced abomasa, several aspects are important: maintenance of proper levels of fiber, maximization of dry matter intake, and limiting the energy density of the diet.
- Facilities and cow comfort play a significant role in the development of displaced abomasum; for example, adequate stall design, heat abatement, bunk space, limiting pen moves, and separating animals from different parity groups.
- Delivering a consistent and properly processed ration daily is a key element to be considered when monitoring feed management in displaced abomasum prevention.

Displaced abomasum (DA) is characterized by the displacement of the abomasum from its normal position on the right ventral aspect of the abdomen to the right or left DA (LDA) side in cattle, with LDA being more frequently diagnosed than right DA. Abomasal displacement is a multifactorial disorder diagnosed almost exclusively in adult dairy cows. In a nationwide survey, it was determined that the DA incidence in United States dairy herds was approximately 3.5%, with occurrence varying from

Disclosure Statement: The authors have nothing to disclose.
[a] Department of Clinical Sciences, Colorado State University, 300 West Drake Road, Fort Collins, CO 80523, USA; [b] Cows Come First, LLC, 14 Bean Road, Ithaca, NY 14850, USA; [c] Department of Population Medicine and Diagnostic Sciences, Cornell University, Veterinary Medical Center, Room C2-554, Ithaca, NY 14853, USA
* Corresponding author. Department of Clinical Sciences, College of Veterinary Medicine and Biomedical Sciences, Colorado State University, Fort Collins, CO 80523.
E-mail address: lcaixeta@umn.edu

2.5% in herds with 500 or more cows to 4.8% in herds having fewer than 500 cows.[1] Moreover, DA is known as an immediate postpartum condition with more than half of LDA cases being diagnosed within 2 weeks after parturition and 80% of the LDA cases occurring within the first month of lactation.[2]

Economic analyses have determined that the average cost per DA diagnosis is more than $700 when accounting for direct (eg, examination, correction, medication, discarded milk, death loss) and indirect (eg, future milk production loss, loss of body weight, decreased reproductive performance, increase risk of removal from the herd) costs.[3] Assuming the 3.5% incidence reported by the US Department of Agriculture survey with the estimated 9 million dairy cows in United States, it is reasonable to approximate that the annual losses to the dairy industry from DA exceed 150 million dollars. Thus, monitoring and managing dairy herds to decrease the incidence of DA is of extreme importance for the sustainability of dairy production and to improve animal health and wellbeing.

The diagnoses, medical therapy, methods for surgical correction, and posttreatment consequences of DA in an individual cow have been reported by various investigators.[4–8] However, the evaluation and management of DA at the herd level have not been explored as consistently. Therefore, the objectives of this review article are to discuss the possible nutritional and nonnutritional factors involved in DA development and provide suggestions on evaluation and management strategies at the herd level to decrease its occurrence.

NONNUTRITIONAL RISK FACTORS FOR DISPLACED ABOMASUM AND NUTRITIONAL RISK FACTORS FOR DISPLACED ABOMASUM
Disturbances of the Abomasal Motor Activity

Abomasal atony has been reported as a key factor in the development of DA. Moreover, it has been hypothesized that abomasal hypomotility occurs before the distention and displacement of the abomasum. Mechanistically, this abomasal stasis contributes to the inflation of this organ because the gas produced during digestion is not pushed out and cannot escape.

Geishauser and colleagues[9] demonstrated in vitro motility disorders in abomasal wall tissue collected from DA cases. During this experiment, tissue samples from DA cases presented normal spontaneous activity of smooth muscle in response to myogenic activity stimulus, whereas nerve-mediated contractile responses were diminished and sensitivity to acetylcholine was significantly decreased. Taken together, these findings suggest that the impaired emptying of the abomasum due to abomasal atony might be determined by a malfunction of the enteric nervous system in addition to an impaired cholinergic muscle responses. Further, decreased concentration of motility-stimulating neurotransmitters in the abomasal wall[10,11] and decreased electrical response activity measured via electromyography have been reported in association with LDA.[12] Further investigations are needed to compare the levels of such neurotransmitters between animals affected by DA and healthy counterparts within the same breed to confirm its relationship with DA development. Nonetheless, in addition to the neurologic factors associated with abomasal hypomotility, factors such as mineral imbalances, endotoxemia, decreased concentrations of glucose and insulin, and elevated β-hydroxybutyrate (BHB), among others, have been reported as possible factors associated with abomasal atony preceding the development of DA.

Calcium is extremely important for proper smooth muscle contractility and neuromuscular transmission. Hence, low-serum or plasma calcium concentration, hypocalcemia, has been implicated as among the main metabolic factors associated with the decreased abomasal motility preceding DA development. Multiple epidemiologic studies have reported the association between hypocalcemia within the first 2 weeks postpartum and the development of DA.[13–17] In a controlled study in which hypocalcemia was induced, decreased abomasal and ruminal motility were reported.[18] Notably, complete abomasal atony was observed in 2 animals even when plasma calcium concentrations were within the normal ionized calcium levels.[18]

Potassium is an important electrolyte regulating appropriate physiologic functioning of muscle cells. In humans, low-plasma concentration of potassium, hypokalemia, is associated with decreased small intestine motility.[19] Similarly in dairy cattle, decreased potassium concentrations were shown to impair abomasal smooth muscle tone in vitro.[20] In vivo, hypokalemia was shown to be present preceding the development of uncomplicated cases of DA by various groups.[21–24] Fortunately, the use of a balanced total mixed ration (TMR) during the periparturient period has virtually eliminated the occurrence of hypokalemia cases in the modern dairy industry, thus the current influence of isolated hypokalemia in the development of DA is close to negligible.

Endotoxemia has been suggested as another factor influencing in the etiopathology of periparturient metabolic diseases. Zebeli and colleagues,[25] and Verheijden and colleagues,[26] reported a disruption of abomasal and ruminal smooth muscle contraction when endotoxemia was experimentally induced in dairy cows under controlled environments. Endotoxemia was also reported to decrease feed intake after parturition.[25] Therefore, endotoxemia might play a role in the development of DA by directly decreasing the smooth muscle contraction, as well as indirectly decreasing abomasal motility due to the associated decrease in feed intake. Nonetheless, the link between endotoxemia and the development of DA is not completely understood.

In addition to feed intake, tonicity of the vagal nerve is important to sustain normal abomasal motility. Increased glucose and insulin levels in blood, characteristic of postprandial states, increase vagal tonicity, leading to increased abomasal motility. Dairy cows that develop DA have been reported to have significantly lower feed intake and lower blood concentrations of glucose and insulin when compared with their healthy counterparts.[27] Thus, suboptimal abomasal motility due to decreased stimulation of the autonomic nervous system might make these animals more susceptible to DA development. Low-glucose and insulin concentrations lead to increased blood concentrations of ketone bodies, including BHB, due to the increased mobilization of lipids to support energy demands.[28] Even though BHB has been directly associated with increased oxidative stress and proapoptotic effects in in vitro studies using bovine abomasum smooth muscle cells,[29] hyperketonemia most likely decreases abomasal motility indirectly by decreasing feed intake.

Collection of Gas and Dilation of the Abomasum

Excessive production and accumulation of gas within the abomasum have also been described as essential for DA development. The gas produced by excessive fermentation of feed material in the abomasum can directly cause the abomasum to inflate and displace. Furthermore, the decreased abomasum emptying rate associated with hypomotility previously described might contribute to accumulation of gas in the abomasum and consequently displacement.

High-concentrate and low-fiber diets have been associated with increased DA incidence.[10,30] It has been previously reported that feeding proper amounts of effective fiber is essential to ensure the establishment of a healthy rumen fiber mat, which is important to sustain normal rumen function.[30] The absence of a healthy rumen fiber mat changes rumen motility and fill, therefore contributing to the development of DA. On the other hand, high-concentrate diets increase the production of gas in the abomasum. These diets also increase the production of volatile fatty acids (VFAs) in the rumen, resulting in decreased ruminal pH and increased osmotic pressure. The increased osmotic pressure will cause an osmotic draw of water into the rumen, which in turn increases the flow rate of the ingesta through the forestomachs. Thus, the amount of VFA that is absorbed in the rumen and omasum is decreased, which increases the quantity of VFA and fluids that reach the abomasum.[31] Ultimately, the increased volume of ruminal content and VFA reaching the abomasum leads to an elevation of luminal pH in the abomasum. This marked change in abomasal pH enables ruminal microbial flora to continue the fermentation process in the abomasum unabated, which further contributes to the production of methane and carbon dioxide, leading to the dilation of the abomasum.[32] Additionally, the excessive water and electrolytes moving into the abomasum from the rumen further distend the abomasal walls.

Mechanical and Anatomic Aspects Determining the Displacement of the Abomasum

In dairy cattle, the rumen occupies the left side of the abdominal cavity almost in its entirety, creating a physical barrier preventing the movement of the abomasum. Other organs, including the gravid uterus, will aid in normal abomasal placement. However, in the days immediately postpartum, the uterus dramatically decreases in size, creating additional space in the abdominal cavity. Moreover, the decrease in dry matter intake (DMI) common during the periparturient period leads to a decrease in ruminal fill that, in turn, contributes to the maintenance of empty space in the abdominal cavity and allows for abnormal movement of the abomasum.[33] Anatomically, the depth of the abdominal cavity of the modern dairy cow is significantly greater than the abdominal depth of dairy cows from the early years of the twentieth century.[34] The larger framed size of the modern dairy cows has been associated with an increased likelihood to develop DA.[35]

Taken together, the larger frame size of the modern dairy cow and decreased ruminal volume during early lactation play a role in the increased incidence of DA in the last 70 years. In the face of this challenge, nutritional management strategies have been developed by various research groups to prevent the development of DA (see later discussion).[30,36–40]

ETIOLOGIC NUTRITIONAL RISK FACTORS IN THE DISPLACED ABOMASUM
Ration Formulation and Physical Form: Early Lactation Nutrition

As discussed previously, DA is often a sequela of other diseases common in the transition period. Considering this factor, early lactation rations should be formulated following the National Research Council's guidelines to reduce and prevent other metabolic diseases common to the periparturient period, which will in turn help reduce DA incidence. The goal of formulating a diet should be to meet, but not exceed, the nutritional requirements of the animal. Feeding high-energy diets has been shown to increase the rate of DA.[36,39] Interestingly, Janovick and colleages[39] also demonstrated that by limiting the amount of cows' high-energy diet, the incidence of DA was reduced when compared with their counterparts receiving normal amounts of the same ration. Therefore, feeding high-energy diets to dry cows is not advised because limiting the individual feed intake in commercial production settings is virtually impossible. On the other hand, limiting feed and energy intake below recommended levels during the periparturient period will not only decreased rumen fill but also trigger excessive mobilization of adipose tissue to fulfill energy requirements, leading to the development of other diseases that are associated with increased incidence of DA, such as ketosis.[41]

Along with energy requirements, it is also necessary to fulfill the requirement of physically effective fiber when formulating diets for early lactation dairy cows. Adequate levels of physically effective fiber stimulate chewing and saliva secretion.[42,43] Saliva secretion is the main buffering solution entering the rumen[44] and is an essential factor for the neutralization of the VFA produced in the rumen. Ultimately, this increased saliva secretion determined by increased dietary roughage will lead to an increase in the ruminal pH, preventing the development of ruminal acidosis. Physically effective fiber in the rumen is important not only for the establishment of a healthy fiber mat and maintenance of normal function and pH but also for the physical expansion of this organ within the abdominal cavity, thereby decreasing the likelihood of abomasal displacement.

Ration Formulation and Physical Form: Dry Cow Nutrition

Although the formulation of early lactation diets with adequate fiber and energy contents is important to prevent DA, following nutritional recommendations for late-lactation and dry cows can greatly improve the results of any nutritional management strategy used to reduce and prevent the occurrence of DA in early lactation. For instance, the use of diets balanced to maintain a consistent body condition score (BCS) before parturition (ie, late lactation and dry period) is extremely important to prevent metabolic disorders in early lactation. Cows that are overconditioned at parturition have an increased risk for developing DA when compared with thin cows.[30] Maintaining late gestation cattle at BCS less than or equal to 4.0 (using a 5-point scale[45]) may lessen the risk of DA because high-BCS cattle are at greater risk of intake depression and negative energy balance, which is associated with the development of DA postpartum.[36,39]

In addition to excessive BCS, other factors, such as low-fiber diets and poor bunk management, contribute to the increased risk of DA in periparturient dairy cattle. Identification of these risk factors can aid in developing measures that prevent periparturient metabolic disorders that may contribute to DA incidence. For example, DMI can decline up to 35% in the final week of gestation, thus prepartum feeding strategies in the dry cow pen are an important area to consider these measures.[30] A common strategy used in commercial dairy farms to address this issue is to add straw (low-energy and high-fiber ingredient) for 4 to 8 weeks before the expected calving date. This strategy helps with limiting energy intake while still allowing for daily maintenance energy consumption as recommended by the National Research Council.

Feeding and Bunk Management

One of the most important aspects to reduce DA incidence within a herd is to maintain a consistent diet available 24 hours for cattle to consume. Commercial dairy operations that are able to meet this goal are often able to overcome other social and overcrowding issues. Conversely, research has shown that reducing the hours of feed availability and increasing the stocking density each have a negative effect on DMI and feeding rate that is compounded when both are present.[46]

TMRs are commonly used in the dairy industry because they enable producers to offer consistent and balanced diets to their animals, thus improving the efficiency of nutrient utilization while decreasing selection within the ration.[40] Even though TMR diets are mixed and delivered to provide a consistent diet throughout the entire day, cattle will sort against longer particles and, over time, the neutral detergent fiber (NDF) of the TMR will increase.[37] To prevent this sorting behavior, high-fiber ingredients such as straw should be processed so that the longest particles are approximately 5 cm (2 in) in length. Additionally, water is often added to the TMR to try and reduce sorting.[38] However, in diets with less than 60% dry matter, additional water increased sorting behavior against long particles, leading to increased variation in diet NDF and increased heating of feed in the bunk.[47]

Apart from the ration formulation and physical form, management of the feed delivered to dairy cattle can significantly affect the incidence of DA. Cleaning bunks daily and providing cattle with at least 60 cm (24 in) of bunk space per animal throughout the periparturient stage of lactation can help reduce DA incidence.[36] A typical 3-row freestall barn will need to be stocked at 85% to 88% stocking density per stall to provide 60 cm (24 in) of bunk space to all cattle in the pen.

Separating primiparous animals from multiparous animals may reduce the incidence of metabolic disease in primiparous animals. Primiparous animals housed with multiparous animals were more likely to be reacted on and displaced from the feed bunk than multiparous cattle.[48,49] This behavior can have several negative effects on primiparous animals, such as increased nonesterified fatty acids (NEFA) concentration[48] and reduced DMI, even when adjusted for body weight and milk production.[49]

Feed bunk design can also affect eating behavior. For example, headlocks reduced displacements due to aggressive behavior between cows when compared with a post and rail system,[50] so feeding in headlocks allows nondominant cows to consume enough feed to fulfill their nutritional requirements without slug feeding. Additionally, proper cooling and providing well-designed stalls are important to improve cow comfort and indirectly decrease the occurrence of DA.[51–53] Bunk and feeding management practice goals are summarized in **Box 1**.

Assessing Ration Physical Form: Penn State Particle Separator

As previously described, the proper particle size in the TMR affects DMI, chewing activity, rumen fermentation, and is important to fulfill fiber requirements.[54] Moreover, delivering diets with optimal particle size can decrease sorting and is a key factor within the nutritional management strategies used to prevent metabolic disorders. Quantitative measurements of particle sizes in TMR were challenging to assess until the development of the Penn State Particle Separator (PSPS).

The PSPS consists of 4 boxes (upper sieve, middle sieve, lower sieve, bottom pan) with different pore sizes. To use the separator, the 4 boxes should be stacked on top of each other with the box with larger holes on top, followed by the box with medium-sized holes, then the box with the smallest holes, and finally the solid pan on the bottom. The technique to use the PSPS has been previously described by others.[55–57] Briefly, approximately 200 g (3 pints) of TMR is placed on the upper sieve. On a flat surface, vigorously shake the sieves horizontally in the same direction 5 times, rotate

---

Box 1
Recommended feeding, bunk management, and management practices

Management Practice	Goal
Removal of old feed from bunk	Daily
Availability of feed	≥23 h/d
Feed push-up	Every 4 h
Eating space	≥60 cm/head (24 in)
Water availability	≥10 linear cm/head (4 in)
Prepartum DMI	
Primiparous	≥10 kg (22 lb)/d
Multiparous	≥12 kg (26.5 lb)/d
Social groupings	Separate primiparous animals

the separator box one-quarter turn, and repeat this process 7 times (40 shakes in total). After shaking, weigh the material in each sieve and bottom pan and compute the percentage of the material by weight under each sieve. Recommendations for sufficient particle size using the PSPS when evaluating lactating TMR diets[56,57] and dry cow diet straw distribution, and the pore sizes for the different sieves of the PSPS are presented in **Table 1**.

Diets without sufficient material on the top 2 screens of the PSPS will most likely be deficient in physically effective NDF (peNDF), which can increase the incidence of DA due to lack of an effective rumen mat, as previously discussed. However, diets with excessive material on the top (19 mm) screen can be equally as problematic for several reasons. The longer particle material on the top screen will be selectively sorted against by cattle,[37,58] and this sorting behavior can lead to a decreased intake of peNDF and a significant increase of peNDF in refusals. It has also been shown that, regardless of particle length of feed presented to the cow, they will chew feed to a uniform length of 10 to 11 mm before swallowing the bolus.[59] Thus, increasing the amount of long particles in the TMR will increase eating time per meal without changing the length of material presented into the rumen.[59] There is no minimum amount of material required to be in the bottom pan; however, by default, most lactating diets containing 40% to 50% concentrate will have 25% to 30% material in the bottom pan. Dry cow TMR will have a different percentage of particle size compared with a lactating diet, typically due to higher forage and fiber content.

Dry cow TMR will have a different percentage of particle size compared with a lactating diet. The degree of sorting against long particles is approximately 15% to 20% over the first 4 hours after feed delivery, with almost no change in sorting 4 to 12 hours after feed delivery.[58] A useful approach in determining sorting behavior in dry cows would be to analyze the diet using a PSPS and then repeat the analysis 4 hours later to determine the change in percent material present on the top screen.

MONITORING DISPLACED ABOMASUM AND OTHER FACTORS ASSOCIATED WITH ITS OCCURRENCE

Creating strategies to prevent the occurrence of DA by monitoring only the incidence of this morbidity is practically impossible. If the multifactorial nature of the pathogenesis of DA is considered (**Fig. 1**), the delay between the diagnosis and

Table 1
Recommendations of total mixed ration particle sizes for lactating dairy cow diets and straw particles size distribution in dry cow diets when analyzing feed material using a Penn State particle separator

Screen Size	Pore Size in cm (in)	Percent (%) of TMR[a]	Percent (%) of Straw or Dry Hay[b]	Percent (%) of TMR[c]
Upper Sieve	2.0 (0.75)	2–8	20	<5
Middle Sieve	0.8 (0.31)	30–50	40	>50
Lower Sieve	0.1 (0.05)	30–50	20	10–20
Bottom Pan	—	<20	20	25–30

[a] Data based on 2 experiments using early lactation. *Data from* Kononoff PJ, Heinrichs AJ. The effect of reducing alfalfa haylage particle size on cows in early lactation. J Dairy Sci 2003;86(4):1445–57; and Kononoff PJ, Heinrichs AJ. The effect of corn silage particle size and cottonseed hulls on cows in early lactation. J Dairy Sci 2003;86(7):2438–51.
[b] Dann H, Miner Institute, Chazy, NY, personal communication, 2016.
[c] *Adapted from* Kotanch K. Miner Institute Farm Report, 2017.

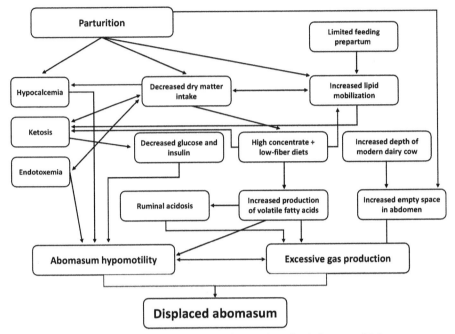

Fig. 1. Schematic representation of the multifactorial etiologic factors of DA.

recording of DA, and the emergence of the previously mentioned risk factors, herd-level monitoring and prevention strategies relying solely in the occurrence of DA as a standalone morbidity are of little significance to veterinarians and dairy producers. However, despite its association with other comorbidities, the determination of a herd alarm level for DA incidence is important, and further investigation should be performed when DA incidence exceeds the thresholds established for each particular farm (**Box 2**).

Displaced Abomasum Alarm Levels

The incidence of DA in the United States dairy herds was determined to be approximately 3.5%,[1] yet a considerable discrepancy was observed when comparing different size herds. Based on the data presented in this nationwide survey and rates observed in well-managed dairy farms, a reasonable goal would be to have less than 3% of cows freshening within a month develop a DA. Well-managed dairy farms, with excellent transition period management, high-quality nutrition, and good cow comfort have reported DA risks to be lower than 1% in the month following parturition.

As previously discussed, the development of DA is generally preceded by the occurrence of several comorbidities and/or nonideal feeding conditions. Therefore, to successfully prevent the occurrence of DA, it is important for farmers, veterinarians, and nutritionists to routinely monitor dairy cows' health and nutrition during the transition period. The appropriate use of a reliable and effective data recording system, from which trustworthy data can be extracted, is essential for monitoring any disease incidence on a dairy farm, including DA.

Box 2
Monitoring displaced abomasum and other factors associated with its occurrence

- Determine a herd alarm level for DA incidence
  - Goal: DA less than 3% of cows freshening within a month

Note: Well-managed dairy farms report DA less than 1% during the month following parturition.

- Routinely monitor dairy cow's health and nutrition during the transition period
  - Monitor and treat infectious diseases
    - Metritis
      - Herd alarm: greater than 15%
    - Mastitis
      - Herd alarm: greater than 5%
    - Retained fetal membranes
      - Herd alarm: greater than 5%
  - Monitor and treat metabolic diseases
    - Hypocalcemia
      - Herd alarm
        - Clinical: greater than or equal to 5%
        - Subclinical: greater than or equal to 30%
    - Hyperketonemia (ketosis)
      - Herd alarm: greater than 15%

Note 1: The prevalence of metritis and retained fetal membranes should be calculated as number of cases divided by the number of fresh cows within a month, whereas the prevalence of mastitis is normally calculated as the number of clinical cases divided by the number of milking cows within a month.

Note 2: Reliable and effective data recording system are paramount.

- Assess nutritional status of dairy cows by monitoring BCS
  - Determine BCS at
    - Dry-off
    - Calving
    - Peak milk production ($\sim$60 days in milk)
    - Midlactation ($\sim$180 days in milk)

Infectious Diseases and Endotoxemia

Animals suffering from metritis, mastitis, and retained fetal membranes in early lactation have been reported to have a significantly higher risk of developing DA when compared with their healthy counterparts.[60,61] Endotoxins and inflammatory mediators released in response to these infectious diseases coupled with other challenges common during the transition period have been directly involved in the pathophysiology of DA by impairing abomasal motility.[32] Additionally, both the inflammatory response and associated fever diminish DMI, which further decreases gastrointestinal tract motility and ruminal fill, enabling abomasum displacement. Thus, monitoring, early diagnosing, and treating infectious diseases, such as metritis, mastitis, and retained placenta, is significant to mitigate their influence in the occurrence of DA.

Mineral and Energy Deficiencies

Mineral imbalances are also common during the transition period in dairy cows and have been identified as predisposing factors to the development of DA in early lactation. Among the mineral imbalances, hypocalcemia should be highlighted due to several reports associating this imbalance with an increased likelihood of DA occurrence.[17,21,62] Even though clinical hypocalcemia can be easily monitored based on the occurrence of pathognomonic clinical signs, monitoring subclinical cases is challenging because of the lack of an inexpensive and reliable method for the analysis of blood calcium concentration on-farm. However, when blood calcium concentrations are measured, animals with serum total calcium less than or equal to 2.0 mmol/L (8 mg/dL) are considered to be hypocalcemic.[15,63] Hypocalcemic dairy cows have been reported to be between 3.1 and 4.8 times more likely to develop DA than their eucalcemic counterparts.[13,17] Despite the current challenges to measure serum calcium concentration in commercial dairy farms, it has been suggested that reasonable alarm levels for subclinical hypocalcemia should be set at greater than or equal to 30%,[62,63] and greater than or equal to 5% for clinical hypocalcemia in multiparous Holstein dairy cows.

Similar to mineral imbalances, energy deficiencies are hallmarks of the transition period in dairy cows and have been associated with the development DA in early lactation. During this period, dairy cows need to mobilize body reserves, especially adipose tissue, to fulfill the energy demands of early lactation.[64–66] As a consequence of increased lipid mobilization, a higher concentration of circulating NEFAs is observed.[28] Elevated concentrations of NEFA can overwhelm liver's capacity to completely oxidize this molecule, resulting in elevated rates of partial oxidation into ketone bodies, producing a state of hyperketonemia, also known as ketosis.[28,66] Although an elevation of NEFA and ketone bodies is normal in the immediate postpartum period, excessively elevated concentrations of NEFA and ketosis have been reported to increase the risk of DA.[13,67–69]

Ketosis has been reported as a proxy of negative energy balance during early lactation and can be monitored by measuring concentrations of BHB in blood, milk, or urine.[69–71] Animals with blood BHB concentrations greater than or equal to 1.2 mmol/L, deemed positive for hyperketonemia, were 7 to 8 times more likely to develop DA in early lactation when compared with their healthy counterparts.[72] Similarly, a study measuring milk BHB within the first 2 weeks of lactation determined that animals with elevated milk BHB concentration greater than or equal to 500 mmol/L were 19 times more likely to be diagnosed with LDA.[71] Finally, when analyzing protein to fat ratio in milk, it was observed that animals with protein-to-fat ratio less than or equal to 0.72 were 8.2 times more likely to be diagnosed with DA in the first 30 days in milk.[73] Frequency of hyperketonemia within each herd determines the recommended intervention: if less than 15%, herd level prevalence should be monitored; if 15% to 40%, all animals should be monitored twice between 3 and 9 DIM and all positive individuals should be treated with 300 mL of propylene glycol for 5 days; and, if more than 40%, all cows should be treated with propylene glycol starting on 3 DIM for 5 days. Management and nutritional protocols should be revised to achieve acceptable prevalence rates in herds with elevated hyperketonemia prevalence; disease prevalence should be reassessed within a month.[74,75]

Body Condition Score

BCS has also been used to assess the nutritional status of dairy cows. During early lactation, a loss of BCS is expected because dairy cows are mobilizing their body reserves to support the increased energy demands of milk production. It has been previously reported that animals losing substantial BCS during the first month postpartum are more likely to develop DA, whereas animals that do not lose BCS in early lactation have a lower risk of developing DA.[76,77] By consistently monitoring BCS, dairy farmers, veterinarians, and nutritionists are able to determine if transition-period nutritional management is optimal. It is advised to determine BCS at dry-off, calving, peak milk production (around 60 days into lactation), and another time during midlactation to monitor BCS dynamics throughout lactation. Thus, if excessive loss or gain of BCS is observed, nutritional interventions can take place to overcome this challenge.

Automated Health-Monitoring Systems

With the recent development and popularization of precision farming technologies, activity and rumination monitors have been used to assist with identification of animals with digestive disorders. Daily walking activity, as well as milk yield, was altered in animals that developed DA 5 to 6 days before diagnosis.[78] Additionally, it has been reported that automated health-monitoring systems that combine rumination and activity information are capable of identifying animals with metabolic and digestive disorders earlier than clinical diagnosis by farm personnel.[79] Thus, the use of activity and rumination monitors may present as an interesting tool for monitoring and preventing DA and other diseases.

PREVENTION OF DISPLACED ABOMASUM AND OTHER FACTORS ASSOCIATED WITH ITS OCCURRENCE

Management strategies that facilitate an efficient transition into lactation are essential to determine the success of any approach used to prevent displaced abomasa. The transition period has been traditionally defined as the period 3 weeks before and after parturition.[80] Nevertheless, metabolic changes can start earlier and have carryover effects beyond this period; hence, the importance of proper management of dairy cows beyond this 6-week period (**Box 3**).

The nutritional management of dairy cows to decrease the incidence of DA must start during the late stages of the previous lactation and dry period even though the occurrence of DA is more common during early lactation. As previously discussed, feeding long-stemmed or coarsely chopped forage in the close-up dry pen helps limit the energy intake prepartum and, consequently, contributes to the maintenance of adequate BCS. By increasing the effective fiber content of prefresh

---

Box 3
Prevention of displaced abomasum and other factors associated with its occurrence

- Use of automated health-monitoring systems for early diagnosis of comorbidities
- Use of anionic salts during the dry period to minimize the occurrence of hypocalcemia
  - Goal: urine pH between 6.0 and 7.0
- Test-and-treat strategy to monitor hyperketonemia
- Routine comprehensive TMR audits
  - Particle length
  - Consistency of the delivered diet
  - Feeding routine
  - Bunk management
- Assess cow comfort
  - Appropriate stocking density for different periods of lactation
  - Bunk space
  - Access to water
  - Stall design
  - Comfortable and sanitary bedding material
  - Heat abatement
- Manage early lactation cows in fresh cow pens

diets, the healthy fiber mat can be maintained and also contribute to a physical expansion of the rumen.

Mineral and Energy Deficiencies

To further reduce the frequency of DA in early lactation, nutritional and management strategies to decrease the occurrence of metabolic diseases, such as hypocalcemia and ketosis, are important. The use of anionic salts to produce a negative dietary cation-anion difference (DCAD) during the dry period has been reported to minimize the occurrence of clinical hypocalcemia in early lactation.[81–83] The degree of acidification caused by the use of anionic salts during the dry period can be determined by measuring individual animal urine pH, with optimal urine pH of dairy cattle consuming anionic salts during the dry period being between 6.0 and 7.0.[84] Additionally, the use of oral calcium supplementation in early lactation has been proposed as an alternative strategy to overcome calcium deficiencies.[85,86] Thus, herd-level monitoring of the effectiveness of the DCAD diet diets during the dry period and supplementing calcium to animals that are more likely to develop hypocalcemia may decrease the likelihood of DA development.

Different nutritional strategies have been studied to minimize negative energy balance and excessive lipid mobilization in early lactation. Even so, ineffective adaptation of fresh cows to the changing physiologic state remains common, leading to the occurrence of ketosis. Fortunately, it has been determined that ketosis can be efficiently monitored by using a combined testing-and-treating strategy.[74] Additionally, it has also been reported that ketotic animals treated with propylene glycol are 40% less likely to develop DA when compared with their nontreated counterparts.[87] Ultimately, monitoring and treating ketosis in early lactation is an effective way to prevent the occurrence of DA.

Diet, Transition Cow Management, and Cow Comfort

Comprehensive TMR audits should be performed on a regular basis to determine if the feed delivered to the cows on a daily basis is in accordance to the recommended diets for each particular group of cows. Oelberg and Stone[88] have described methods to evaluate TMR consistency and provided practical solutions to improve TMR quality to enhance production and health in dairy farms. To efficiently monitor and improve the measure, these audits should be tailored to each dairy farm.

Cow comfort during the transition period also has a remarkable impact on DMI and, consequently, DA development. Aspects such as proper stocking density, sufficient bunk space, free access to water, correct stall designs with comfortable and sanitary bedding material, heat abatement systems, and frequent and adequate delivered feed management cannot be overlooked during this time. Finally, managing cows in a transition or fresh cow pen for 3 to 4 weeks postpartum facilitates the monitoring of the metabolic and infectious diseases associated with the development of DA, enabling farmers, veterinarian, and nutritionists to act quickly when problems arise.

SUMMARY

DA is a multifactorial disorder usually diagnosed in early lactation dairy cows. Various components of cow health, including infectious and metabolic diseases, physical form and composition of diets during the transition period, and cow comfort, are factors linked to the pathogenesis of DA. It is important to understand how these factors play a role in the development of DA to establish herd-level strategies to monitor and reduce the occurrence of this clinical disorder.

REFERENCES

1. NAHMS-USDA. National Animal Health Monitoring System: dairy cattle management practices in the United States. In: Agriculture UDo, ed. Available at: https://www.aphis.usda.gov/aphis/ourfocus/animalhealth/monitoring-and-surveillance/nahms/nahms_dairy_studies2007. Accessed on May 22, 2017.
2. Trent A. Surgery of the abomasum. In: Fubini SL, Ducharme NG, editors. Farm animal surgery. St Louis (MO): Saunders; 2004. p. 196–239.
3. McArt JA, Nydam DV, Overton MW. Hyperketonemia in early lactation dairy cattle: a deterministic estimate of component and total cost per case. J Dairy Sci 2015; 98(3):2043–54.
4. Sterner KE, Grymer J, Bartlett PC, et al. Factors influencing the survival of dairy cows after correction of left displaced abomasum. J Am Vet Med Assoc 2008; 232(10):1521–9.
5. Fubini SL, Ducharme NG, Erb HN, et al. A comparison in 101 dairy cows of right paralumbar fossa omentopexy and right paramedian abomasopexy for treatment of left displacement of the abomasum. Can Vet J 1992;33(5):318–24.
6. Niehaus AJ. Surgical management of abomasal disease. Vet Clin North Am Food Anim Pract 2016;32(3):629–44.
7. Gabel AA, Heath RB. Treatment of right-sided torsion of the abomasum in cattle. J Am Vet Med Assoc 1969;155(4):642–4.
8. Pentecost RL, Niehaus AJ, Anderson DE, et al. Outcome following surgical correction of abomasal displacement in lactating dairy cattle: a retrospective study of 127 cases (1999-2010). J Vet Sci Anim Husb 2014;1(4):1.
9. Geishauser T, Reiche D, Schemann M. In vitro motility disorders associated with displaced abomasum in dairy cows. Neurogastroenterol Motil 1998;10(5): 395–401.
10. Doll K, Sickinger M, Seeger T. New aspects in the pathogenesis of abomasal displacement. Vet J 2009;181(2):90–6.
11. Sickinger M, Leiser R, Failing K, et al. Evaluation of differences between breeds for substance P, vasoactive intestinal polypeptide, and neurofilament 200 in the abomasal wall of cattle. Am J Vet Res 2008;69(10):1247–53.
12. Nelson D, Petersen G, Huhn J, et al. Electromyography of the reticulum, abomasum and duodenum in dairy cows with left displacement of the abomasum. Transbound Emerg Dis 1995;42(1–10):325–37.
13. Chapinal N, Carson M, Duffield TF, et al. The association of serum metabolites with clinical disease during the transition period. J Dairy Sci 2011;94(10): 4897–903.
14. Curtis CR, Erb HN, Sniffen CJ, et al. Association of parturient hypocalcemia with eight periparturient disorders in Holstein cows. J Am Vet Med Assoc 1983;183(5): 559–61.
15. Goff JP. The monitoring, prevention, and treatment of milk fever and subclinical hypocalcemia in dairy cows. Vet J 2008;176(1):50–7.
16. Seifi HA, Leblanc SJ, Leslie KE, et al. Metabolic predictors of post-partum disease and culling risk in dairy cattle. Vet J 2011;188(2):216–20.
17. Massey C, Wang C, Donovan G, et al. Hypocalcemia at parturition as a risk factor for left displacement of the abomasum in dairy cows. J Am Vet Med Assoc 1993; 203(6):852–3.
18. Daniel R. Motility of the rumen and abomasum during hypocalcaemia. Can J Comp Med 1983;47(3):276.

19. Chen JZ, Deng AW, Xu JF. Electroenterogram manifestations and significance in hypokalemia. Di Yi Jun Yi Da Xue Xue Bao 2005;25(1):7–9.
20. Turck G, Leonhard-Marek S. Potassium and insulin affect the contractility of abomasal smooth muscle. J Dairy Sci 2010;93(8):3561–8.
21. Delgado-Lecaroz R, Warnick LD, Guard CL, et al. Cross-sectional study of the association of abomasal displacement or volvulus with serum electrolyte and mineral concentrations in dairy cows. Can Vet J 2000;41(4):301–5.
22. Zadnik T. Review of anterior displacement of the abomasum in cattle in Slovenia. Vet Rec 2003;153(1):24–5.
23. Constable P, Grunberg W, Staufenbiel R, et al. Clinicopathologic variables associated with hypokalemia in lactating dairy cows with abomasal displacement or volvulus. J Am Vet Med Assoc 2013;242(6):826–35.
24. Wallace C. Left abomasal displacement, a retrospective study of 315 cases. Bovine Pract 1975.
25. Zebeli Q, Sivaraman S, Dunn SM, et al. Intermittent parenteral administration of endotoxin triggers metabolic and immunological alterations typically associated with displaced abomasum and retained placenta in periparturient dairy cows. J Dairy Sci 2011;94(10):4968–83.
26. Verheijden JH, Van Miert AS, Schotman AJ, et al. Pathophysiological aspects of E. coli mastitis in ruminants. Vet Res Commun 1983;7(1–4):229–36.
27. Van Winden SC, Jorritsma R, Muller KE, et al. Feed intake, milk yield, and metabolic parameters prior to left displaced abomasum in dairy cows. J Dairy Sci 2003;86(4):1465–71.
28. Herdt TH. Ruminant adaptation to negative energy balance. Influences on the etiology of ketosis and fatty liver. Vet Clin North Am Food Anim Pract 2000;16(2): 215–30, v.
29. Tian W, Wei T, Li B, et al. Pathway of programmed cell death and oxidative stress induced by beta-hydroxybutyrate in dairy cow abomasum smooth muscle cells and in mouse gastric smooth muscle. PLoS One 2014;9(5):e96775.
30. Shaver RD. Nutritional risk factors in the etiology of left displaced abomasum in dairy cows: a review. J Dairy Sci 1997;80(10):2449–53.
31. Sarashina T, Ichijo S, Takahashi J, et al. Origin of abomasum gas in the cows with displaced abomasum. Nihon Juigaku Zasshi 1990;52(2):371–8.
32. Van Winden SC, Muller KE, Kuiper R, et al. Studies on the pH value of abomasal contents in dairy cows during the first 3 weeks after calving. J Vet Med A Physiol Pathol Clin Med 2002;49(3):157–60.
33. Constable PD, Miller GY, Hoffsis GF, et al. Risk factors for abomasal volvulus and left abomasal displacement in cattle. Am J Vet Res 1992;53(7):1184–92.
34. Wittek T, Sen I, Constable PD. Changes in abdominal dimensions during late gestation and early lactation in Holstein-Friesian heifers and cows and their relationship to left displaced abomasum. Vet Rec 2007;161(5):155–61.
35. Becker JC, Heins BJ, Hansen LB. Costs for health care of Holstein cows selected for large versus small body size. J Dairy Sci 2012;95(9):5384–92.
36. Cameron RE, Dyk PB, Herdt TH, et al. Dry cow diet, management, and energy balance as risk factors for displaced abomasum in high producing dairy herds. J Dairy Sci 1998;81(1):132–9.
37. Endres MI, Espejo LA. Feeding management and characteristics of rations for high-producing dairy cows in freestall herds. J Dairy Sci 2010;93(2):822–9.
38. Fish JA, DeVries TJ. Short communication: varying dietary dry matter concentration through water addition: effect on nutrient intake and sorting of dairy cows in late lactation. J Dairy Sci 2012;95(2):850–5.

39. Janovick NA, Boisclair YR, Drackley JK. Prepartum dietary energy intake affects metabolism and health during the periparturient period in primiparous and multiparous Holstein cows. J Dairy Sci 2011;94(3):1385–400.
40. Coppock C, Bath D, Harris B. From feeding to feeding systems. J Dairy Sci 1981; 64(6):1230–49.
41. Grummer RR, Mashek DG, Hayirli A. Dry matter intake and energy balance in the transition period. Vet Clin North Am Food Anim Pract 2004;20(3):447–70.
42. Zebeli Q, Tafaj M, Weber I, et al. Effects of varying dietary forage particle size in two concentrate levels on chewing activity, ruminal mat characteristics, and passage in dairy cows. J Dairy Sci 2007;90(4):1929–42.
43. Lechartier C, Peyraud JL. The effects of forage proportion and rapidly degradable dry matter from concentrate on ruminal digestion in dairy cows fed corn silage-based diets with fixed neutral detergent fiber and starch contents. J Dairy Sci 2010;93(2):666–81.
44. Kay RN. The influence of saliva on digestion in ruminants. World Rev Nutr Diet 1966;6:292–325.
45. Ferguson JD, Galligan DT, Thomsen N. Principal descriptors of body condition score in Holstein cows. J Dairy Sci 1994;77(9):2695–703.
46. Collings LK, Weary DM, Chapinal N, et al. Temporal feed restriction and overstocking increase competition for feed by dairy cattle. J Dairy Sci 2011;94(11): 5480–6.
47. Felton CA, DeVries TJ. Effect of water addition to a total mixed ration on feed temperature, feed intake, sorting behavior, and milk production of dairy cows. J Dairy Sci 2010;93(6):2651–60.
48. Huzzey JM, Grant RJ, Overton TR. Short communication: Relationship between competitive success during displacements at an overstocked feed bunk and measures of physiology and behavior in Holstein dairy cattle. J Dairy Sci 2012; 95(8):4434–41.
49. Neave HW, Lomb J, von Keyserlingk MA, et al. Parity differences in the behavior of transition dairy cows. J Dairy Sci 2017;100(1):548–61.
50. Huzzey JM, DeVries TJ, Valois P, et al. Stocking density and feed barrier design affect the feeding and social behavior of dairy cattle. J Dairy Sci 2006;89(1): 126–33.
51. do Amaral BC, Connor EE, Tao S, et al. Heat-stress abatement during the dry period: does cooling improve transition into lactation? J Dairy Sci 2009;92(12): 5988–99.
52. Mader TL, Griffin D. Management of cattle exposed to adverse environmental conditions. Vet Clin North Am Food Anim Pract 2015;31(2):247–58.
53. Krawczel PD, Hill CT, Dann HM, et al. Short communication: effect of stocking density on indices of cow comfort. J Dairy Sci 2008;91(5):1903–7.
54. National Research Council. Nutrient requirements of dairy cattle: 2001. National Academies Press; 2001.
55. Lammers BP, Buckmaster DR, Heinrichs AJ. A simple method for the analysis of particle sizes of forage and total mixed rations. J Dairy Sci 1996;79(5):922–8.
56. Kononoff PJ, Heinrichs AJ. The effect of reducing alfalfa haylage particle size on cows in early lactation. J Dairy Sci 2003;86(4):1445–57.
57. Kononoff PJ, Heinrichs AJ. The effect of corn silage particle size and cottonseed hulls on cows in early lactation. J Dairy Sci 2003;86(7):2438–51.
58. Hosseinkhani A, Devries TJ, Proudfoot KL, et al. The effects of feed bunk competition on the feed sorting behavior of close-up dry cows. J Dairy Sci 2008;91(3): 1115–21.

59. Schadt I, Ferguson JD, Azzaro G, et al. How do dairy cows chew?–particle size analysis of selected feeds with different particle length distributions and of respective ingested bolus particles. J Dairy Sci 2012;95(8):4707–20.

60. Detilleux JC, Grohn YT, Eicker SW, et al. Effects of left displaced abomasum on test day milk yields of Holstein cows. J Dairy Sci 1997;80(1):121–6.

61. Rohrbach BW, Cannedy AL, Freeman K, et al. Risk factors for abomasal displacement in dairy cows. J Am Vet Med Assoc 1999;214(11):1660–3.

62. Chapinal N, Leblanc SJ, Carson ME, et al. Herd-level association of serum metabolites in the transition period with disease, milk production, and early lactation reproductive performance. J Dairy Sci 2012;95(10):5676–82.

63. Oetzel GR. Monitoring and testing dairy herds for metabolic disease. Vet Clin North Am Food Anim Pract 2004;20(3):651–74.

64. Bauman DE, Currie WB. Partitioning of nutrients during pregnancy and lactation: a review of mechanisms involving homeostasis and homeorhesis. J Dairy Sci 1980;63(9):1514–29.

65. Bell AW. Regulation of organic nutrient metabolism during transition from late pregnancy to early lactation. J Anim Sci 1995;73(9):2804–19.

66. Drackley JK. ADSA Foundation Scholar Award. Biology of dairy cows during the transition period: the final frontier? J Dairy Sci 1999;82(11):2259–73.

67. Duffield TF, Lissemore KD, McBride BW, et al. Impact of hyperketonemia in early lactation dairy cows on health and production. J Dairy Sci 2009;92(2):571–80.

68. Ospina PA, Nydam DV, Stokol T, et al. Association between the proportion of sampled transition cows with increased nonesterified fatty acids and beta-hydroxybutyrate and disease incidence, pregnancy rate, and milk production at the herd level. J Dairy Sci 2010;93(8):3595–601.

69. McArt JA, Nydam DV, Oetzel GR. Epidemiology of subclinical ketosis in early lactation dairy cattle. J Dairy Sci 2012;95(9):5056–66.

70. Ospina PA, Nydam DV, Stokol T, et al. Evaluation of nonesterified fatty acids and beta-hydroxybutyrate in transition dairy cattle in the northeastern United States: critical thresholds for prediction of clinical diseases. J Dairy Sci 2010;93(2):546–54.

71. Geishauser T, Leslie K, Duffield T, et al. An evaluation of milk ketone tests for the prediction of left displaced abomasum in dairy cows. J Dairy Sci 1997;80(12):3188–92.

72. McArt JA, Nydam DV, Oetzel GR, et al. Elevated non-esterified fatty acids and beta-hydroxybutyrate and their association with transition dairy cow performance. Vet J 2013;198(3):560–70.

73. Geishauser TD, Leslie KE, Duffield TF, et al. An evaluation of protein/fat ratio in first DHI test milk for prediction of subsequent displaced abomasum in dairy cows. Can J Vet Res 1998;62(2):144–7.

74. Ospina PA, McArt JA, Overton TR, et al. Using nonesterified fatty acids and beta-hydroxybutyrate concentrations during the transition period for herd-level monitoring of increased risk of disease and decreased reproductive and milking performance. Vet Clin North Am Food Anim Pract 2013;29(2):387–412.

75. McArt JA, Nydam DV, Oetzel GR, et al. An economic analysis of hyperketonemia testing and propylene glycol treatment strategies in early lactation dairy cattle. Prev Vet Med 2014;117(1):170–9.

76. Gearhart MA, Curtis CR, Erb HN, et al. Relationship of changes in condition score to cow health in Holsteins. J Dairy Sci 1990;73(11):3132–40.

77. Hoedemaker M, Prange D, Gundelach Y. Body condition change ante- and postpartum, health and reproductive performance in German Holstein cows. Reprod Domest Anim 2009;44(2):167–73.
78. Edwards JL, Tozer PR. Using activity and milk yield as predictors of fresh cow disorders. J Dairy Sci 2004;87(2):524–31.
79. Stangaferro ML, Wijma R, Caixeta LS, et al. Use of rumination and activity monitoring for the identification of dairy cows with health disorders: part I. Metabolic and digestive disorders. J Dairy Sci 2016;99(9):7395–410.
80. Grummer RR. Impact of changes in organic nutrient metabolism on feeding the transition dairy cow. J Anim Sci 1995;73(9):2820–33.
81. Oetzel GR, Olson JD, Curtis CR, et al. Ammonium chloride and ammonium sulfate for prevention of parturient paresis in dairy cows. J Dairy Sci 1988;71(12): 3302–9.
82. Ramos-Nieves JM, Thering BJ, Waldron MR, et al. Effects of anion supplementation to low-potassium prepartum diets on macromineral status and performance of periparturient dairy cows. J Dairy Sci 2009;92(11):5677–91.
83. Grunberg W, Donkin SS, Constable PD. Periparturient effects of feeding a low dietary cation-anion difference diet on acid-base, calcium, and phosphorus homeostasis and on intravenous glucose tolerance test in high-producing dairy cows. J Dairy Sci 2011;94(2):727–45.
84. Oetzel GR. Management of dry cows for the prevention of milk fever and other mineral disorders. Vet Clin North Am Food Anim Pract 2000;16(2):369–86, vii.
85. McArt JA, Oetzel GR. A stochastic estimate of the economic impact of oral calcium supplementation in postparturient dairy cows. J Dairy Sci 2015;98(10): 7408–18.
86. Oetzel GR, Miller BE. Effect of oral calcium bolus supplementation on early-lactation health and milk yield in commercial dairy herds. J Dairy Sci 2012; 95(12):7051–65.
87. McArt JA, Nydam DV, Oetzel GR. A field trial on the effect of propylene glycol on displaced abomasum, removal from herd, and reproduction in fresh cows diagnosed with subclinical ketosis. J Dairy Sci 2012;95(5):2505–12.
88. Oelberg TJ, Stone W. Monitoring total mixed rations and feed delivery systems. Vet Clin North Am Food Anim Pract 2014;30(3):721–44.

Diagnosis and Treatment of Infectious Enteritis in Neonatal and Juvenile Ruminants

Meera C. Heller, DVM, PhD*, Munashe Chigerwe, BVSc, MPH, PhD

KEYWORDS

- Ruminant • Enteritis • Infection • Juvenile • Neonate • Diarrhea

KEY POINTS

- Common causes of infectious enteritis in neonate and juvenile ruminants include viral, bacterial, and protozoal pathogens.
- The most common presenting sign in ruminants with infectious enteritis is diarrhea.
- Diagnosis of the cause of enteritis has important zoonotic and herd health implications.
- Severity of clinical signs with similar pathogens may differ between calves and small ruminants.
- Treatment of enteritis involves supportive care to correct fluid and electrolyte imbalances, provision of nutritional support for the neonate, prevention and treatment of endotoxemia or sepsis, and pathogen-specific treatments when relevant and available.

PATHOPHYSIOLOGY

Several mechanisms of diarrhea are possible in ruminant neonates. This article summarizes the various mechanisms:

- Malabsorption
  - It is important to remember that, under physiologic conditions, more fluid is secreted into the intestinal lumen, and reabsorbed, compared with the ingested amount. Therefore, impaired reabsorption of fluids has a major impact on the fluid balance of the patient. Several diarrheal pathogens interfere with digestion and absorption by blunting intestinal villi, as observed with rotavirus and coronavirus infections.
- Osmotic
  - Increased solutes within the intestinal lumen osmotically pull more water into the lumen, thereby resulting in dehydration of the patient. Osmotic particles

Disclosure: The authors have nothing to disclose.
Department of Veterinary Medicine and Epidemiology, University of California Davis, One Shields Avenue, Davis, CA 95616, USA
* Corresponding author.
E-mail address: mcheller@ucdavis.edu

include maldigested disaccharides, and increased D-lactate levels from bacteria fermentation of unabsorbed nutrients that enter the colon.

- Secretory
  - Specific pathogens, such as enterotoxigenic *Escherichia coli* (ETEC), stimulate cyclic AMP, thus increasing secretion of chloride (Cl), sodium (Na), and potassium (K) into the intestinal lumen, thereby drawing water into the intestinal lumen.
  - In addition, some pathogens denude the intestinal surface and cause villous blunting, resulting in maldigestion and malabsorption. This damage to the villous leads to proliferation of secretory crypt cells and increased secretory capacity of the intestinal wall.
- Abnormal intestinal motility
  - Decreasing intestinal transit time may lead to maldigestion and malabsorption because of inadequate time for digestion and absorption of the ingested feed material. This process further contributes to osmotic retention of fluid in the intestinal tract.
- Increased hydrostatic pressure
  - Disease conditions, including heart failure, renal disease, and liver disease, may result in increased hydrostatic pressure within the intestinal tract causing movement of water from extracellular tissues into the intestinal lumen, resulting in diarrhea.
- Gastrointestinal (GI) inflammation
  - Inflammation of the GI tract or the peritoneum (peritonitis) can exacerbate all of the above mechanisms of diarrhea. Increasing intestinal permeability or increasing hydrostatic pressure within the intestinal wall can increase fluid loss into the lumen. In addition, prostaglandin production stimulates fluid secretion into the lumen. Infiltration of the intestinal wall by inflammatory cells can also disrupt intestinal motility, increase intestinal secretion, and decrease absorptive function.

Diarrhea often results in fluid and electrolyte losses for the patient. As long as the ruminant neonate can compensate for losses, it will remain hemodynamically stable, and continue to nurse. However, if losses exceed intake, systemic effects will be observed on clinical examination. Fluid loss from the vascular compartment leads to hypovolemia (dehydration), hypotension, and shock. Metabolic acidosis develops as a result of intestinal and fecal loss of sodium bicarbonate, increased L-lactate from hypoperfused tissues, and increased absorption of L-lactate and D-lactate produced by bacterial fermentation in the intestinal tract.[1] As dehydration and acidosis worsen, clinical signs progress, leading to weakness, loss of suckle reflex, and recumbency. Vascular collapse and electrolyte imbalances can lead to heart failure, whereas death can also result from malnutrition and hypoglycemia in neonates. In addition, endotoxemia from gram-negative bacterial infection, such as *Salmonella* or *E coli*, can directly cause circulatory failure.

PATIENT HISTORY

Patient history should include information regarding the age and use of the animal (eg, dairy, beef, show animal), history of colostrum ingestion, duration and progression of diarrhea, age, and number of animals affected or dead in the herd. Assessment of housing, management, feeding, sanitation practices, and preventive health measures is also important. On-farm standard operating procedures regarding treatment protocols are important to obtain and review, especially when approaching outbreaks of diarrhea. It is also important to ascertain whether there have been any recent dietary or husbandry changes (weaning), transportation, on-farm treatments, or addition of new animals.

PHYSICAL EXAMINATION

In clinic settings, ruminant patients should be examined in an area that can be isolated from other patients according to infectious disease control protocols. In farm settings, care should be taken to minimize cross-contamination between animals and particularly minimizing exposure to younger animals. In either scenario, the facility should be cleaned and disinfected following the examination. The examiner should wear personal protective equipment (eg, gloves, boots that can be disinfected, and coveralls) that are cleaned or discarded after handling the patient.

Although it is necessary to perform a complete physical examination in ruminant patients with enteritis, this article focuses on the techniques that are specific for organ examination in ruminants with enteritis. These techniques include the following:

- Assessment of hydration status: tacky or dry mucous membranes, decreased skin turgor, and eyeball recession (sunken eyes) indicate dehydration. Parameters for assessing dehydration in neonates are presented in **Table 1**.[2] Also, a previous issue (March 2009) covers this topic as well.[3] **Fig. 1** shows a calf with eyeball recession caused by dehydration.
- Signs of endotoxemia or septicemia: assess mucous membranes for color and capillary refill time. Assess the sclera for injected, dilated blood vessels. Septicemic calves may show evidence of hypopyon (**Fig. 2**) in the anterior chamber of the eyes, swollen joints, omphalophlebitis, or meningitis on physical examination. Evidence of sepsis negatively affects prognosis.
- Posture: the posture of the patient may indicate evidence of abdominal pain; for instance, abdominal distension, arching of the back (kyphosis), treading of the hind feet, and lying down with hind legs outstretched. In cases of overt abdominal pain, the possibility of surgical conditions should be investigated and ruled out. In primary cases of neonatal enteritis that do not show evidence of septicemia or endotoxemia, the attitude and posture of the animal can provide evidence of dehydration and metabolic acidosis. Recumbent animals with greater mentation deficits in general have more severe metabolic acidosis.

Table 1								
Estimation of dehydration in calves with diarrhea by eyeball recession, skin tent, and increase in total protein								
	Dehydration (% Body Weight)							
Factor	0	2	4	6	8	10	12	14
Eyeball Recession (mm)	0	1	2	3	4	6	7	8
Neck Skin Tent (s)	2	3	4	5	6	7	8	9
Increase in TP (g/dL)	0	0.2	0.5	0.7	1.0	1.2	1.4	1.7

Abbreviation: TP, total protein.

Adapted from Constable PD, Walker PG, Morin DE, et al. Clinical and laboratory assessment of hydration status of neonatal calves with diarrhea. J Am Vet Med Assoc 1998;212(7):991-6; with permission.

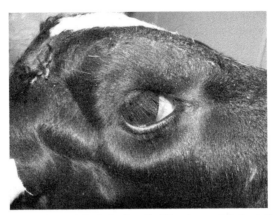

Fig. 1. Eyeball recession in a dehydrated calf. (*Courtesy of* Robert Callan, DVM, PhD, Colorado State University, Fort Collins, CO)

- Rectal temperature: body temperature may be either pyrexic, normal, or hypothermic in neonates with enteritis. Hypothermia generally indicates that the patient's body is decompensating. It may also be an indication of hypoglycemia. The presence of hypothermia is often a poor prognostic indicator.
- Body condition: poor body condition may indicate chronicity or malnutrition, which could be a compounding factor and worthy of further herd investigation with the client.
- Oral examination: examination for oral ulceration and hypersalivation (ptyalism) is important because some viral causes of enteritis can also cause oral lesions. The presence of a suckle reflex is important and helps to determine the most appropriate fluid therapy strategy. The presence of a suckle reflex makes oral nutritional support much easier and allows a more cost-effective treatment plan.
- Abdominal palpation, auscultation, percussion and succussion: abdominal palpation may help identify evidence of pain or allow palpation of abdominal viscera. Simultaneous auscultation and percussion (pinging) on the left and right abdominal walls aids in identification of viscera filled with fluid and air under

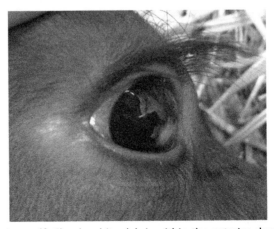

Fig. 2. Hypopyon in a calf. Cloudy white debris within the anterior chamber is consistent with hypopyon in this septic calf.

pressure. Intestinal structures that may ping in a neonate include the abomasum, small intestine, and cecum. Succussion of the abdomen is used to evaluate for the presence of excessive fluid in abdominal viscera, including the abomasum, small intestine, cecum, and rumen. The presence of sloshing fluid sounds in the abdomen (succussion splash) is an indication of fluid distension of the viscera caused by decreased intestinal motility and fluid accumulation.

- Characteristics of the diarrhea: patients should be evaluated for color, odor and volume of feces, presence of tenesmus, blood, and mucus.

DIFFERENTIAL DIAGNOSES

- Important differential diagnoses for infectious enteritis can be broadly classified into bacterial, viral, and protozoal. There is a strong correlation between age and the observation of particular pathogens. Common differential diagnoses associated with age in calves and small ruminants are shown in **Table 2**.
- For an in-depth discussion of clostridial enteritis, please see Simpson KM and colleagues' article, "Clostridial Abomasitis and Enteritis in Ruminants," in this issue; nematodiasis can be seen in Craig TM article, "Gastrointestinal Nematodes, Diagnosis and Control," in this issue; coccidiosis can be seen in Keeton STN and Navarre CB's article, "Coccidiosis in Large and Small Ruminants," in this issue; and herd assessment and control of *Salmonella* can be seen in Holschbach CL and Peek SF's article, "Salmonella in Dairy Cattle," in this issue. This article provides an overview of the salient features of the various infectious enteritis diseases in ruminant neonates (less than 6 months of age).

BACTERIAL ENTERITIS
Escherichia coli

Enterotoxigenic Escherichia coli

- Fimbria (pili) confer the ability of ETEC to attach to immature enterocytes. Fimbria antigens identified in pathogens causing disease in livestock include F4 (K88), F5 (K99), F6 (987P), F41, F42, F165, F17, and F18.

Table 2		
Timeline for calf diarrhea agents		
Agent	**Typical Age at Infection**	**Small Ruminants**
E coli (ETEC, K99)	0–7 d	—
E coli (EHEC)	2 d–4 wk	—
Rotavirus	5–14 d	Up to 16 wk; may differ depending on serogroup
Coronavirus	5 d–1 mo	—
Cryptosporidium	1–4 wk	1–4 wk
Clostridium perfringens	Varies with type	Varies with type
Salmonella	5–14 d, anytime	1–7 d, anytime
Giardia	2 wk–2 mo	—
BVDV	First month of life, anytime	—
Nematodiasis	After 3 wk of life	After 3 wk
Coccidia (*Eimeria*)	After 1 mo of life, weaning	2 wk–5 mo, weaning

Abbreviations: BVDV, bovine viral diarrhea virus; EHEC, enterohemorrhagic *E coli*; ETEC, enterotoxigenic *E coli*.

- Enterotoxins produced by ETEC stimulate increased secretion by intestinal crypt cells, causing a severe secretory diarrhea.
- Expression of the enterocyte surface proteins that allow for ETEC pili attachment decreases with age. Thus, affected ruminants are usually less than 7 days of age and often less than 4 days of age.
- Necropsy findings include fluid-filled intestines with a lack of mucosal damage or hemorrhage.
- Diagnosis is through fecal culture followed by immunoassay for the fimbria antigen or polymerase chain reaction (PCR) to detect the specific fimbria virulence factor gene.
- PCR can also be used to identify the specific toxin virulence factor genes.

Attaching and effacing /Shiga toxin–producing, enterohemorrhagic Escherichia coli

- Belong to the "O" labeled serogroups.
- Cause cytotoxic damage to the intestinal mucosa, producing a mucohemorrhagic colitis. Calves experience diarrhea, dysentery, and abdominal pain.
- Clinical signs generally occur in calves 2 days to 4 weeks of age; however adult cattle may have subclinical disease and serve as a source of infection.
- Common necropsy findings include mucosal damage, mucosal petechiation, and GI hemorrhage.
- Diagnosis is through fecal culture followed by PCR for bacterial virulence-associated genes.

Salmonella

- There are many subtypes of Salmonella species. Cattle disease is mainly caused by serogroups B, C, D, and E.
- Infection can result in a wide range of clinical disease, from subclinical shedders to acute bacteremia, endotoxemia, and death.
- The most common clinical signs in young ruminants are fever, diarrhea, anorexia, depression, and dehydration. Affected animals frequently show signs of endotoxemia or sepsis. Infection results in severe inflammation of the mucosa. Rapid emaciation occurs in clinically affected animals because of cachexia stimulated by systemic inflammation coupled with malabsorption and protein loss from the inflamed gut.
- Septic calves require more intensive treatment, including systemic antibiotics.
- Diagnosis is based on fecal culture with increased sensitivity achieved by using an enrichment broth, followed by PCR.
- Necropsy findings usually include fibrinous to fibrinonecrotic enteritis, and there may be signs of bacterial embolization to other organs such as the kidneys.
- Some Salmonella serotypes are zoonotic (eg, Salmonella Typhimurium, Salmonella Newport).[4] Salmonella Dublin is host adapted in cattle, meaning that a nonclinical carrier status can exist in infected cattle.[3]
- For further details, please refer to Holschbach CL and Peek SF's article, "Salmonella in Dairy Cattle," in this issue.

Clostridium perfringens

- Clostridia species are present in the soil and can be cultured from the intestinal tract of normal livestock. Clostridium perfringens proliferates quickly postmortem, making definitive diagnosis difficult. Diagnosis is usually based on history, rapidly progressing clinical signs, necropsy findings, culture results, and the presence of toxins. C perfringens types A, B, C, D, and E can cause abomasitis or enteritis in young ruminants. **Table 3** lists common diseases caused by each type and the specific toxins produced. The different types produce different toxin profiles, and the actions of these various toxins largely dictate the clinical signs observed.

- *C perfringens* type A causes hemorrhagic abomasitis and enteritis in calves.
- Clinical signs include pasty feces, which may progress to hemorrhagic diarrhea, accompanied by a painful distended abomasum. Clinical signs progress quickly and calves can be found dead without previously observed clinical signs.
- The alpha toxin is a phospholipase that causes endothelial damage, resulting in hemorrhagic and necrotic intestinal lesions. Normal abomasal pH and GI motility reduce the likelihood of clostridial overgrowth. Bacterial proliferation and toxin production are usually associated with decreased abomasal motility and increased abomasal pH.
- *C perfringens* types B and C both cause severe necrotic enterocolitis and enterotoxemia in lambs, kids, calves, piglets, and foals. The disease is characterized by diarrhea that swiftly becomes hemorrhagic and contains sloughed GI mucosa. Systemic signs progress rapidly from weakness, dehydration, and depression to toxemia and death. Progression may be so swift that overt signs of diarrhea may not be observed. Types B and C produce beta toxin, which is highly pathogenic but readily inactivated by proteolytic enzymes present in the intestinal tract, such as trypsin. Neonates are predisposed because of the presence of trypsin inhibitors in colostrum. The disease is generally seen in neonatal ruminants most commonly less than 10 days of age but can occur up to 1 month of age if trypsin inhibitors are still present in the diet. Diagnosis should be suspected based on rapidity and severity of disease, necropsy findings that include severe mucosal ulceration of the small intestine and colon, and identification of the bacteria in intestinal contents. Beta toxin assays are not generally available from diagnostic laboratories in the United States.
- *C perfringens* type D is associated with overeating disease and is most commonly seen in fast-growing lambs and kids. Bottle-raised animals and animals consuming large amounts of readily fermentable carbohydrates are most susceptible. The epsilon toxin may cause local intestinal necrosis but is also absorbed and results in systemic disease related to disruption of endothelial cells in affected organs.
- Please refer to Simpson KM and colleagues', "Clostridial Abomasitis and Enteritis in Ruminants," in this issue.

Table 3
Diseases caused by *Clostridium perfringens*

C perfringens Type	Toxin Produced	Disease
A	Alpha	• Hemorrhagic enteritis of cattle • Abomasal tympany and ulcers in neonatal calves • Gas gangrene • Yellow lamb disease
B	Alpha, beta, epsilon	• Lamb dysentery • Enterotoxemia (overeating disease) of foals
C	Alpha, beta	• Necrotic hemorrhagic enterotoxemia of calves, lambs, kids, foals, and piglets
D	Alpha, epsilon	• Enterotoxemia of sheep, goats, and cattle
E	Alpha, iota	• Abomasal tympany and ulcers in calves • Enteritis in rabbits

VIRAL ENTERITIS
Rotavirus

- Rotavirus is a common cause of diarrhea in neonatal calves and is often involved in coinfections with other diarrheal pathogens.
- The virus invades small intestine villous epithelial cells, and replicates in the cytoplasm. Infection is usually self-limiting because enterocytes undergo cytolysis faster than they can be replaced by the host. This infection causes intestinal villi to become blunted as villous epithelial cells are replaced by squamous/cuboidal epithelial cells. Small intestinal villus atrophy results in maldigestion and malabsorption.
- Rotavirus also elaborates an enterotoxin, NSP4, which causes calcium influx into the cell resulting in a secretory component to the diarrhea. Damaged epithelial cells also release vasoactive components, increasing permeability and fluid loss. As villous epithelium is lost, hyperplasia of crypt cells with increased secretory capacity also exacerbates the secretory component of diarrhea in these animals.
- Clinical signs are usually seen 1 to 3 days after infection, and can last for 5 to 9 days.
- Adult cows may shed the virus at the time of parturition, facilitating transmission to calves.
- Rotaviral enteritis can be diagnosed by submitting fecal samples for immunofluorescence, electron microscopic examination, or PCR. Other immunoassays exist but may not be readily available for clinical diagnostics. Feces collected early in the disease, during the first 24 to 48 hours, generally have a higher diagnostic value, because signs of diarrhea frequently continue after fecal shedding of viral particles has ceased.

Coronavirus

- Infection by coronavirus can occur via the oral or respiratory route. Corona virus causes 3 clinical syndromes: calf diarrhea, winter dysentery in adult ruminants, and respiratory disease.
- Viral infection begins in the small intestine but can spread to the colon. Viral S protein facilitates attachment and fusion with host cells. Mature villous epithelial cells are the primary target; however, crypt cells can also be affected. The virus replicates within the enterocytes and causes cell lysis. Disease caused by coronavirus is generally more severe than rotaviral enteritis and the disease manifests as a mucohemorrhagic enterocolitis, with clinical signs persisting longer than rotavirus because of crypt cell involvement. As with rotavirus, the loss of villous epithelial cells causes a maldigestive and malabsorptive diarrhea with secondary secretory component from crypt cell proliferation. The maldigestion results in accumulation of undigested lactose causing an osmotic diarrhea.
- Coronavirus can be transmitted to calves by carrier cows with virus shedding increased at parturition and during winter months.
- Diagnosis of coronavirus is through PCR of feces, electron microscopic examination of feces, virus isolation, or immunoassays.

BOVINE VIRAL DIARRHEA

- Diarrhea caused by peracute bovine viral diarrhea virus (BVDV) infection can occur in immunocompetent, non–persistently infected calves.[4]
- Morbidity rates of peracute bovine viral diarrhea (BVD) may reach up to 40% with mortalities reported at 20%.[4]

- Clinical signs associated with peracute BVD include severe diarrhea, pyrexia, thrombocytopenia, hemorrhagic disease, and death.
- Persistently infected calves may have severe enteritis as part of mucosal disease syndrome or may be more susceptible to diarrhea caused by other diarrheal agents because of their immunocompromised status.

Other Viruses

- Other zoonotic viruses that may be associated with diarrhea in calves are Noro-virus (bovine Norovirus) and Torovirus (bovine Torovirus [BToV])
- Norovirus is a major cause of acute gastroenteritis in humans; however, the virus isolated from cattle is phylogenetically distinct from human viruses, which may indicate that it has a low zoonotic potential. Experimental infections in newborn calves showed that the virus infects small intestinal epithelial cells causing villous blunting.[5] Norovirus has also been detected in the feces of clinically healthy calves.
- Toroviruses cause acute enteric infection in piglets and children, and BToV has been found in feces of diarrheic calves.[6] It causes a mild to moderate diarrhea in calves less than 3 weeks of age. The virus causes damage to villous and cryptic enterocytes in the upper small intestine. The virus isolated from cattle has antigenic cross reactivity with human toroviruses.
- Many other viruses have been associated with enteric disease in small ruminants, including adenoviruses, astroviruses, bunyaviruses, and paramyxoviruses.[7] However, the relevance of these viruses to clinical practice in North America is unknown.

PARASITIC GASTROENTERITIS
Protozoa

Cryptosporidium

- There are currently 13 species of *Cryptosporidium* with varying degrees of host specificity. Multiple genotypes of *Cryptosporidium parvum* have been identified and can cause enteritis in sheep, goats, and humans.[8] Although it can infect all ages of ruminants, clinical signs are typically seen in preweaning animals. *Cryptosporidium hominis* infects humans, and *Cryptosporidium andersoni* has been found in the abomasum of cattle but its clinical significance is unknown.
- Infection occurs via ingestion of an encysted sporulated oocyst. The parasite invades intestinal epithelium but remains extracytoplasmic, residing in the cell membrane cleft.
- Epithelial destruction causes mild to moderate villous atrophy, resulting in a malabsorptive diarrhea.
- Small infective doses can result in prolonged infection and high parasite burdens because of the phenomenon known as autoinfection, in which the parasite replicates within the host and is directly reinfective without exiting the body.
- The organism is extremely hardy in the environment and is resistant to most chemical disinfectants, including bleach and alcohol. Ammonia-based or peroxide-based products are effective. Care should be taken to avoid contamination of watersheds, which can result in significant environmental and public health issues.
- Diagnosis is through fecal smear or sugar floatation; however, the parasite is very small and may be missed by less experienced technicians. Acid-fast staining of samples increases sensitivity. In areas where acid-fast stain may not be readily

available, there is also a technique for using more typical Ziehl-Neelsen stain to identify *Cryptosporidium* oocysts.[9]

- On-farm control of cryptosporidiosis is difficult because of the extremely high levels of oocytes shed and the environmental hardiness of oocytes resulting in a high environmental burden. The infective dose is small because of the replication and autoinfection that take place within the host.
- Several drugs have been tested and found to have limited activity against *Cryptosporidium*, including paromomycin,[10] decoquinate,[11] and halofuginone. Of these, halofuginone is considered the most promising but is not available or labeled in all countries and has limited efficacy in cases of multipathogen diarrhea complex.[12]

Giardia

- *Giardia duodenalis* (also called *Giardia lamblia*, *Giardia intestinalis*) is classified into different assemblages based on genotypes. Assemblages A and B are zoonotic, and assemblage E is livestock associated.
- All 3 assemblages have been reported in cattle.[8]
- Young calves are most often affected within the first 2 months of life, and infection is often asymptomatic or subclinical. However, giardia infection can cause acute or chronic diarrhea, reduced weight gain, and general ill thrift in young calves. *Giardia* is commonly found in coinfections with coccidia or *Cryptosporidium*.
  - Infection occurs via ingestion of cysts from the environment. After ingestion, each cyst releases 2 trophozoites in the upper small intestine. The trophozoites can either attach to epithelial cells via their ventral disk or live freely in the intestinal lumen. Trophozoites multiply in the lumen by binary fission.
  - Exposure to bile salts causes encystation.
  - Excreted cysts are immediately infective (entire cycle in humans, 72 hours).
  - The prepatent period in ruminants ranges from 3 to 10 days.
- Diagnosis is through fecal smear or floatation; however, fecal examination for *Giardia* requires relevant expertise. Diagnosis can also be achieved by antigen detection in feces via indirect fluorescent antibody test, enzyme-linked immunosorbent assay, or SNAP test, or by PCR. In areas where diagnostic laboratories are difficult to access, staining fecal smears with a Romanowsky stain can aid in identifying organisms.[13]

Coccidiosis

- Coccidia are fairly host specific, and most do not cause clinically relevant disease. Ruminants are affected by species of the genus *Eimeria*. At least 13 *Eimeria* species infect cattle, 16 infect sheep, and 15 have been reported in goats. Only a few *Eimeria* species are pathogenic and cause significant disease. In cattle, life-threatening disease is most commonly caused by *Eimeria bovis* and *Eimeria zuernii*.[14]
- Infected animals shed unsporulated oocysts, which sporulate in the environment to become infective. Oocysts are resistant to environmental changes and persist, especially in cool, moist environments. Once ingested, the oocysts are degraded to allow excystation to occur. Schizonts and gamonts replicate within cells of the lower ileum, cecum, and large intestine, rupturing the host cells.
- The life cycle length differs depending on species, but in general the prepatent period ranges from 15 to 20 days.

- Disease is usually seen in older calves, kids, and lambs, and is usually associated with a stressor such as weaning.
- Typical clinical signs are diarrhea with tenesmus. Mucus and blood may be observed in the feces. In some cases, severe bloody diarrhea is a significant cause of blood loss. Neurologic signs (nervous coccidiosis) are also possible and are associated with toxin production by the coccidia in the GI tract.
- Animals raised in contaminated environments can experience chronic reinfections.
- Chronic subclinical infections can present as ill thrift and poorly growing juvenile animals that are susceptible to other diseases. These animals may also show anemia and hypoproteinemia.
- Diagnosis is through fecal floatation, McMaster, or modified Stoll techniques.

For detailed information, please refer to Keeton STN and Navarre CB's article, "Coccidiosis in Large and Small Ruminants," in this issue.

NONINFECTIOUS DIFFERENTIAL DIAGNOSES FOR ENTERITIS

Differential diagnoses of noninfectious causes of diarrhea in neonatal and juvenile ruminants include the following:

- Improper mixing of milk replacer
- Improper handling of milk or milk replacer
- Grain overload (lactic acidosis)

DIAGNOSTICS

Laboratory diagnostic tests are important for guiding therapy, but they are poor predictors of prognosis in calves with diarrhea.[15] Physical examination findings are more sensitive predictors of outcome and should be the primary consideration when making clinical decisions.[15]

Packed Cell Volume and Serum Total Protein

- Packed cell volume (PCV) and serum total protein (STP) aid in the assessment of the level of anemia and hypoproteinemia, respectively. PCV and STP can be determined using a hematocrit centrifuge and refractometer.
- Assessment of these parameters is useful in guiding the initiation and continuation of fluid therapy. Increased PCV and STP levels generally indicate dehydration at the time of initial presentation. However, PCV and STP levels decrease in severely dehydrated neonates treated with large volumes of intravenous fluids and can be detrimental to the survival of the patient if not monitored so that fluid therapy can be adjusted appropriately.
- Low STP level is associated with protein loss via the GI tract or failure of passive transfer of immunity in neonatal animals. In cases of infectious enteritis, low hematocrit can be caused by blood loss from the GI tract or anemia of chronic disease. In cases of blood loss from the GI tract, both hematocrit and STP are decreased simultaneously. Coccidiosis is a frequent cause of whole-blood loss via the GI tract. Diarrheal diseases also causing blood loss in neonates include salmonellosis, enterohemorrhagic *E coli*, and clostridial enteritis.

Blood Gas Analysis

- Blood gas analysis provides an assessment of blood pH and acid/base status. Metabolic acidosis is common in neonatal and juvenile ruminants with enteritis.

Debilitated animals who are not ventilating adequately because of weakness may also have evidence of respiratory acidosis. Portable point-of-care blood analyzers (i-STAT, epoc) are available for use in ruminants and can perform blood gas analysis.

- These blood analyzers frequently include major electrolytes in their analysis, allowing assessment of potassium, sodium, and chloride status. In acidotic patients, it is important to consider the extracellular shift of potassium when assessing blood potassium levels. Hyperkalemia may be observed in patients with metabolic acidosis, increasing the risk of cardiac arrhythmias and potential cardiac arrest. Hyperkalemia generally resolves on initiation of appropriate fluid therapy.
- Blood lactate levels can be helpful in assessing systemic perfusion. Severely dehydrated calves can have markedly increased blood L-lactate levels. Note that most lactate analyzers only report L-lactate and not D-lactate. D-Lactate is produced by microbial flora in the colon and is exacerbated in conditions resulting in maldigestion and malabsorption. D-Lactate is an important cause of metabolic acidosis in calves with enteritis and contributes to the weakness and decreased mentation often observed in these patients.[16]

Complete Blood Count and Serum Biochemical Analysis

- A complete blood count provides information to appropriately classify the anemia present (smear evaluation) and assess inflammation (leukocytes with differential counts, and fibrinogen).
- Leukopenia characterized by neutropenia with a left shift, and the presence of cellular toxic changes are evidence of systemic sepsis and might be the result of systemic endotoxemia, bacteremia, or salmonellosis.
- Leukopenia and thrombocytopenia may be observed with acute BVDV type II infection. Marked leukopenia may also be observed with BVDV mucosal disease.
- Serum biochemical analysis assesses concentrations of albumin and globulin, identifies electrolyte derangements, and provides evidence of organ dysfunction secondary to the infectious agent.
- Portable serum biochemical analyzers may be useful in identifying electrolyte imbalances but may not be equipped to assess albumin, globulin, and organ enzyme activities.

TREATMENT
Principles of Treatment of Infectious Enteritis in Neonatal Ruminants

Infectious enteritis causes diarrhea and associated fluid and electrolyte losses. Thus, fluid therapy is an important part of management of infectious enteritis. Oral fluid therapy, if instituted early in the disease process, can be highly successful and cost-effective in treating animals with enteritis and diarrhea. Oral electrolyte solutions should be evaluated for their sodium composition, pH buffering capacity, energy content, and osmolarity.[3] Guidelines for electrolyte replacers are provided in **Table 4**.

In animals with severely compromised intestinal motility, intravenous fluid therapy can be more effective at correcting the electrolyte imbalances and fluid loss than oral administration. Physical examination findings and diagnostic results should be used to guide treatment decisions, and some published algorithms exist to help clinicians in the decision process.[17] Blood and protein loss should also be considered and treated accordingly. Please refer to the March, 2009 issue for an in-depth discussion of fluid therapy in calves.

Table 4
Recommendations for electrolyte, carbohydrate, buffering capacity, and osmolality of oral electrolyte replacement fluids used to treat enteritis and diarrhea in neonatal ruminants

Component	Recommendation
Na^+ concentration	90–130 mEq/L
K^+ concentration	10–30 mEq/L
Cl^- concentration	40–80 mEq/L
Glucose + glycine concentration	100–280 mM/L
Buffering capacity (SID = $[Na^+] + [K^+] - [Cl^-]$)	50–80 mEq/L
[Glucose + glycine]/[Na] ratio	1:1–3:1
Total osmolality	400–600

Abbreviation: SID, strong ion difference, measured.

Intravenous Crystalloid Fluids

- These include 1.3% sodium bicarbonate, 0.9% sodium chloride, and balanced electrolyte solutions such as lactated Ringer or Plasma-Lyte.
- The choice of the crystalloids may depend on the test results of a serum biochemical analysis.
- When serum biochemical analysis test results are not available, a balanced electrolyte solution such as lactated Ringer or Plasma-Lyte should be considered for intravenous fluids.
- Both the level of dehydration at presentation and ongoing fluid losses caused by diarrhea must be considered when calculating fluid administration rates. Administration rates greater than maintenance are often necessary to treat hypovolemic shock caused by dehydration and account for continued losses from diarrhea. The patient's STP status must also be considered. Intravenous fluids should be administered with caution in patients with albumin levels less than 2 g/dL.
- Initial treatment of shock with intravenous fluid replacement may be indicated in severely compromised patients. A typical shock fluid therapy plan is to provide 90 mL/kg of intravenous fluids at a maximum rate of 40 to 50 mL/kg/h.[18] Slower rates should be used for small ruminants and in animals with low total protein levels. Signs of appropriate response include improved mentation and activity, decreased skin tent or eyeball recession, improved suckle response, decreased capillary refill time, and improved peripheral perfusion noted by warming of distal extremities. Signs of fluid overload include wet cough, harsh lung sounds, increased respiratory rate, and edema.
- General maintenance fluid rates for juvenile ruminants range from 4 to 6 mL/kg/h (100–150 mL/kg/d). Additional fluid losses from diarrhea may increase fluid needs by 50% to 100%. Thus, total fluid rates in ruminants with active diarrhea are in the range of 1.5 to 2 times maintenance. Any oral fluid administration also contributes to the daily fluid requirement and should be taken into account when calculating fluid volume to correct dehydration and when calculating maintenance requirements.
- Most neonates with enteritis have decreased nutritional intake and absorption. They benefit from additional intravenous dextrose supplementation. Dextrose may safely be added to intravenous fluids at a concentration of 2.5% to 5% when administered at a maintenance fluid rate. This concentration should be decreased proportionally when increasing fluid rate to more than

maintenance, or if blood glucose measurements are greater than the normal range (6.5 ± 1.2 mmol/L, 117 ± 21.6 mg/dL).[19,20] Note that neonatal ruminants are effectively monogastrics and normally have higher blood glucose levels than adults, so adult reference ranges should not be applied to them. A reasonable goal for blood glucose management in calves is to keep blood glucose within 80 to 120 mg/dL.

- Correction of hyperkalemia can be accomplished by administering small volumes of hypertonic (8.4%) sodium bicarbonate, followed by oral electrolytes.[21] Hypertonic sodium bicarbonate can safely be administered at a rate of 6.4 mL/kg body weight (equivalent to 6.4 mEq HCO_3^-/kg body weight) as a bolus over 5 minutes in calves with diarrhea and evidence of metabolic acidosis.
- A recent issue (March, 2009) covered fluid therapy in calves extensively.

Colloids

- Plasma transfusion should be considered in ruminants with severe hypoproteinemia (albumin levels <1.5 g/dL) on serum biochemical analysis.
- Dosage rates for plasma administration range from 10 to 20 mL/kg.[22]
- Blood transfusion (particularly in coccidiosis) should be considered when PCV is less than 12%[22] with associated clinical signs of compromise, including tachycardia, tachypnea, weakness, and poor appetite.
- Following plasma or blood transfusion administration, fluid therapy may be continued with crystalloid fluids.

Antimicrobial and Nonsteroidal Antiinflammatory Therapy

- Enteritis can predispose neonates to bacteremia and secondary infections because of compromised gut barrier and bacterial translocation.
- Broad-spectrum antibiotics, with special attention to adequate gram-negative coverage, should be instituted in patients showing signs of endotoxemia or sepsis. Although the choice of antibiotics should be based on susceptibility of the isolate cultured, broad-spectrum antibiotics may be initiated while awaiting these results. Susceptibility of *Salmonella* to tetracyclines, ampicillin, and amoxicillin is variable, whereas resistance to penicillin, erythromycin, and tylosin is highly likely.[23] Florfenicol should be considered for treatment of salmonellosis.[23] Use of aminoglycosides should be avoided because of prolonged tissue residues in animals intended for food. Cephalosporins and fluoroquinolones may not be used in an extralabel manner in the United States. Tetracyclines should be avoided in dehydrated neonates until fluid hydration and renal perfusion are restored to minimize the risk of nephrotoxicity.
- Use of nonsteroidal antiinflammatory drugs (NSAIDs; eg, flunixin meglumine) may be considered to control pyrexia and inflammation. Flunixin meglumine (1.1 mg/kg intravenously) or meloxicam (0.5 mg/kg intravenously or subcutaneously) were reported to improve outcome in calves with nonspecific diarrhea.[24,25] The use of NSAIDs should be restricted in dehydrated ruminants and only administered once the patient has been sufficiently hydrated.
- Metaphylactic use of antimicrobials can only be recommended for outbreaks caused by a specific bacterial pathogen. Prophylactic treatment with antimicrobials has been shown to increase the risk of diarrhea in neonatal calves.[26]

Prevention

- Appropriate colostrum handling and administration are instrumental in preventing neonatal diarrhea in ruminants. Few clinicians dispute a link between inadequate colostrum consumption and an increased risk for diarrhea in neonates. Supplementing calves with colostrum orally past the traditional 24 hours after birth decreases diarrhea and diarrheal treatments in preweaned calves[26,27]

- A minimum of 150 to 200 g of immunoglobulin G (IgG) in colostrum or a colostrum replacer should be fed to calves within the first 24 hours (Chigerwe and colleagues, 2008)[28] to provide adequate transfer of passive immunity. The concentration of IgG in colostrum can be estimated before feeding calves using a hydrometer or a Brix refractometer.
- Evaluation of the passive transfer status of neonates provides valuable risk assessment, husbandry, and epidemiologic information in both individual cases and herd outbreaks. Passive transfer status can be assessed using STP, sodium sulfite precipitation, immunocrit test, or radial immunodiffusion.
- Other factors associated with an increased risk of diarrhea include hygiene of the maternity area and neonate housing, stocking density, and disinfection practices. Attention should be paid to maternal health prepartum as well.
- Vaccination of the dams before parturition with a K99 *E coli*, rotavirus, coronavirus product can reduce the diarrhea associated with that pathogen.[29,30] Vaccination for other diarrheal agents is of varying efficacy.
- In beef operations, a method known as the Sandhills Calving System can be used to prevent calf diarrhea in a herd or to break a herd of a recurring neonatal diarrhea problem.[31] In this method, cows are continually calving on new ground, reducing contamination and reducing mixing of calves of different ages.

SUMMARY

Causes of infectious enteritis in adult ruminants are bacterial, viral, and parasitic. The most consistent clinical sign of infectious enteritis is diarrhea. Specific causes of infectious enteritis in adult ruminants cannot be distinguished easily based on clinical examination alone. Laboratory diagnostic tests are required to differentiate the causes. Most of the causes have herd implications, thus identification of the cause is recommended. Management of infectious enteritis in adult ruminants includes administration of oral electrolyte fluids or intravenous fluids such as crystalloids and colloids, NSAIDs, antibiotics, anthelmintics, and anticoccidiosis treatments.

REFERENCES

1. Lorenz I, Gentile A, Klee W. Investigations of D-lactate metabolism and the clinical signs of D-lactataemia in calves. Vet Rec 2005;156(13):412–5.
2. Constable PD, Walker PG, Morin DE, et al. Clinical and laboratory assessment of hydration status of neonatal calves with diarrhea. J Am Vet Med Assoc 1998; 212(7):991–6.
3. Smith GW. Treatment of calf diarrhea: oral fluid therapy. Vet Clin North Am Food Anim Pract 2009;25(1):55–72, vi.
4. Constable PD, Hinchcliff KW, Done SH. Diseases of the alimentary tract, in veterinary medicine: a textbook of the diseases of cattle, horses, sheep, pigs and goats. St Louis: Elsevier; 2017. p. 436–621.
5. Di Felice E, Mauroy A, Pozzo FD, et al. Bovine noroviruses: a missing component of calf diarrhoea diagnosis. Vet J 2016;207:53–62.
6. Cho YI, Han JI, Wang C, et al. Case-control study of microbiological etiology associated with calf diarrhea. Vet Microbiol 2013;166(3–4):375–85.
7. Martella V, Decaro N, Buonavoglia C. Enteric viral infections in lambs or kids. Vet Microbiol 2015;181(1–2):154–60.

8. Olson ME, O'Handley RM, Ralston BJ, et al. Update on cryptosporidium and giardia infections in cattle. Trends Parasitol 2004;20(4):185–91.

9. Aghamolaie S, Rostami A, Fallahi SH, et al. Evaluation of modified Ziehl-Neelsen, direct fluorescent-antibody and PCR assay for detection of Cryptosporidium spp. in children faecal specimens. J Parasit Dis 2016;40(3):958–63.

10. Grinberg A, Markovics A, Galindez J, et al. Controlling the onset of natural cryptosporidiosis in calves with paromomycin sulphate. Vet Rec 2002;151(20):606–8.

11. Moore DA, Atwill ER, Kirk JH, et al. Prophylactic use of decoquinate for infections with Cryptosporidium parvum in experimentally challenged neonatal calves. J Am Vet Med Assoc 2003;223(6):839–45.

12. Almawly J, Prattley D, French NP, et al. Utility of halofuginone lactate for the prevention of natural cryptosporidiosis of calves, in the presence of co-infection with rotavirus and Salmonella Typhimurium. Vet Parasitol 2013;197(1–2):59–67.

13. Brar APS, Sood NK, Singla LD, et al. Validation of Romanowsky staining as a novel screening test for the detection of faecal cryptosporidial oocysts. J Parasit Dis 2017;41(1):260–2.

14. Jolley WR, Bardsley KD. Ruminant coccidiosis. Vet Clin North Am Food Anim Pract 2006;22(3):613–21.

15. Trefz FM, Lorenz I, Lorch A, et al. Clinical signs, profound acidemia, hypoglycemia, and hypernatremia are predictive of mortality in 1,400 critically ill neonatal calves with diarrhea. PLoS One 2017;12(8):e0182938.

16. Lorenz I. D-Lactic acidosis in calves. Vet J 2009;179(2):197–203.

17. Trefz FM, Lorch A, Feist M, et al. Construction and validation of a decision tree for treating metabolic acidosis in calves with neonatal diarrhea. BMC Vet Res 2012; 8:238.

18. Berchtold J. Treatment of calf diarrhea: intravenous fluid therapy. Vet Clin North Am Food Anim Pract 2009;25(1):73–99, vi.

19. Doornenbal H, Tong AK, Murray NL. Reference values of blood parameters in beef cattle of different ages and stages of lactation. Can J Vet Res 1988;52(1): 99–105.

20. Knowles TG, Edwards JE, Bazeley KJ, et al. Changes in the blood biochemical and haematological profile of neonatal calves with age. Vet Rec 2000;147(21): 593–8.

21. Trefz FM, Constable PD, Lorenz I. Effect of intravenous small-volume hypertonic sodium bicarbonate, sodium chloride, and glucose solutions in decreasing plasma potassium concentration in hyperkalemic neonatal calves with diarrhea. J Vet Intern Med 2017;31(3):907–21.

22. Balcomb C, Foster D. Update on the use of blood and blood products in ruminants. Vet Clin North Am Food Anim Pract 2014;30(2):455–74, vii.

23. Smith BP. Salmonellosis in ruminants. In: Smith BP, editor. Large animal internal medicine 5th Edition. St Louis (MO): Elsevier Mosby; 2015. p. 830–4.

24. Todd CG, Millman ST, McKnight DR, et al. Nonsteroidal anti-inflammatory drug therapy for neonatal calf diarrhea complex: effects on calf performance. J Anim Sci 2010;88(6):2019–28.

25. Barnett SC, Sischo WM, Moore DA, et al. Evaluation of flunixin meglumine as an adjunct treatment for diarrhea in dairy calves. J Am Vet Med Assoc 2003;223(9): 1329–33.

26. Berge AC, Moore DA, Besser TE, et al. Targeting therapy to minimize antimicrobial use in preweaned calves: effects on health, growth, and treatment costs. J Dairy Sci 2009;92(9):4707–14.

27. Berge AC, Besser TE, Moore DA, et al. Evaluation of the effects of oral colostrum supplementation during the first fourteen days on the health and performance of preweaned calves. J Dairy Sci 2009;92(1):286–95.
28. Chigerwe M, Tyler JW, Middleton JR, et al. Comparison of four methods to assess colostral IgG concentration in dairy cows. J Am Vet Med Assoc 2008;233(5): 761–6.
29. Moon HW, Bunn TO. Vaccines for preventing enterotoxigenic *Escherichia coli* infections in farm animals. Vaccine 1993;11(2):213–20.
30. Wilson WD, Pusterla N, Plummer PJ, et al. Use of biologics in the prevention of infectious diseases. In: Smith BP, editor. Large animal internal medicine. St Louis (MO): Elsevier Mosby; 2015. p. 1437–95.
31. Smith DR, Dale M, Groteleuschen DM, et al. Strategies for controlling neonatal diarrhea in cow-calf herds–the Sandhills calving system. AABP Proc 2006;39: 94–8.

Diagnosis and Treatment of Infectious Enteritis in Adult Ruminants

Munashe Chigerwe, BVSc, MPH, PhD*, Meera C. Heller, DVM, PhD

KEYWORDS

- Ruminant • Enteritis • Infection • Adult • Diarrhea • Treatment

KEY POINTS

- Viral, bacterial, and protozoal pathogens are the most significant causes of infectious enteritis in adult ruminants.
- The most common consistent presenting sign in ruminants with infectious enteritis is diarrhea.
- Diagnosis of etiology of enteritis has important zoonotic and herd implications.
- Severity of clinical signs with similar pathogens may differ between large and small ruminants.
- Treatment of enteritis is symptomatic to correct fluid and electrolyte imbalances and, when relevant, pathogen-specific treatment.

INTRODUCTION

Enteritis refers to the inflammation of the intestine. Several bacterial, protozoal, and viral diseases cause infectious enteritis in adult cattle and small ruminants. Diagnosis of specific pathogens is warranted, particularly when herd implications or zoonotic implications are considered. This review summarizes the most important differential diagnoses, diagnosis, and management of infectious enteritis in adult ruminants. Important diagnostic samples, diagnostic tests, supportive therapy, and specific treatments for infectious enteritis are discussed.

PATHOPHYSIOLOGY OF INFECTIOUS ENTERITIS IN ADULT RUMINANTS

The pathophysiology of diarrhea secondary to enteritis in adult ruminants is similar to young ruminants. In adult ruminants, diarrhea is more likely to develop due to

Disclosure Statement: The authors have nothing to disclose.
Department of Veterinary Medicine and Epidemiology, University of California Davis, One Shields Avenue, Davis, CA 95616, USA
* Corresponding author.
E-mail address: mchigerwe@ucdavis.edu

maldigestion and malabsorption secondary to infectious enteritis, whereas osmotic diarrhea is likely to develop secondary to carbohydrate engorgement. Detailed pathophysiologic mechanism of diarrhea in young ruminants please see Meera C. Heller and Munashe Chigerwe's article "Diagnosis and treatment of infectious enteritis in neonatal and juvenile ruminants," in this issue.

PATIENT HISTORY

The most common presenting clinical sign associated with enteritis in ruminants is diarrhea. Patient history should include information regarding the age and use of the animal (eg, dairy, beef, or show), presence of hyporexia or anorexia, duration and progression of diarrhea, number of animals affected or dead in the herd or flock, vaccination history, deworming history, recent dietary or husbandry changes, recent transportation, reproductive status (eg, pregnant), characteristics of the diarrhea (eg, color, odor, and volume of feces and presence of tenesmus, blood, mucus, or gravel), and evidence of abdominal pain (eg, arching of back, treading of hind feet, or lying down).

PHYSICAL EXAMINATION

In clinic settings, ruminant patients should be should be examined in the isolation area according to infectious disease control protocols. In farm settings, a cow may be examined in a sick pen or handling facilities when applicable. In either scenario, the examination room or facility should be cleaned and disinfected after the examination. The examiner should wear personal protective equipment (eg, gloves, boots that can be disinfected, and coveralls).

Although it is necessary to perform a full physical examination in a ruminant patient with enteritis, this review focuses on the specific organ examination for ruminants with enteritis. This includes the following:

- Body condition — enteritis may be associated with weight loss.
- Posture — posture of the patient may indicate evidence of abdominal pain, for instance, abdominal distension, arching of back, treading of hind feet, or lying down.
- Rectal temperature — enteritis is an inflammatory condition, which may cause pyrexia.
- Oral examination — checking for evidence of oral ulceration and hypersalivation (ptyalism). This is important because some viral causes of enteritis also cause oral lesions.
- Assessment of hydration status and mucous membrane color — hydration status and color of mucous membranes (ocular, oral, and or vulva), including capillary refill time should be assessed.
- Abdominal palpation, auscultation, percussion, and succussion — abdominal palpation is practical in adult sheep and goats but unrewarding in adult cattle. Abdominal palpation may help identify evidence of pain or allow palpation of abdominal viscera. Simultaneous auscultation and percussion on the left and right abdominal wall help identify viscera filled with air, including the intestine. Succussion of the abdomen confirms the presence of excessive fluid in abdominal viscera, including the small intestine.
- Rectal examination — rectal examination is practical in cattle but may be delayed in cases of presence of a rectal prolapse (secondary to diarrhea). Rectal examination aids in identifying distended abdominal viscera, including small intestine, rumen, colon, or cecum. If not performed already, characteristics of the diarrhea (eg, color,

odor, and volume of feces and presence of tenesmus, blood, mucus, or gravel) should be evaluated during the rectal examination and by evaluating feces on the rectal sleeve.

DIFFERENTIAL DIAGNOSES

- Important differential diagnoses for infectious enteritis can be broadly classified into bacterial (salmonellosis, paratuberculosis, and *Clostridium perfringens* type A), viral (bovine viral diarrhea [BVD]virus, malignant catarrhal fever, and bovine coronavirus [BCoV]), and parasitic (coccidiosis and nematodiasis).
- Differential diagnoses, species affected, recommended samples, and diagnostic tests to be requested for infectious causes of enteritis in adult ruminants are summarized in **Table 1**.
- An in-depth discussion of paratuberculosis (see Marie-Eve Fecteau's article "Para-tuberculosis in Cattle," in this issue), coccidiosis and nematodiasis (see Sarah

Table 1
Important differential diagnoses, species affected, recommended samples, and diagnostic tests to be requested for infectious causes of enteritis in adult ruminants

Differential Diagnosis	Species Affected	Samples	Tests
Bacterial			
Salmonellosis	Bovine, caprine, ovine	Feces	Culture, PCR
		Blood	Culture
		Intestinal tissues	Culture
Paratuberculosis	Bovine, caprine, ovine	Feces	Culture, PCR
		Serum	ELISA or AGID
		Intestinal tissues	Culture
			Histopathology
		Milk	ELISA or AGID
		Mesenteric lymph node	Culture
			Histopathology
C perfringens	Bovine, caprine, ovine	Feces or intestinal contents	Anaerobic culture
			Genomic-type testing
			Immunohistochemistry
			ELISA—toxin testing for types A, B, C, and D
Viral			
BVD virus	Bovine	EDTA blood, milk, serum, tissue	PCR for acute infections
		Tissue (ear notch)	Antigen capture ELISA, IHC
Malignant catarrhal fever	Bovine	EDTA blood, lung, spleen	PCR
BCoV	Bovine	Feces	PCR
Parasitic			
Coccidiosis	Bovine, caprine, and ovine	Feces	Fecal flotation
Nematodiasis	Bovine, caprine, and ovine	Feces	Fecal flotation

Abbreviations: AGID, agar gel immunodiffusion; IHC, immunohistochemistry; PCR, polymerase chain reaction.

Tammy Nicole Keeton and Christine B. Navarre's article "Coccidiosis in Large and Small Ruminants," in this issue), clostridial enteritis (see Robert Callan's article "Clostridial Abomasitis and Enteritis in Ruminants," in this issue), and herd assessment and control of *Salmonella* are reviewed. This article briefly describes the salient features of the various diseases causing infectious enteritis in adult ruminants.

Bacterial Enteritis

Salmonellosis

- *Salmonella enterica* subsp *enterica* serovars (serotypes) are of clinical importance in adult ruminants. Examples of important serovars include Typhimurium, Dublin, and Newport.[1]
- Transmission is through the fecal-oral route in all ages. Transmission via milk or colostrum is a possible route of infection for neonates.
- Clinical signs associated with salmonellosis in adult ruminants include pyrexia and diarrhea.[2] The diarrheic feces may vary from watery to mucoid and may contain fibrin and blood.[3] Due to the presence of significant concentrations of proteins, the diarrheic feces have a putrid, foul odor.[3]
- Endotoxemia may occur in part due to the damaged intestinal mucosa, leading to pyrexia, depressed attitude, and shock. Bacteremia is also possible secondary to the enteritis. The enteritis causes an acute protein-losing enteropathy.
- Some *Salmonella* serotypes are potentially zoonotic (eg, *Salmonella* Typhimurium and *Salmonella* Newport)[4] whereas *Salmonella* Dublin is host-adapted (serotypes found in the host species and long-term carriers exist) in cattle.[3]

Paratuberculosis

- Paratuberculosis (Johne disease) is a chronic enteric disease of ruminants caused by the bacterium, *Mycobacterium avium* subsp *paratuberculosis*.
- Transmission of the bacterium is through the fecal-oral route in all ages of ruminants. Additionally, transmission through milk orcolostrum or transplacentally is possible in neonates.[5]
- Infection generally occurs at a young age; however, clinical signs are seen only in adult animals due to the long incubation period.
- Clinical signs include watery diarrhea, submandibular edema due to hypoproteinemia, and weight loss in the face of a good appetite.[6] Hypoproteinemia is secondary to chronic protein-losing enteropathy (due to maldigestion and malabsorption).
- Diarrhea is an inconsistent sign in goats and sheep, which may only exhibit chronic weight loss.[6]
- **Fig. 1** depicts a 5-year-old mixed breed bull showing clinical signs of paratuberculosis, including thin body condition and profuse diarrhea.

Clostridium perfringens type A

- Although *Clostridium* infections occur more commonly in young ruminants, *C perfringens* type A has been associated with highly fatal hemolytic hemorrhagic enteritis in adult cattle and sheep and hemolytic enterotoxemia in goats.[7]
- Clinical signs include acute onset of depression, dyspnea, pyrexia, diarrhea, pale or jaundiced mucous membranes, abdominal pain, and hemoglobinuria.
- The disease is often fatal and animals are likely to die within 12 hours after onset of clinical signs.[7]
- *C perfringens* type A has also been associated with jejunal hemorrhagic syndrome in adult dairy cattle.[8]

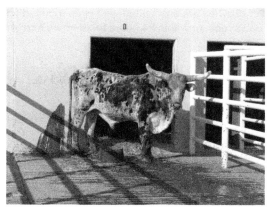

Fig. 1. A 5-year-old mixed breed bull showing clinical signs of paratuberculosis, including thin body condition and profuse diarrhea.

Viral Enteritis

Bovine viral diarrhea

- Peracute diarrhea due BVD virus infection can occur in immunocompetent, non-persistently infected adult ruminants.[7]
- Morbidity rates of peracute BVD may reach up to 40% with mortality rates reported at 20%.[7]
- Clinical signs associated with peracute BVD include severe diarrhea, pyrexia, thrombocytopenia, hemorrhagic disease, agalactia, and death.[7]
- Reproductive disorders associated with peracute disease include decreased conception rates, abortion, stillbirth, congenital defects, and weak calves.[7]

Malignant catarrhal fever

- In North America, sheep-associated malignant catarrhal fever caused by ovine herpes virus type 2 affects cattle and other wild ruminants. Sheep and goats are asymptomatic carriers.[9]
- Wildebeest-associated malignant catarrhal fever, caused by alcelaphine herpes virus type 1, may occur outside Africa in zoologic establishments where domestic or wild ruminants are in contact with wildebeest.
- Transmission from sheep to cattle is presumably through direct or indirect contact, aerosols, and nasal or ocular secretions from infected sheep.[10]
- Clinical signs include diarrhea, oral and nasal erosions, corneal opacity, hyperemic coronary bands with lameness, hematuria, dermatitis, and encephalitis.[11]
- The disease has a low morbidity but high mortality rates.

Winter dysentery

- The etiologic agent of winter dysentery is BCoV.
- Transmission is through fecal-oral route and outbreaks occur more commonly in adult lactating dairy cows in winter.[12] Occurrence of disease in the herd may coincide with a rise in respiratory disease also caused by BCoV.
- Outbreaks are associated with high morbidity (30%–50%) but low mortality (2%).[7]
- Clinical signs associated with BCoV include acute onset of decreased appetite, decreased milk production, diarrhea, and pyrexia.[7]

- Clinical signs of diarrhea are associated with virus-induced enterocolitis.[7]
- A majority of cows recover within 24 hours to 36 hours after the onset of clinical signs.[7]

Parasitic Gastroenteritis

Nematodiasis

- Nematodes in the genera *Haemonchus*, *Trichostrongylus*, *Ostertagia*, *Cooperia*, and *Nematodirus* cause gastroenteritis in ruminants.
- The life cycle of the nematodes is direct and transmission is through ingestion of infective larval stages (third larval stage).
- Although all young ruminants are more susceptible to nematodiasis compared with adult ruminants, adult goats do not build an effective immunity against trichostrongylid-type nematodes and are susceptible throughout their life span.[7]
- Grazing adult goats are more susceptible to ingestion of high larval loads compared with browsing goats.[7]
- Risk factors for occurrence of clinical nematodiasis include ingestion of high larval loads, overcrowding on pasture, wet weather, lush pastures, and low plane of nutrition.[7]
- Clinical signs associated with nematodiasis in adult ruminants include diarrhea, weight loss, decreased production, pale mucous membranes (*Haemonchus* spp), submandibular edema, and death.
- **Fig. 2** depicts a Boer buck showing clinical signs of haemonchosis.

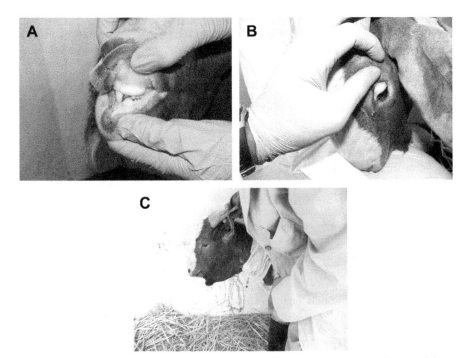

Fig. 2. A Boer buck with haemonchosis. (*A*) Depicts pale oral mucous membranes. (*B*) Depicts pale ocular mucous membranes. (*C*) Depicts submandibular edema. Note the diarrhea stained wall.

Coccidiosis

- Coccidial parasites of the genus *Eimeria* are important in ruminants. The life cycle of coccidia is direct, and infection occurs via ingestion of the infective oocysts.
- Coccidiosis is commonly a disease of young, nonimmune ruminants.
- Other risk factors for clinical coccidiosis other than young age include nutritional status of the animal, high stocking density, other concurrent diseases such as helminthiasis, and environmental or management stressors.
- Coccidiosis is uncommon in adult sheep and cattle because of acquired immunity after infection[13] but an important disease of adult goats.[14]
- Additionally, outbreaks of coccidiosis have been reported in adult beef cattle.[15]
- Clinical signs include inappetence and acute diarrhea, with foul-smelling feces containing blood and mucus.
- Pale mucous membranes might be present depending on the degree of blood loss in the feces.
- In cattle, muscle tremors, hyperesthesia, and seizures are associated with nervous coccidiosis.[16]

NONINFECTIOUS DIFFERENTIAL DIAGNOSES FOR ENTERITIS IN ADULT RUMINANTS

Differential diagnoses of noninfectious causes of diarrhea in adult ruminants include the following:

- Copper deficiency
- Lactic acidosis/grain overload
- Renal amyloidosis
- Liver and cardiac disease
- Ragwort (*Senecio jacobaea*) poisoning
- Arsenic poisoning

DIAGNOSTICS

Table 1 summarizes the specific samples and diagnostic tests for consideration in diagnosing causes of enteritis in adult ruminants. Ancillary diagnostic test may help differentiate causes of infectious enteritis and help with clinical management of ruminants while waiting for other specific test results. The following tests are performed in clinical practice without the need to send samples to a specialty laboratory.

Fecal Flotation

1. Saturated solutions of sodium chloride, sugar (sucrose), or magnesium sulfate are inexpensive and easy to use.
2. To make a saturated float solution, mix 400 g of sodium chloride, or 400 g of magnesium sulfate, with 1 L of warm tap water. For the sucrose solution, mix 454 g of granulated sugar with 355 mL of warm of tap water.[17]
3. The saturated solution of sodium chloride, sugar, or magnesium sulfate is sufficient to float common helminths eggs and coccidia oocysts in ruminants.
4. Mix 1 g of feces with 10 mL to 12 mL of the saturated float solution. Mixing of the fecal sample is easy in cases of diarrhea.
5. Pour the mixture through a strainer or gauze into a 15-mL centrifuge tube. Add the float solution into the centrifuge tube so that the liquid is level with the top of the tube (forms a meniscus).

6. Place a coverslip on top of the tube and centrifuge the tube at 1500 rpm for 5 minutes to 10 minutes. If the centrifuge does not have free-swinging buckets, the coverslip must be placed on the tube after centrifugation (otherwise it falls off during centrifugation). If a centrifuge is not available, the sample in step 5 is allowed to sit with coverslip in place for 30 minutes.
7. Remove the coverslip and place on a glass slide and examine under the microscope at ×100 [magnification] (×10 ocular and ×10 objective).
8. For qualitative assessments of microscopy of the coverslip, using routine slides is sufficient. For quantitative assessments, McMaster chambers are required.
9. Other quantitative method techniques without the use of McMaster chambers have been described as follows: in step 4, mix 2 g of feces with 30 mL of the saturated sugar solution and follow through step 5. Follow step 6 but without placing the coverslip on top of the tube. Collect 0.15 mL of the centrifuged solution (solution making the meniscus), drop it on a routine slide, and place a coverslip. Count all the eggs under the coverslip at ×100, then multiply by 200. This represents the approximate number of eggs per gram in the sample.

Packed Cell Volume and Serum Total Protein

- Determination of packed cell volume (PCV) and serum total protein (STP) assesses the levels of anemia and hypoproteinemia, respectively.
- PCV and STP assessment is determined using a hematocrit centrifuge and refractometer, respectively.
- Heamonchosis is consistently associated with severe anemia whereas salmonellosis, *Clostridium*, and coccidiosis might cause mild anemia due to blood loss in the feces.
- Paratuberculosis may be associated with mild anemia due the chronicity of the disease.
- Paratuberculosis, helminthiasis, and coccidiosis are consistently associated with hypoproteinemia.

Other Ancillary Diagnostics

Complete blood cell count and serum biochemical analysis

- A complete blood cell count further classifies the anemia present (smear evaluation) and assesses inflammation (leukocytes with differential counts and fibrinogen).
- Leukopenia characterized by neutropenia with a left shift and presence of cellular toxic changes might be present in salmonellosis due to endotoxemia and bacteremia.
- Leukopenia and thrombocytopenia might be present with BVD virus infection.
- Serum biochemical analysis assesses concentrations of albumin and globulin and identifies electrolyte derangements and evidence of organ insufficiency secondary to the infectious agent.
- Portable serum biochemical analyzers may be useful in identifying electrolyte imbalances but may not be equipped to assess albumin, globulins, and enzyme activities.

Plasma pepsinogen levels

- Acidic pH in the abomasum is required for conversion of pepsinogen to pepsin.
- When parietal cells (responsible for abomasal acid production) are damaged secondary to abomasal parasites, conversion of pepsinogen to pepsin (active enzyme) is impaired and thus protein digestion is impaired.

- Elevated plasma plasminogen levels are used to aid in diagnosis of ostertagiosis.[7] Plasma pepsinogen levels are also elevated in haemonchosis.
- Plasma pepsinogen level reference ranges differ among laboratories.

TREATMENT
Principles of Treatment of Infectious Enteritis in Adult Ruminants

Infectious enteritis causes diarrhea and associated fluid and electrolyte losses. Thus, fluid therapy is an important part of management of infectious enteritis. Maldigestion and malabsorption are the dominant underlying pathophysiologic mechanisms; hence, intravenous therapy is more effective (at least initially) at correcting the electrolyte imbalances and fluid loss compared with oral administration. Blood and protein loss should also be considered and treated accordingly. The following type of fluids should considered as part of the fluid therapy.

Crystalloids

- Crystalloids include 0.9% sodium chloride, lactated Ringer solution, and other balanced crystalloid fluids, such as Plasma-Lyte.
- The choice of the crystalloids may depend on the test results of serum biochemical analysis.
- When serum biochemical analysis test results are not available, balanced electrolytes, such as Plasma-Lyte (Baxter Healthcare Corporation, Deerfield, IL), should be considered.
- The level of dehydration at presentation and ongoing losses due to diarrhea must be considered when calculating fluid administration rates. Administration rates above maintenance must be considered. The patient's STP status must also be considered; intravenous fluids should be administered with caution in patients with albumin levels less than 2 g/dL.

Colloids

- Plasma transfusion or hetastarch should be considered in ruminants with submandibular edema on clinical examination or those that have severe hypoproteinemia (albumin levels <1.5 g/dL) on serum biochemical analysis.
- Dosage rates for plasma and hetastarch administration range from 15 mL/kg to 20 mL/kg[18] and 10 mL/kg to 20 mL/kg (based on equine doses),[19] respectively.
- Whole-blood transfusion (particularly in haemonchosis) should be considered when PCV is less than 12%.[20]
- After plasma, hetastarch, or blood transfusion administration, fluid therapy may be continued with crystalloids.

Antimicrobial and Nonsteroidal Anti-Inflammatory Therapy

- Diarrhea can predispose ruminants to secondary bacterial infections.
- Prophylactic antibiotic therapy is usually considered. Broad-spectrum antibiotics, including tetracyclines, macrolides (nonlactating ruminants), and florfenicol (nonlactating animals), may be considered. Tetracyclines should be avoided in dehydrated patients if normal hydration and renal perfusion cannot be reestablished within several hours due to the risk of nephrotoxicity.
- Use of nonsteroidal anti-inflammatory drugs (NSAIDs) (eg, flunixin meglumine) may be considered to control pyrexia and inflammation. NSAIDs are contraindicated, however, in dehydrated patients if normal hydration and renal perfusion cannot be reestablished within several hours due to the risk of nephrotoxicity.

SPECIFIC TREATMENTS
Bacterial Pathogens

Salmonellosis

- Use of antibiotics in salmonellosis is controversial due to concerns of their effectiveness and selection of antimicrobial resistance. This concern, however, is based on human studies where invasive salmonella infections are uncommon and antimicrobial therapy is not recommended.[21]
- Successful treatment of bacteremia due to salmonellosis may rely on early administration of appropriate antibiotics, fluid and electrolyte therapy, and NSAID.[3]
- Bacteremia is common in calves with salmonellosis; hence, antibiotics are recommended.[21] Likewise, bacteremia might occur in adult ruminants.
- Although the choice of antibiotics should be based on susceptibility of the isolate cultured and antibiotic sensitivity test, broad-spectrum antibiotics should be considered while awaiting test results. Susceptibility of *Salmonella* to tetracyclines, ampicillin, and amoxicillin is variable whereas resistance to penicillin, erythromycin, and tylosin is highly likely.[3] Florfenicol may be considered for treatment of salmonellosis.[3] Use of aminoglycosides is discouraged because they have prolonged tissue residues in ruminant animals intended for food. Sulfonamides, cephalosporins, and fluoroquinolones have extralabel restrictions in the United States.
- Flunixin meglumine (1.1–2.2 mg/kg intravenously) was reported to improve outcome in calves with nonspecific diarrhea and should be considered in adult ruminants.[22] The use of NSAIDs should be withheld in dehydrated ruminants until the patient is sufficiently hydrated.
- Intravenous fluids, as previously described, are important as part of therapy in adult ruminants with salmonellosis.

Paratuberculosis

- Treatment of paratuberculosis is uncommon in adult ruminants used for production.
- In instances where the animal's genetic or sentimental value is important to the client, treatment may be considered.
- Most chemotherapeutic agents recommended for treatment of paratuberculosis are not labeled for use in ruminants. Thus, animals treated with these chemotherapeutic agents should not be used for milk or meat production or have greatly extended drug withdrawal times to ensure no detectable residues in meat or milk.
- A majority of ruminants with clinical paratuberculosis maintain a good appetite until the terminal stages. Hence, intravenous fluids (crystalloids or colloids) may not be warranted until submandibular edema develops.

Clostridium perfringens type A

- The disease has an acute onset and swift progression of clinical signs.
- For therapy to be effective, it must be instituted immediately. Supportive intravenous fluid therapy and administration of antibiotics to halt the production of *C perfringens* toxins and decrease pathogen numbers in the intestinal tract are the cornerstones of successful treatment.
- In cases of hemorrhagic bowel syndrome, laparotomy with manual massage to break down obstructing blood clots or removal by enterotomy may be necessary to clear intraluminal blood clots and restore intestinal function.

Viral Pathogens

- There is no specific treatment of viral pathogens causing enteritis in adult ruminants.
- Supportive treatment, including intravenous fluids, NSAIDs, and prophylactic antibiotics, should be considered, as indicated previously (principles of treatment of infectious enteritis in adult ruminants).

Parasitic pathogens

Helminths and coccidiosis

- Intravenous fluids (at least twice maintenance) is recommended in parasitic gastroenteritis to correct dehydration and ongoing losses.
- In cases of submandibular edema present, plasma (15–20 mL/kg)[18] or hetastarch (10–20 mL/kg) is recommended.[19]
- When severe anemia is present (PCV <12%), whole-blood transfusion is warranted.
- To control pain associated with the diarrhea, NSAIDs may administered (flunixin meglumine at 1.1–2.2 mg/kg) once the patient is hydrated.
- Administration of antibiotics to treat helminthiasis and coccidiosis may not be necessary but should be considered based on other concurrent diseases or evidence of systemic sepsis.
- Specific anthelmintic and anticoccidiosis therapeutic agents are summarized in **Tables 2** and **3**, respectively.[13,23]
- The choice of the anthelmintic may depend on the withdrawal time for meat and milk, safety of the drug, spectrum of activity, ease of administration, cost, and evidence of anthelmintic resistance.

Table 2
Summary of commonly used anthelmintics for management of helminthiasis in cattle, sheep, and goats

Drug	Species	Dose and Route
Ivermectin	Cattle	0.2 mg/kg SC or po
		0.5 mg/kg topical
	Sheep	0.2 mg/kg SC or po
	Goats	0.2 mg/kg SC or po
		0.5 mg/kg topical
Doramectin	Cattle (beef)	0.2 mg/kg SC or IM
		0.5 mg/kg topical
Moxidectin	Cattle	0.2 mg/kg po or SC
		0.5 mg/kg topical
	Goats	0.2 mg/kg po or SC
		0.5 mg/kg topical
	Sheep	0.2 mg/kg po or SC
Eprinomectin	Cattle	0.5 mg/kg topical
Albendazole	Cattle and goats	10 mg/kg po
	Sheep	7.5 mg/kg po
Fenbendazole	Cattle, goats, and sheep	5 mg/kg po
Levamisole	Cattle and sheep	7.5 mg/kg po
	Goats	12 mg/kg po

Abbreviations: IM, intramuscularly; SC, subcutaneously.
Data from Baynes RE, Payne M, Martin-Jimenez T, et al. Extralable use of ivermectin and moxidectin. J Am Vet Med Assoc 2000;217:668–71.

Table 3
Summary for drugs used to treat coccidiosis in cattle, goats, and sheep

Drug	Species	Dose and Route
Amprolium	Cattle	10 mg/kg po for 5 d
	Goats and sheep	20–40 mg/kg po for 5 d or 65 mg/kg po once
Monensin	Sheep	2 mg/kg po for 20 d
Sulfadimethoxine	Cattle, goats, and sheep	55 mg/kg po on day 1 followed by 27.5 mg/kg on days 2–5
Sulfamethazine	Cattle	(1). 247 mg/kg po on day 1 and 123 mg/kg on days 2–5
		(2). 140 mg/kg for 3 d
		(3). 140 mg/kg once then 70 mg/kg for 5–7 d

Extralabel use of sulfonamides in dairy cattle greater than 20 mo of age is prohibited in the United States.
Data from Ballweber LR. Coccidiosis in food animals. In: Smith BP, editor. Large animal internal medicine. 5th edition. St Louis (MO): Elsevier Mosby; 2015. p. 1516–7.

- A detailed review of helminthiasis can be seen in Thomas M. Craig's article, "Gastrointestinal Nematodes, Diagnosis and Control," in this issue; and coccidiosis is reviewed in detail in Sarah Tammy Nicole Keeton and Christine B. Navarre's article "Coccidiosis in Large and Small Ruminants," in this issue .

SUMMARY

Causes of infectious enteritis in adult ruminants are bacterial, viral, and parasitic. The most consistent clinical sign of infectious enteritis is diarrhea. Specific etiologies causing infectious enteritis in adult ruminants cannot be distinguished easily based on clinical examination alone. Laboratory diagnostic tests are required to differentiate the etiologies. A majority of the etiologies have herd implications; thus, identification of the etiology is recommended. Management of infectious enteritis in adult ruminants includes administration of intravenous fluids, such as crystalloids and colloids; NSAID; antibiotics; anthelmintics; and coccidiostats.

REFERENCES

1. Salmonellosis. The Center For Food Security and Public Health. Institute for International Cooperation in Animal Biologics. Iowa State University. 2005-2013. Available: http://www.cfsph.iastate.edu/Factsheets/pdfs/nontyphoidal_salmonellosis.pdf. Accessed June 23, 2017.
2. Gibson EA. Salmonella infection in cattle. J Dairy Res 1965;32:97–134.
3. Smith BP. Salmonellosis in ruminants. In: Smith BP, editor. Large animal internal medicine. 5th edition. St Louis (MO): Elsevier Mosby; 2015. p. 830–4.
4. Cobbold RN, Rice DH, Davis MA, et al. Long-term persistence of multi-drug-resistant Salmonella enterica serovar Newport in two dairy herds. J Am Vet Med Assoc 2006;288:588–91.
5. Seitz SE, Heider LE, Heuston WD, et al. Bovine fetal infection with mycobacterium paratuberculosis. J Am Vet Med Assoc 1989;194:1423–6.
6. Sweeney RW. Paratuberculosis (Johne's disease). In: Smith BP, editor. Large animal internal medicine. 5th edition. St Louis (MO): Elsevier Mosby; 2015. p. 834–7.

7. Constable PD, Hinchcliff KW, Done SH, et al. Diseases of the alimentary tract. In: Veterinary medicine: a textbook of the diseases of cattle, horses, sheep, pigs, and goats. 11th edition. St Louis (MO): Elsevier; 2017. p. 436–621.

8. Elhanafy MM, French DD, Braun U. Understanding jejunal hemorrhage syndrome. J Am Vet Med Assoc 2013;243:352–8.

9. Metzler AE. The malignant catarrhal fever complex. Comp Immunol Microbiol Infect Dis 1991;14:107–24.

10. Taus NS, Oaks JL, Gailbreath K, et al. Experimental aerosol infection of cattle (Bos taurus) with ovine herpesvirus 2 using nasal secretions from infected sheep. Vet Microbiol 2006;116:29–36.

11. Callan RJ. Malignant catarrhal fever. In: Smith BP, editor. Large animal internal medicine. 5th edition. St Louis (MO): Elsevier Mosby; 2015. p. 759–62.

12. Boileau MJ, Kapil S. Bovine coronavirus associated syndromes. Vet Clin North Am Food Anim Pract 2010;26:123–46.

13. Ballweber LR. Coccidiosis in food animals. In: Smith BP, editor. Large animal internal medicine. 5th edition. St Louis (MO): Elsevier Mosby; 2015. p. 1516–7.

14. Chhabra RC, Pandy VS. Coccidia of goats in Zimbabwe. Vet Parasitol 1991;39: 199–205.

15. Reddy BS, Sivajothi S, Rayulu VC. Clinical coccidiosis in adult cattle. J Parasit Dis 2015;39:557–9.

16. Jolley WR, Bardsley KD. Ruminant coccidiois. Vet Clin North Am Food Anim Pract 2006;22:613–21.

17. Foreyt WJ. Veterinary parasitology reference manual. 5th edition. Ames (IO): Iowa State University Press; 1997. p. 3–10.

18. Barrington GM, Parish SM. Ruminant immunodeficiency diseases. In: Smith BP, editor. Large animal internal medicine. 3rd edition. St Louis (MO): Mosby; 2002. p. 1600–2.

19. Radostits OM, Gay CC, Hinchcliff KW, et al. Drug doses and intervals for horses and ruminants. In: Veterinary medicine: a textbook of the diseases of cattle, horses, sheep, pigs, and goats. 10th edition. St Louis (MO): Elsevier; 2007. p. 2057.

20. Balcomb CB, Foster D. Update on the use of blood products in ruminants. Vet Clin North Am Food Anim Pract 2014;30:455–74.

21. Mohler VL, Izzo MM, House JK. Salmonella in calves. Vet Clin North Am Food Anim Pract 2009;25:47–54.

22. Barnett SC, Sischo WM, Moore DA, et al. Evaluation of flunixin meglumine as an adjunct treatment for diarrhea in dairy calves. J Am Vet Med Assoc 2003;223: 1329–33.

23. Baynes RE, Payne M, Martin-Jimenez T, et al. Extralable use of ivermectin and moxidectin. J Am Vet Med Assoc 2000;217:668–71.

Salmonella in Dairy Cattle

Chelsea L. Holschbach, DVM[a], Simon F. Peek, BVSc, PhD[b],*

KEYWORDS

- *Salmonella* • Dairy cattle • *Salmonella* Dublin • Diagnostic tests • Prevention
- Public health

KEY POINTS

- *Salmonella* Dublin, the host adapted serotype in cattle, has the ability to establish lifelong infection in cattle, characterized by an asymptomatic carrier status with intermittent periods of bacteremia and shedding.
- Enteric, septicemic, and reproductive diseases are all possible manifestations of *Salmonella* infection, with pneumonia being a common manifestation of *Salmonella* Dublin infection in calves.
- Definitive diagnosis is based on detection of the organism through aerobic culture of feces or detection of genetic material from the bacteria via polymerase chain reaction techniques.
- Fluid therapy is the mainstay of treatment for cattle with enteric salmonellosis; antimicrobial therapy remains controversial.
- Larger herd size, crowded husbandry, free stall housing, and purchase of replacement animals contribute to an increased propensity for exposure to contaminated manure, the major source of infection on dairies.

INTRODUCTION

As an infectious, contagious pathogen *Salmonella* is probably rivalled by only bovine viral diarrhea virus in its ability to cause such a variety of clinical problems in dairy cattle. Enteric, septicemic, and reproductive diseases are all possible manifestations of *Salmonella* infection and, although reproductive losses are only of concern in sexually mature females, enteric disease can be seen in susceptible cattle at any age from true neonates through adulthood. The increasing prevalence in recent years of the host adapted serotype *Salmonella enterica* serotype Dublin, conventionally referred to by the abbreviated title of *Salmonella* Dublin, has added a new, and highly challenging,

Disclosure Statement: The authors have nothing to disclose.
[a] Large Animal Medicine, Department of Medical Sciences, UW-School of Veterinary Medicine, University of Wisconsin-Madison, 2015 Linden Drive West, Madison, WI 53706, USA;
[b] Department of Medical Sciences, UW-School of Veterinary Medicine, University of Wisconsin-Madison, 2015 Linden Drive West, Madison, WI 53706, USA
* Corresponding author.
E-mail address: simon.peek@wisc.edu

facet to salmonellosis on many modern dairies. The ability to establish lifelong infection, characterized by an asymptomatic carrier status, with intermittent periods of bacteremia and intermittent shedding, challenges control of this serotype. Enteric infection with other non–host-adapted serotypes, particularly in calves, can also be associated with true bacteremia, sepsis, and high mortality rates. No current discussion of bovine salmonellosis could be complete without acknowledging the increasing public health concern regarding its relevance as an important zoonosis, the risk that contaminated dairy and dairy beef products can pose to human health, and, just as important, the reality that increasing antimicrobial resistance among zoonotic enteric pathogens such as *Salmonella* brings the use of antimicrobials by veterinarians and producers under ever stricter scrutiny.

ETIOLOGY AND TAXONOMY

Salmonella is a genus of gram-negative, facultative anaerobic bacteria that belong to the family of Enterobacteriaceae. There are 2 recognized species within the genus: *S enterica* and *Salmonella bongori*. *S enterica* can be further divided into 6 subspecies, *S enterica* subspecies *enterica* being the most relevant in dairy cattle.[1] More than 2500 serovars (serotypes), differentiated by their antigenic composition, have been identified. Serovars are based on the somatic (O), flagellar (H), and capsular (Vi) antigens.[2] Most human and veterinary diagnostic laboratories have phenotypically divided *Salmonella* isolates into serogroups based on detection of the O lipopolysaccharide and H flagellar antigens, historically by agglutination methods.[2,3] Although these traditional serotyping techniques have formed the basis of human and veterinary diagnostic practice for salmonellosis for several decades, they are labor intensive and time consuming, typically taking at least 48 hours.[4]

With the advent of more advanced molecular diagnostic methods, genetic approaches to serotyping are beginning to supercede traditional tests. In general, these methods use 1 of 2 types of targets for serotype determination, the first are indirect targets, which use random surrogate genomic markers known to be associated with certain serotypes, and the second method uses direct targets requiring the use of highly specific genetic determinants of a particular serotype.[5] The latter typically involve the *rfb* gene cluster responsible for O somatic group antigen synthesis[6] and the *fliC* and *fliB* genes encoding the 2 flagellar antigens of *Salmonella*.[7] Genomic sequencing is becoming increasingly common for the identification and serotyping of *Salmonella* isolates.[4,5] The hope is that, with diminishing costs and continued refinement, more rapid, accurate genoserotyping will improve diagnostic and surveillance efforts for both public health and veterinary purposes.[8]

Most commonly, clinical bovine isolates have been divided by their O antigens, and serovars are further grouped into serogroups assigned to an early letter of the alphabet (eg, A, B, C, D, and E).[9] By current convention, *Salmonella* isolates are referred to by their serovar/serogroup classification (eg, *S enterica* subspecies *enterica* serovar Typhimurium, is abbreviated to *Salmonella* Typhimurium). Despite the diversity of serovars, relatively few are of clinical importance among cattle. The majority of cattle isolates are *Salmonella* of types B, C, and E, which are non–host specific, or *Salmonella* Dublin (type D), which is the host-adapted serovar in cattle.[9]

PREVALENT SEROTYPES IN DAIRY CATTLE

The isolation of *Salmonella* from the feces of dairy cows or calves as well as the environment on dairy farms is increasingly common. As part of the United States Department of Agriculture's National Animal Health Monitoring System (NAHMS) Dairy 2007 study,[10] fecal samples were collected from approximately 30 healthy cows on each of 121 dairy operations across 17 states. Forty percent of the dairy operations had at least 1 cow that was *Salmonella* positive on fecal culture. Of the roughly 3800 healthy cows sampled, 14% were fecal culture positive. Compared with the Dairy 1996 NAHMS study,[11] the percentage of *Salmonella*-positive operations had doubled and the percentage of positive cows had more than doubled.[10] For the 2007 study, when environmental sampling was performed in conjunction with individual cow sampling, the number of dairies with a positive *Salmonella* culture increased to nearly 50%.[10] Within the 2007 study, the most frequently isolated *Salmonella* serotypes included *Salmonella* Cerro, *Salmonella* Kentucky, *Salmonella* Montevideo, and *Salmonella* Muenster. These serotypes fall within groups K, C3, C1, and E, respectively.

In a comprehensive study of more than 800 dairy herds in the northeastern United States in 2009, fecal samples were collected from female dairy cattle for *Salmonella* culture based on a suspicion of clinical disease.[12] *Salmonella* was found in 11% of the dairy herds monitored for approximately 1 year over the course of the study. The herd-level incidence rate was approximately 9 positive herds per 100 herd-years; however, just 17% of the positive study herds accounted for more than 70% of the clinical *Salmonella* cases.[12] The predominate serotype identified was *Salmonella* Newport, accounting for 41% of the cases, followed by *Salmonella* Typhimurium, accounting for nearly 20% of cases.[12] Clustering of disease among herds was consistent with another US prevalence study that found that 25% of the enrolled dairy farms accounted for more than 75% of the *Salmonella*-positive fecal and environmental samples.[13] In this study, sampling of conventional and organic herds on 5 occasions over a period of 1 year resulted in detection at least 1 *Salmonella*-positive fecal sample on more than 90% of farms (100/110). Serogroup E1 was the most commonly identified serogroup in fecal samples, although serogroup B was the most common isolate across farms, with 43% of fecal-positive farms having at least 1 serogroup B isolate.

Data from a more recent 2013 study demonstrated that of the nearly 1800 *Salmonella* isolates identified at the National Veterinary Services Laboratory from clinical and nonclinical case submissions, the most common serotype was *Salmonella* Dublin (18%) followed by *Salmonella* Cerro (16%) and *Salmonella* Typhimurium (13%).[14] A retrospective study of *S enterica* isolates submitted to the Wisconsin Veterinary Diagnostic Laboratory from 2006 to 2015 parallels the findings from the National Veterinary Services Laboratory. Of the nearly 5000 isolates identified, *Salmonella* Dublin was the most prevalent serotype identified, accounting for a total of 1153 isolates (23% of total). Along with Dublin, *Salmonella* Cerro (16%), Newport (14%), Montevideo (8%), Kentucky (8%), and Typhimurium (4%) comprised the top 6 most commonly isolated sertotypes.[15] The emergence of *Salmonella* Dublin as one of the most commonly isolated serotypes is of major concern for the dairy industry. As the host-adapted strain of *Salmonella* in cattle, animals infected with *Salmonella* Dublin can become chronic, subclinical carriers that have the potential to shed large numbers of organisms into the environment. These carriers also play an important role in maintaining infection within a herd by shedding not only in feces, but also in milk and colostrum.

PATHOGENESIS

Salmonella infections are well-known for their association with clinical signs of enterocolitis, septicemia, and abortion in dairy cattle.[9] Pneumonia is an increasingly common manifestation of *Salmonella* Dublin infection in calves[16,17] and worth bearing in mind when dealing with mild, moderate, or severe respiratory disease on heifer rearing facilities. Whether or not this merely represents hematogenous localization of the organism to the lungs in much the same way that is seen with septic arthritis, for example, or a more specific organ tropism for the lungs by this serovar is uncertain. However, personal observations by one of the authors and many others suggest that this particular clinical manifestation of *Salmonella* Dublin infection is increasingly common during the late nursing and postweaning period.

Salmonella infection is most commonly transmitted by fecal–oral contamination from other livestock, rodents, birds, or by feeding contaminated protein source animal byproducts.[1] Given the increased frequency with which the organism can be isolated on dairy farms, from both symptomatic and asymptomatic cattle, it is reasonable to assume that fecal–oral spread from other cattle is the most common means of spread on modern dairies. Older literature establishing that aerosol transmission was possible in closely confined, penned calves would also seem to be currently relevant with respect to the spread of certain *Salmonella* serotypes, especially *Salmonella* Dublin, on endemic heifer rearing facilities.[18,19] In both calves and adults, those factors that determine pathogenicity and whether or not clinical disease is seen include virulence of the serotype, dose of inoculum, degree of immunity (passive or adaptive) or previous exposure of host to the serotype, and other stressors currently affecting the host.[20] The organism will less frequently penetrate ocular or nasal mucous membranes.

The most detailed studies of the pathogenesis of bovine salmonellosis infection come from the literature describing enteric infection via the oral route, mainly in calves.[21–23] Once ingested, *Salmonella* attaches to mucosal cells and is capable of destroying enterocytes. Attachment is increased if gastrointestinal stasis is present or the normal flora has been disturbed or is not yet established, as is the case in neonates.[1] The organism penetrates through the enterocytes to the lamina propria of the distal small intestine and colon, where they stimulate an inflammatory response or are engulfed by macrophages and neutrophils.[1] Once salmonellae have gained entry to mononuclear phagocytes, they can be rapidly disseminated throughout the body. Salmonellae have a predilection for lymphoid tissues, invading through M-cells, and are found in the highest numbers in the Peyer patches and mesenteric lymph nodes. From here, the organism often enters the lymphatics and may eventually lead to bacteremia.[9,23] Experimental studies have also shown that oral exposure can lead to infection and systemic dissemination via pharyngeal lymphoid tissue (tonsils) without the need for true enteric infection.[24] Salmonellae are capable of surviving and multiplying in numerous host tissues, often as facultative intracellular bacteria in macrophages and reticuloendothelial cells.[1] These characteristics guard them against the hosts' normal defense mechanisms and potentially facilitate true bacteremia.

The virulence mechanisms of salmonellae are, therefore, composed of their ability to invade the intestinal mucosa, locate to and multiply within the lymphoid tissues, and to evade host defense mechanisms. Enterocolitis caused by *Salmonella* spp. is due to inflammation with subsequent maldigestion and malabsorption, and to a lesser extent from secretory mechanisms.[9,23] Inflammation in the colon leads to the commonly observed fresh blood in the feces of both adults and calves. The diarrhea caused by *Salmonella* spp. is principally mediated by the host inflammatory reaction to the infection.

To establish infection, enteropathogens such as *Salmonella* must first be able to overcome those host factors that resist colonization of the gut, principle among these being a fairly dense gut microbiota,[25] which secrete a variety of bacteriocins, antibiotics, and colicins that hinder enteropathogen growth.[26] There is increasing evidence that many enteropathogens, including salmonellae, are not able to colonize the gut in the face of a normal microbiota[25] and hence factors that negatively influence this key component of resistance are important in the predisposition to enteric disease. Once *Salmonella* density reaches a critical threshold (about 10^8 colony-forming units per gram in the case of *Salmonella* Typhimurium in mice), then a sufficient number of organisms can invade the gut epithelium by first docking with and then invading the epithelial cells.[25] At a molecular level, *Salmonella* Typhimurium does this by specific bacterial adhesins for attachment and then a secretion system that injects a cocktail of bacterial toxins (the type III secretion system) that enables the bacterium to reach the lamina propria.[27] Damaged gut cells are expelled into the lumen, as part of the host defense system, giving rise to some of the clinical signs of salmonellosis and a profound inflammatory response is initiated via interleukin-18 within 10 to 18 hours after infection.[27]

There are molecular reasons that underscore the clinical observation that differences in pathogenicity between serotypes exist. Some strains of *Salmonella* Dublin and *Salmonella* Typhimurium, for example, have a virulence plasmid (carrying the SpV gene) that facilitates survival of the organism within phagocytes, partly perhaps explaining the increased association of these 2 serotypes with clinical disease in calves and adults. The ease with which genes can be transferred between *Salmonella* and other members of the *Enterobacteriaceae* also provides a rational explanation for the transfer of antimicrobial resistance.[20]

Precise and eloquent experimental data on the mechanisms by which *Salmonella* infection can lead to reproductive loss and abortion are hard to find. Clinically, abortions are most common when serotypes B, C, or D are involved and it makes intuitive sense that abortion in cattle infected with *Salmonella* spp. could arise through several different mechanisms. Septicemia could lead to seeding of the fetus and uterus, causing fetal infection and death.[1,9] The fact that diagnostic post mortem investigations of aborted fetuses can often recover the organism from fetal samples supports this possibility. Endotoxemia leading to inflammatory mediator release might also cause luteolysis secondary to prostaglandin release. High fevers or hyperthermia could also play a role in prostaglandin release or cause abortion through more direct fetal injury. Cows may abort at any stage of gestation, but expulsion of the fetus is most common at 5 to 9 months of gestation.[1,9]

DIAGNOSTICS
Live Animal

A definitive diagnosis of *Salmonella* infection in the live animal involves detection of the organism, most commonly by aerobic culture. Although a clinical history of febrile illness accompanied by hemorrhagic enteritis and anorexia may be suggestive in either calves or adults, there is a sufficient differential diagnosis list in both age groups that diagnostic sampling must be performed. When reproductive losses are encountered in pregnant cattle, unless there are concurrent cases of bloody diarrhea, the clinical signs are even less definitive for salmonellosis and the differential list even longer. For hemorrhagic enteritis in adults, the differential list principally includes winter dysentery and bovine viral diarrhea virus infection; in calves, depending on age, such a presentation merits consideration of several viral (rotavirus, coronavirus), protozoal (*Cryptosporidium*, *Eimeria*), and bacterial causes (*Escherichia coli*, *Clostridium perfringens*). However, one should not rely on the presence of blood in the stool; many cases of enteric salmonellosis present without this clinical finding. Remarkable variation in clinical severity will occur based on serovar virulence, host immunologic status, and inoculating dose. In calves, death may occur owing to septicemia before diarrhea becomes obvious or a significant clinical abnormality. In large free stall dairies, it is increasingly common to encounter *Salmonella* infection as an endemic challenge with clinical presentations that are highly variable, ranging from the classic textbook description of reproductive losses and enteric disease in adult cattle through to lower impact problems with fevers of unknown origin, little to no diarrhea, and only modest consequences in terms of appetite and milk yield reduction.

Because *Salmonella* organisms are easily and rapidly out competed by other fecal gram negatives, the majority of diagnostic laboratories use enrichment media such as tetrathionate or selenite broth to improve the chances of *Salmonella* growth and then plate these enriched samples onto selective media such as brilliant green or xylose lysine deso-oxycholate agar.[28] Veterinarians working in the field are advised to contact their local diagnostic laboratory for assistance with sample handling, processing, and submission before investigating either individual or group problems with enteric disease suspicious for *Salmonella* infection. It is frequently worthwhile to place samples directly into enrichment media before submission to improve the chances of positive culture and to keep samples chilled until they arrive at the diagnostic laboratory.

Disadvantages of fecal culture include the fact that shedding can be sporadic, even in true infections (certainly when one considers the sensitivity of bacterial culture) and that, in the face of an ongoing outbreak, one can occasionally encounter clinically normal calves and adults who shed the organism but never develop any clinical signs.[20] The latter situation may still provide useful information, however, both from the perspective of deciding which animals merit treatment but also from the broader standpoint of identifying an enteric pathogen that should never be trivialized or considered a commensal. However, the general pattern is that subclinically or persistently infected cattle shed low numbers of organisms, whereas clinically ill or acutely infected animals may excrete higher numbers in feces.[17] When the clinical suspicion of *Salmonella* is high, a single negative culture is not sufficient to rule out infection. As mentioned, fecal samples should be submitted to qualified diagnostic laboratories that are equipped to culture enteric pathogens and with careful attention to sample handling.[9] Although culturing of individual cow fecal samples is the most common method used to assess individual and herd *Salmonella* status, it can be expensive and time consuming, especially in larger herds. In a study comparing individual, pooled, and composite fecal samples, it was found that composite fecal sampling was more sensitive at the sample level than the other 2 methods, primarily because of the increased number of cattle sampled indirectly through this method.[29] Hence, if one is merely trying to obtain a yes or no answer or identify and track specific serovars, or antimicrobial susceptibility patterns over time, composite fecal samples are typically collected from areas on dairy operations where manure accumulates from a majority of adult animals, such as holding pens, alleyways, and lagoons.[29]

Newer techniques for diagnosing *Salmonella* are based on detection of genetic material from the bacteria, that is, polymerase chain reaction (PCR) techniques.[30,31] These techniques are generally thought to be more sensitive than culture, but have the disadvantage that subsequent serotyping is not always possible.[17] Both species-specific (*S enterica*) and individual serotype PCR tests are available at some, but not all, veterinary diagnostic laboratories within the United States. There are 2 main PCR methods: the traditional PCR and the real-time PCR. In the traditional PCR method, the test result is qualitative (yes or no). In real-time PCR, a threshold cycle (Ct-value) gives a quantitative value of DNA in the sample; the Ct-value is inversely correlated with the starting concentration of the target DNA; hence, the lower the Ct number the more *Salmonella* DNA there will be in the sample. At the current point in time, only a few veterinary diagnostic laboratories offer both species-specific and serotype (usually *Salmonella* Dublin) assays for use with biological samples such as feces, milk, or tracheal and bronchoalveolar lavage fluid. The advantage is a quicker turnaround time and the potential for greater sensitivity, although parallel cultures are still necessary for in vitro antibiograms to be performed to aid treatment decisions (Dr Keith Poulsen, Wisconsin State Veterinary Diagnostic Laboratory, personal communication, 2017). It is possible that, in the near future, PCR assays may become used for environmental samples although these can contain so many potential PCR inhibitors and out-competing organisms that sensitivity and specificity may be lost.[32] The use of PCR methodology to investigate contamination of milk is also of increasing relevance, potentially for veterinarians, but also from the public health perspective. Certain serovars, notoriously *Salmonella* Dublin, but also to include *Salmonella* Typhimurium and Newport, can be found in the milk or colostrum of infected lactating animals.[9] Although conventional pasteurization should kill the organism, there is an understandable desire for food safety reasons to use highly sensitive methods to detect the organism after harvest.[33]

Although fecal culture remains the gold standard at most laboratories, blood culture, a culture of transtracheal wash or bronchoalveolar lavage fluid, and joint fluid may all be useful choices for individuals experiencing bacteremic salmonellosis. The propensity for bacteremia in neonatal calves with salmonellosis makes aseptically obtained aerobic blood cultures a particularly useful diagnostic sample to consider in valuable animals.[1,9] Culture of these nonfecal samples is far less likely to be diagnostically valuable in adults, although PCR methods on such samples may potentially improve sensitivity in the future.

Post Mortem Sampling

Although gross post mortem findings of severe, diffuse, fibrinonecrotic ileotyphlocolitis with watery, often bloody content are highly suggestive, they are neither consistent enough or definitive for enteric *Salmonella* infection in calves or adults.[20] However, in both calves and adults, necropsy material can provide excellent diagnostic material for the definitive diagnosis of *Salmonella* infection. In all age groups, it is advised to obtain numerous samples from the gastrointestinal tract (ileum, cecum, colon), mesenteric lymph node, and gall bladder (bile is a particularly useful sample), as well as lung tissue, especially when consideration of *Salmonella* Dublin is warranted, as increasingly is the case. Because veterinarians are rarely only interested in the diagnosis of *Salmonella* infection during a field necropsy, one may need to take multiple samples from such sites and handle the samples specifically as described to enhance the chances of a positive *Salmonella* culture. Culture remains the most common method used by most diagnostic laboratories to confirm *Salmonella* infection in post mortem samples.

Samples from abortion cases that may have been caused by *Salmonella*, should include fluid or tissue from both the dam and the fetus. Most *Salmonella*-associated abortions are in the last trimester so there will be a fetus to work with, preferably relatively fresh depending on the delay before the fetus is discovered. Samples from the dam might include milk or colostrum, serum, and feces. Feces and milk can be screened via culture or PCR, whereas the serum sample can be used for *Salmonella* Dublin serology (described elsewhere in this article). Providing the fetus is not severely autolyzed, heart blood, abomasal contents, and intestinal or biliary samples might be useful but diagnostically veterinarians are all too commonly challenged by the "freshness" of an abortus. As is true of many enteritis investigations, with abortion cases veterinarians are typically attempting to submit samples that might reveal one of many possible infectious etiologies and it may be simpler to submit the entire fetus if this can be done in a timely manner.

Environmental Sampling

Environmental sampling on dairy farms and heifer rearing facilities has largely been a research tool rather than a clinically applicable procedure. However, quite a lot of information has been learned regarding areas of large free stall facilities where positive *Salmonella* cultures can often be repeatedly obtained either in herds with or without known clinical disease.[34,35] Not surprisingly, areas of high traffic use and density and where sick cows and cows soon to calve are located are frequently discovered to yield positive cultures.[34] Just as was discussed under individual cow fecal sampling, veterinarians are advised to seek the input of the laboratory to which they are going to submit samples before obtaining on-farm environmental specimens. The use of buffered peptone water or more specific enrichment broths before submission may improve chances of *Salmonella* being isolated from heavily contaminated samples.[34] Drag swabs, milk filters, and even absorbent socks worn over shoes, as have been used for environmental sampling in poultry houses, can be used.

Diagnostic Testing for Salmonella Dublin

Proof of current infection with *Salmonella* Dublin can be achieved via conventional culture with serotyping or PCR methodologies if available.[9,17] In addition, both in the United States and several countries in Europe it is also currently possible to use an enzyme-linked immunosorbent assay (ELISA) to measure the level of antibodies directed against O-antigens from *Salmonella* Dublin in blood and milk. In this way, one can measure the humoral immune response as an indicator of current or previous infection.[36,37] Some laboratories report the ELISA result as a semiquantitative percentage value, giving an optical density reading referable to a standard set of controls. In addition, ELISA tests can also be used for individual or bulk tank milk sample screening,[38] and have come to be used quite extensively in countries such as Denmark, where active surveillance programs for this serovar are in effect.[17,39] Sensitivity for the serum ELISA is considerably higher than fecal culture for the identification of *Salmonella* Dublin infected cattle,[17] and as a diagnostic test the serum ELISA is reported to perform best when used in animals between 3 and 10 months of age (**Box 1**).[36]

TREATMENT

Fluid therapy is the mainstay of treatment for cattle with enteric salmonellosis.[40] The type of fluid and route of administration is based on the severity of clinical signs

---

Box 1
Salmonella diagnostic testing options

- Individual animal fecal culture using enrichment and selective media.
- Composite fecal sampling.
- *Salmonella* polymerase chain reaction (feces, milk, tracheal or bronchoalveolar lavage fluid).
- Blood, transtracheal wash, bronchoalveolar lavage, or joint fluid culture when bacteremia is suspected in calves.
- Culture of post mortem samples: gastrointestinal tract, mesenteric lymph node, bile, and lung.
- Environmental cultures.
- *Salmonella* Dublin enzyme-linked immunosorbent assay: serum or milk.

and the economic value of the animal. In calves with acute, severe diarrhea showing signs of hypovolemic shock, intravenous fluid therapy using a balanced electrolyte solution, such as lactated Ringers, is necessary.[20,40] In severely depressed or comatose animals, resuscitative fluids, such as hypertonic saline, are indicated. If administered, hypertonic saline, dosed at 2-4 mL/kg, should always be followed with isotonic crystalloids or water to replace the "borrowed" water from the intracellular space. Dextrose supplementation can be a critical part of the intravenous fluid therapy plan for calves with salmonellosis, not only because of poor feed intake, but because of the increased risk of hypoglycemia that may accompany septicemia. Calves that are ambulatory, have a suckle, and are only moderately dehydrated can often be managed with oral fluids.[40] Calves and even adult cattle can develop severe metabolic acidosis with peracute *Salmonella* infections and intravenous bicarbonate-rich fluids should be considered when profound depression or shocklike signs accompany diarrhea. Oral electrolyte solutions have proven to be helpful in correcting mild to moderate dehydration; however, depending on the degree of bowel inflammation, fluid absorption and digestion may be altered. Fluid therapy for adult cattle in the field setting can prove to be more challenging owing to the sheer volume of fluid needed in cases of severe dehydration. Hypertonic saline followed by at least 10 gallons of oral electrolytes or water, either consumed voluntarily or given by orogastric tube, is a highly efficient method of fluid resuscitation in adult cattle.

In valuable calves or adults, colloids (plasma or hetastarch) are often indicated as a result of hypoproteinemia secondary to albumin loss from the gastrointestinal tract. Synthetic colloids, such as hetastarch, are a more reasonably priced option, but only augment colloidal pressure. Plasma has the added benefit of immunoglobulins and acute phase proteins, which provide therapeutic benefits in septic or inflammatory conditions.[9]

Antimicrobial therapy for the treatment of salmonellosis was, is, and probably always will be, controversial. Of utmost concern is the potential for the creation of antibiotic-resistant strains of *Salmonella* that may present a risk to humans or animals in the future. Although antimicrobial therapy may aid in clinical recovery, it has also been criticized as failing to limit fecal shedding or to impart a positive effect on the duration of fecal shedding. In truth, this criticism is largely extrapolated from research in other species. In cattle, the effect of prior antibiotic use on fecal shedding may be age variable, with research identifying that the risk of fecal shedding after antibiotic treatment is greater for adults and heifers than in calves.[41] However, the risk of true bacteremia in calves with enteric salmonellosis is substantial, justifying the use of antimicrobials in patients of this age.[1] Bacteremic spread of the organism can result in concurrent disease in multiple organs, such as pneumonia, arthritis, and meningitis. The presence of these clinical infections should always merit antimicrobial administration. The comparative risks for such systemic complications in adults are less than in calves, making the routine use of antimicrobials in mature animals less justifiable.

If possible, antimicrobial selection should be based on culture and susceptibility of the *Salmonella* isolate. The dilemma faced by practitioners is frequently that real-time decisions regarding antimicrobial use and selection have to be made in advance of any definitive microbiologic data. Some guidelines regarding *Salmonella* susceptibility can be provided, however. According to the NAHMS 2007 study, isolates were found to be most resistant to tetracycline, streptomycin, ampicillin, and ceftiofur, but were frequently sensitive to aminoglycosides, fluoroquinolones, and trimethoprim-sulfas.[10] To the US readership, these lists will not provide much comfort because of restrictions on antimicrobial use under the current Animal Medicinal Drug Use Clarification Act. Fluoroquinolones and certain sulfonamides may not be used extra-label in the United

States. Additionally, there is a voluntary ban on the use of aminoglycosides, such as gentamicin and amikacin, in food-producing animals because of long-term tissue residues. As of 2012, the extra-label use of ceftiofur in regard to dose, route, and frequency of administration is also prohibited. Owing to the facultative intracellular nature of the organism, it is also worth bearing in mind that antimicrobial penetration into the cell can be limited, even for antimicrobials that show in vitro efficacy. When chosen, antibiotic therapy should be continued for at least 5 to 7 days in cases of acute or peracute salmonellosis.[9] Appropriate withdrawal times should be observed for all antimicrobial usage and Animal Medicinal Drug Use Clarification Act guidelines followed at all times. For questions regarding extended withdrawal times and extra-label use of antimicrobials, US readers are advised to contact the Food Animal Residue Avoidance Database.

In addition to crystalloid fluid therapy, colloid administration when indicated by hypoproteinemia, and responsible, legal, and signalment appropriate selection of antibiotics, the third and final component of therapy for salmonellosis is antiinflammatory use. The inflammatory cascade triggered by local or systemic infection with *Salmonella* is a critical component of the pathogenesis of this organism and culminates in many of the clinical signs observed. Direct endotoxin-mediated effects alongside the host systemic inflammatory response are major components of many calf and adult *Salmonella* infections that can be mitigated, at least in part, by the use of nonsteroidal antiinflammatory drugs.[1] Cattle may be dosed with flunixin meglumine at 1.1 mg/kg of body weight intravenously every 24 hours and then tapered to 0.5 mg/kg every 24 hours, or the medication discontinued after the patient stabilizes.[9] Label use of flunixin meglumine includes dosages of up to 2.2 mg/kg in the United States. Prolonged administration of nonsteroidal antiinflammatory drugs, particularly at the higher dose or in the face of dehydration, can lead to abomasal ulceration and renal papillary necrosis.[1,9,20] In rare circumstances, some clinicians elect to administer "shock" doses of corticosteroids, but this measure would be uncommon in either general or referral practice. Soluble prednisolone sodium succinate would be the preferred agent in such circumstances.

PREVENTION AND CONTROL
Adult Cows

From both the literature and personal experience, it seems that not only are herd epidemics becoming more common, but perhaps more worryingly the disease has become endemic on an increasing number of facilities. Endemicity is obviously problematic with any serovar, but is inevitable when the herd prevalence of *Salmonella* Dublin infection increases. Frequently, the disease becomes a cyclical problem responsible for a spectrum of illness that varies from the more classic presentations described through to milder illness perhaps characterized by fever, looser than normal stool, and mild production loss. Depending on the interaction of general cow health, other concurrent stressors, climatologic stress, and the level of fecal–oral challenge at any one time, adult cows may or may not become clinically ill. Transition cow management becomes an important factor in whether or not new infections are acquired and subsequently result in clinical illness in the late dry and early lactation period, a time when cattle may be at their most susceptible to infectious disease.[9]

As with any fecally–orally spread organism, control strategies are broadly speaking simple to describe, but not necessarily so easy to put into place for many dairies. Larger herd size, crowded husbandry, and free stall housing all contribute to an increased propensity for exposure to contaminated manure, and although purchased feedstuffs are still occasionally incriminated as a means by which new *Salmonella* infections are introduced onto farms, as are rodent and bird populations, the major source of infection are other cattle shedding the organism in their feces. The high likelihood of feces being contaminated with *Salmonella* organisms on many diaries should mitigate against the spreading of manure on fields that are to be used for forages, or common use equipment for manure handling and feed distribution. Evidence suggests that heating of manure to greater than 45°C for more than 3 days, alongside aeration of composted manure using straw, markedly and significantly reduces the number of *Salmonella* organisms, although it is uncertain how practical this information is to larger dairies with modern large-volume manure handling systems.[42] Peculiarly, and perhaps rather worryingly, 1 study looking at risk factors for increased antimicrobial resistance among *Salmonella* isolates on dairy farms identified the use of composted manure for bedding as a significant problem.[43] The most directly applicable research regarding modern manure handling systems and survival of *Salmonella* organisms under natural rather than laboratory conditions demonstrated that a multiple-drug–resistant strain of *Salmonella* Newport survived for less than 24 hours in a compost pile at 64°C, but would survive for more than 4 months and more than 9 months in an effluent lagoon and field soil, respectively.[44]

Once salmonellosis has been confirmed in adult cattle, there are a number of further investigative and control measures that may be implemented. These measures do not differ according to serotype, but there are some specific challenges concerning the host adapted serovar *Salmonella* Dublin that will be discussed in a later section.

It is prudent to consider the possible source(s) of the infection. Although commodities, especially protein feed sources, and wild bird and rodent populations have been incriminated in many texts over the years, it seems quite uncommon these days for a single point source event to have introduced the infection onto a dairy de novo. Environmental sampling of feed, water, and storage facilities can be helpful in identifying contamination in this regard, but if, as is commonly the case on larger dairies, management continues to purchase replacement animals or expand from other herds, it seems inevitable from prevalence data that the infection will be introduced via infected cattle and their feces. In all probability, many "new" outbreaks are likely surges in clinical disease and new infections in a herd where the infection already existed but hitherto had remained subclinical. Factors in transition cow management that reduce immunologic competence or increase exposure risk, are likely to contribute to the onset of clinical disease in such circumstances.

The isolation of affected animals and strict attention to hygiene are pieces of advice routinely given but difficult to implement on large dairies. The numbers of affected animals can be overwhelming and lactating cows have to be milked at least twice a day, requiring them to walk and congregate in frequently trafficked areas and holding pens for the parlor into which they release enormous numbers of organism whenever they defecate. Avoidance of common use equipment for manure handling and feed distribution have already been mentioned, but should be in place on well-managed dairies anyway. Sick, transition, and maternity animals should never be housed together, but unfortunately are for convenience on many occasions; this condition merely ensures exposure of the most susceptible animals to those most likely to be contagious.

Cleaning and disinfection of the environment are also important, but again somewhat intimidating in the context of a larger dairy. Proper cleaning and disinfection of the environment and equipment after a *Salmonella* outbreak can, however, be critically important in decreasing the risk of disease transmission to both cattle and humans. Cleaning is defined as the removal of all visible debris and is arguably the most important step in decontamination of animal environments. Even the best disinfectants will be minimally effective when used in the presence of organic matter, such as feces and bedding material.[1] Not only does cleaning remove the physical barrier between disinfectants and the organism, but it also removes a majority of the organisms so that fewer need to be killed by the disinfectants. This is especially helpful with fecally–orally spread infections like *Salmonella*. where the infectious dose is relatively high (often in the order of 10^6–10^8 organisms[9,17]). Livestock trailers, maternity and calf pens, feeding equipment, and other areas suspect of being contaminated with *Salmonella* should be the main focus for cleaning and disinfection. Although high-power washing can be quite helpful in removing organic debris, its use is not recommended because of the risk of cross-contamination of the environment, and splashing and aerosolization of contaminated material, which can lead to human and animal infection.[9,45] Power washing also fails to remove biofilm, which is an essential and vital component to proper cleaning. In place of power washing, hand-held foamers can be used to apply alkaline detergent and acid rinses for cleaning. The Wisconsin Veterinary Diagnostic laboratory has formulated a cleaning and disinfecting protocol specifically for premises with confirmed *Salmonella*, which can be found at www.wvdl.wisc.edu. A recent paper examining disinfection efficacy against several common bacterial pathogens in a large animal hospital environment showed an approximately 90% reduction in colony-forming units per milliliter of *S enterica* when either an accelerated hydrogen peroxide or peroxy monosulfate disinfectant product was used via a mist application technique, provided adequate cleaning was performed first.[46]

As with antimicrobial drugs, disinfectants have a spectrum of activity that can be highly variable between disinfectant classes.[1] Examples of disinfectants commonly used in veterinary medicine include bleach (sodium hypochlorite), quaternary ammonium, phenols, and peroxides. Bleach is rapidly inactivated by organic debris, but has a broad spectrum of activity. Quaternary ammonium has moderate activity in organic debris and is effective against gram-negative bacteria, such as *Salmonella*. The principle advantage of phenols is better activity in organic debris. Peroxides are increasingly used for environmental disinfection, footbaths, and environmental misting and fogging,[1,46] and are perceived as being more environmentally friendly than chemicals such as phenols and bleach. Chlorine dioxide is a powerful oxidant as well as disinfectant, and it can be used to remove and prevent biofilm formation. Its use in the dairy industry is becoming more common. Current recommendations from the Wisconsin State Veterinary Diagnostic Laboratory are for its use in solution at 250 ppm. Although rarely done on farm, the effectiveness of environmental cleaning and subsequent disinfection for *Salmonella* control can be assessed by postdisinfection sampling.

Ongoing efforts at animal isolation and environmental hygiene will be important because shedding of *Salmonella* will continue for many weeks after the initial cases have seemingly resolved. With respect to control, shedding continues periodically for the life of the animal in the case of *Salmonella* Dublin. Once *Salmonella* has been identified on a farm, veterinarians and management should increase awareness of the public health risk among workers and revisit personal hygiene, protective clothing, and appropriate disinfectant footbath use for employees. If time and labor resources are limited, then concentrating cleaning and disinfection efforts toward high-risk groups (transition cows, maternity pen) and high use traffic areas may be a reasonable compromise.

Inevitably, the identification of *Salmonella* infection in adult cows or calves will lead to a conversation about vaccine use as a preventative strategy. Many farms have at one time or another tried a commercially available or autogenous *Salmonella* vaccine as an adjunct component of control. The safety and efficacy of autogenous products are questioned by many academicians, but individual experiences are sometimes compelling, at least in the short term in the face of an outbreak. As with other infectious contagious diseases such as infectious bovine keratoconjunctivitis, when any vaccine product is used during an outbreak it is impossible to know whether improvement was associated with vaccine use or natural immunologic exposure and protective antibody responses. The most commonly used product in the United States currently for the control of salmonellosis in adults is a siderophore receptor/porin vaccine derived from *Salmonella* Newport (*Salmonella* Newport Bacterial Extract, Zoetis Animal Health, Parsippany, NJ). It is administered to dry cows as an initial 2 injection series and boostered annually. It can, however, be given at any stage of lactation or to heifers. It will not prevent infection, but has been associated with an amelioration in disease severity. It does result in demonstrable antibody levels in colostrum when administered twice during the dry period, although the protective effect of these antibodies against challenge postnatally in calves at this time is unknown.[47] The efficacy of other gram-negative core vaccines to prevent or decrease *Salmonella* disease, such as the J5 product (Enviracor, Zoetis Animal Health) or Endovac-bovi (Immvac, Columbia, MO), which are specifically marketed for protection against coliform mastitis, is highly debatable.

The maintenance of good general health, excellent hygiene, and particular attention to the well-being of late gestation and early lactation animals are all critical components of *Salmonella* control. A closed herd is ideal, but rarely achieved, making exposure to the organism inevitable on most dairies. Prompt diagnosis, treatment, and isolation are important during an outbreak in adult cattle and environmental sampling to include bulk tank milk and high-risk housing areas should now be considered a routine part of disease prevention and surveillance.

Calves

Many of the important components of adult cow control programs mentioned in the previous section overlap with specific measures recommended for calves. An article in a previous volume of this journal provided an excellent review of control measures specific to calves.[20]

As in adult herds, endemic disease is increasingly common among calves. Commercial heifer rearing facilities that manage preweaned calves from as young as a few hours of age onward, sourced and transported from multiple farms of origin, create a high-risk environment for the acquisition and spread of neonatal salmonellosis. Adequate passive transfer, although imperative for rearing healthy calves, is not an absolute guarantee for protection from *Salmonella* infection. Fecal–oral transmission is a prime means of spread for enteric and septicemic *Salmonella* infection in calves, but one must be mindful of the risk posed by other secretions such as colostrum, unpasteurized milk, and respiratory secretions, especially in the case of *Salmonella* Dublin.

Hygiene, isolation, and treatment principles for calves, calf housing, and personnel working with calves are very similar to those discussed in the adult section. Special consideration should be given to fecal contamination of milk, milk replacer, colostrum, feeding equipment, and starter rations as a means of cross-infection. Periodic environmental sampling of equipment such as nipple feeders, buckets, and housing can be valuable tools to trouble shoot outbreaks and improve quality control and prevention efforts. Milk and colostrum are effective enrichment media for *Salmonella*, so sampling these sources should be done "as fed" rather than as initially mixed or prepared.[9] The increased availability of colostrum pasteurizers has added a very helpful tool to control not only *Salmonella* Dublin, but also other serotypes that can also be found in colostrum. Maternity area hygiene and management are extremely important in the control of neonatal salmonellosis. Decreasing the postpartum exposure to the dam reduces the chances of immediate infection. A rather alarming recent publication has identified that true vertical transmission in newborn calves is documented with several serovars common to cattle in the United States.[48] If further studies confirm this finding, it would add yet another serious challenge to the control of salmonellosis in calves.

Because exposure of calves to *Salmonella* is very likely in the commercial dairy environment, management efforts should be directed toward limiting dose and maximizing health and disease resistance in the young replacement animal population. There are no revelations within this advice, but just as occurs with adult cattle, the degree to which farms are able to dedicate personnel and time may only be prioritized in the midst of, or immediately after, an outbreak of clinical disease. Prompt diagnosis, separation, and treatment are important, but group housing of calves can quickly create a "perfect storm" for contagious disease spread. As with adults, vaccination and immunization with modified live or killed (autogenous or commercially available) products is often part of the control and prevention measures instituted. There is very little evidence to support effective control of *Salmonella* infection in calves via passive transfer from immunized dams with any type of vaccine although the siderophore/porin product mentioned in the previous section in adults will stimulate colostral antibody.[47] *Salmonella* is predominantly cleared by cellular immune responses and humoral antibody alone may not provide satisfactory protection. Vaccine use in calves is best considered when management efforts at control and prevention have already been put in place, or if these have been implemented but found to make little difference in the pattern or severity of disease. Autogenous products derived from a specific serovar isolated from clinical cases must be used very carefully owing to the risk of anaphylactic reactions, and only from reputable biologic manufacturers. Similarly, caution is advised regarding modified live vaccine use in calves owing to the potential for adverse reactions. Killed vaccines have performed inconsistently in the small number of trials carried out in the past in calves.[49,50]

COMMENTS REGARDING *SALMONELLA* DUBLIN CONTROL

The increasing prevalence of *Salmonella* Dublin infection in the US dairy industry[14,15] and its unique status as the host adapted serovar of *S enterica* subspecies *enterica* in cattle merit some more specific attention. For readers who wish more, and a greater in-depth discussion of this serovar, we refer you to the excellent primary sources and review paper authored by Dr Liza Nielsen from Denmark who, together with her international collaborators, has published a great deal of excellent work, particularly as it applies to disease impact as well as control and surveillance strategies.[17,36,38,39,51–53]

Within the European community, especially within the Scandinavian countries, there are currently several active surveillance and certification programs that are designed to control, and potentially eradicate *Salmonella* Dublin infection in cattle herds. It is doubtful whether the immediate future holds much promise for such coordinated efforts within the US dairy industry, but there are undoubtedly useful lessons to be learned from experiences in other countries. All of the control measures described in this article for adults and calves can be applied to *Salmonella* Dublin infection, just as they can to other serovars. However, the serologic response to *Salmonella* Dublin, and the ability to measure that as a potential surrogate marker of the carrier status, opens up possibilities for identification and control.

Currently within the United States, the serologic test for *Salmonella* Dublin is available commercially through the Animal Health Diagnostic Center at Cornell University and can be applied to either blood (serum) or bulk tank milk samples. It is important to recognize that a single time point positive test result does not confirm the carrier status, but indicates an antibody response owing to previous exposure, current infection, or passively derived antibody in a calf less than 3 months of age.[17] Repeated individual animal sampling at specified intervals can be used during surveillance programs to identify animals that are likely to be carriers based on the persistence of an ELISA positive result with a high optical density reading.[17,36,39] Using the data generated by Nielsen as a guide, the Animal Health Diagnostic Center at Cornell University categorizes a carrier as any animal that has 3 strong positive serum ELISA results over an 8-month period (Dr Belinda Thompson, personal communication).

From the currently available literature it does not seem to be possible to predict or estimate what percentage of infected calves or adults will go on to become true carriers, although the number is probably quite low. In herds classified as being endemic for *Salmonella* Dublin in Denmark, the seroprevalence is highly variable but may only be at 15% of the whole herd, with a higher proportion of infection in young stock compared with adults.[17] Reinfection of previously infected and seemingly recovered animals also seems to be possible when individuals are followed over long periods of time. Some of these subsequent infections may also result in the development of carrier status (Dr Belinda Thompson, personal communication).

Bulk tank samples can be used for periodic milking herd surveillance, or, if applied to selected milking groups, to identify whether *Salmonella* Dublin has been introduced into a herd or is present in a particular population of cattle within the herd.[17] From epidemiologic data, it seems that the risk of becoming a carrier after infection is greater for calves and for adults infected around the time of calving.[54] Another study shows that *Salmonella* Dublin infection in endemic herds can be reduced when an individual employee was dedicated to colostrum administration to newborn calves and calving cows were moved into a specific maternity pen before calving.[51]

A number of epidemiologic investigations in endemic *Salmonella* Dublin herds in Scandinavia have identified risk factors and important control points for eradication of infection.[51,54–57] Many of the risk factors and management tools demonstrated to improve control of *Salmonella* Dublin infection are intuitively sensible and relevant to other *Salmonella* serovars. Improving the likelihood of control is associated with avoiding cattle purchases from other farms and ensuring good calving area management and individual calf-rearing practices with solid, not permeable, barriers between calves.[51] Aggressive culling programs are not practical in situations where prevalence is high and may only become reasonable once new calf infections are serologically proven to decline to very low, or absent, levels.[17,56] It may be difficult for some producers and heifer rearers to instigate all of the management changes and practices that have been successful in European countries, but readers are directed to information available through the Animal Health Diagnostic Center at Cornell University website for very helpful guidelines concerning control of *Salmonella* Dublin.[58]

In the United States, there is a commercial live *Salmonella* Dublin vaccine (Entervene D, Boehringer Ingelheim Vetmedica, St. Joseph, MO) that is being used as a component of *Salmonella* Dublin control on many farms. The product is administered parenterally to newborn calves to stimulate an immune response before initial exposure to the pathogen. The goal is to prevent the serious health consequences of natural infection as well as the development of the carrier status in what is the most susceptible population of animals within endemic herds. However, when given according to label instructions the product will interfere with serologic testing, giving a false-positive result at up to 8 months of life.[9] Furthermore, the product can be associated with fatal anaphylactic reactions in some recipient calves. These reactions seem to be more common in endemic herds than in naïve ones.[9] This product can stimulate colostral antibody production when given to dry cows and was not associated with any adverse reactions when given to late pregnant animals.[59] The vaccinated cohort in this study were from a farm with no clinical history of salmonellosis in recent years.[59] Whether this colostral antibody might provide protection against neonatal infection is currently unknown.

Herd Biosecurity?

Biosecurity Recommendations
- Maintain a closed herd.
- If purchasing cattle, ensure a negative serologic test from individual animals or a negative bulk tank milk test from the herd of origin within the last 6 months.
- Maintain separate maternity and sick cow pens.
- Have separate equipment for feed and manure handling.
- Dedicate personnel to solely work with high-risk or sick cattle versus neonates.

PUBLIC HEALTH CONCERNS WITH *SALMONELLA* AND THE DAIRY INDUSTRY

Salmonellosis not only can cause severe disease in cattle, but also poses a significant zoonotic risk. Farm workers, calf handlers, and their families are clearly at risk of becoming infected by *Salmonella* spp. during outbreaks of clinical illness, but the risk of exposure goes far beyond farm workers or veterinarians with direct animal contact during outbreaks of disease. Asymptomatic shedding of *Salmonella*, a characteristic of *Salmonella* Dublin infection, but also an issue with many other common bovine serovars such as Newport and Typhimurium, creates risk for people in direct contact with the animal, its feces, or milk.[9,60,61] However, the majority of human salmonellosis cases do not derive from direct animal contact, but are instead acquired through foodborne exposure.[62] So-called nontyphoidal salmonellosis is one of the leading causes of acute bacterial gastroenteritis in humans in the United States, responsible for an estimated 1.4 million cases of illness annually.[63] The predominant risk for zoonotic salmonellosis from cattle lies in exposure to contaminated meat from beef, which would include dairy beef and cull dairy cows, typically via fecal contamination of the carcass at the time of slaughter.[63–65]

Although *Salmonella* mastitis is extremely uncommon, shedding of the organism in milk is not, and its presence has been documented in bulk tank milk in several studies.[66–69] A positive bulk tank or milk filter sample may represent fecal contamination, true lactational shedding, or a combination of both. Conventional pasteurization should kill the organism, provided effective temperature and duration are reached. It is important to consider the diagnostic procedure performed to identify the *Salmonella* in bulk tank or milk filter samples when interpreting these studies. Studies using PCR[66,67,69] rather than culture will detect a greater prevalence of *Salmonella*-contaminated samples because of genomic material from both live and dead organisms in the sample. Side-by-side comparisons of conventional culture and PCR using the same samples have been performed and show that approximately one-quarter (2.6% vs 11.2%) of those bulk tank samples that are PCR positive for *S enterica* will be positive by culture. True "dairy" products actually account for only a small percentage of human salmonellosis in the United States, and many of these outbreaks are due to the consumption of raw milk and raw milk products.[67,70]

Bacterial antimicrobial resistance represents an important current and future problem in infectious disease public health. Concerns regarding zoonotic *Salmonella* infections have been amplified in recent years by the emergence of multiple drug-resistant strains of several *S enterica* serovars associated with cattle.[71–74] It is generally accepted that antimicrobial-resistant bacteria are produced, maintained, and disseminated as a result of selection pressure introduced by the use of antimicrobial drugs.[75] Suspected principal foci of selection pressure include use of antimicrobials for the treatment of humans and in food-producing animals for treatment or prevention of disease and growth promotion.[75,76] Modern molecular methods combined with other conventional techniques such as pulse field gel electrophoresis can be used to investigate the origins of foodborne human enteric disease and the role of antimicrobial use in cattle with the occurrence of multiple drug-resistant *Salmonella* infection in humans. At this point in time, there are few published studies establishing such links from "farm to fork."[73] A recent extensive systematic literature review of 858 publications on the effect of antimicrobial use in agricultural animals on drug-resistant foodborne salmonellosis in humans from 2010 to 2014 concluded that, although antibiotic use in cattle increased the likelihood of colonization in the host, there were no studies that traced antimicrobial-resistant *Salmonella* in humans back to the farm.[76]

The antimicrobials of choice for treating bacterial gastroenteritis in humans are generally the fluoroquinolone, ciprofloxacin, for adults and the cephalosporin, ceftriaxone, for children.[63,77] At issue today is whether the veterinary analogs of these drugs may be responsible for the emergence of antimicrobial resistance in foodborne pathogens like *Salmonella*. The mechanism by which *S enterica* typically acquires antimicrobial resistance to fluoroquinolones differs quite markedly and, importantly, from that by which resistance to cephalosporins develops. Specifically, fluoroquinolone resistance is usually acquired through clonal dissemination of *Salmonella* isolates with mutations in chromosomally encoded resistance genes. Cephalosporin resistance usually is obtained via independent acquisition of mobile genetic elements via plasmids and transposons.[78] Further work is needed in this area to determine whether there is a connection between veterinary use of ceftiofur and the emergence of ceftriaxone resistance in *Salmonella* spp.[63] Although ceftriaxone-resistant *Salmonella* Typhimurium has been documented in cattle,[73] other larger studies have demonstrated little to no resistance to this particular third-generation cephalosporin in cattle sourced serovars despite more common resistance to other cephalosporins.[72,79] Although it is now 8 years old, interested readers are directed to the excellent review of antimicrobial resistant *Salmonella* in dairy cattle by Alexander and colleagues.[79] In a more recent publication, a significant decrease was observed in antimicrobial resistance among dairy cattle *Salmonella* isolates in the northeastern United States.[71]

Many practitioners and diagnostic laboratories will be very familiar with the wide variety of antimicrobial sensitivity patterns demonstrated by different *S enterica* serovars obtained from individual animal and environmental samples. Certain serovars seem to be more commonly associated with greater in vitro resistance than others. The paper by Cummings and colleagues[71] demonstrated a decrease in resistance trends between 2004 and 2011. It was postulated that this might have been related to an increase in the prevalence of the serovar Cerro in fecal samples from their study population. The biggest concern arises with serovars that have historically been more common in dairy cattle and that are associated with human disease outbreaks, such as Newport and Typhimurium. In particular, several human foodborne outbreaks caused by *Salmonella* Typhimurium DT104 of dairy or beef origin that are characteristically resistant to the antibiotics ampicillin, chloramphenicol, streptomycin, sulfonamides, and tetracycline have been reported.[63,80]

An interesting and rigorously investigated example of zoonotic multiple drug resistant *Salmonella* from cattle is provided by the Wisconsin experience with *Salmonella* Heidelberg over the last 2 years. Since 2015, the Wisconsin State Veterinary

Diagnostic Laboratory (WVDL), in conjunction with human and veterinary health organizations throughout Wisconsin, have been tracking a multidrug-resistant strain of *Salmonella* Heidelberg, a Group B serovar (Dr Keith Poulsen, WVDL personal communication). As of November 2016, there were 12 confirmed human infections from 7 different Wisconsin counties. Upon questioning, more than 90% of the infected individuals reported purchasing Holstein bull calves from livestock dealers or sale barns. During 2015 and 2016, the WVDL also isolated several multidrug-resistant *Salmonella* Heidelberg isolates from calves located mostly in Wisconsin. Pulse-field gel electrophoresis and whole genome sequencing of isolates indicated that the human and bovine isolates were very closely related. This strain of *Salmonella* Heidelberg is highly pathogenic and multidrug resistant. Only 1 antimicrobial drug is an effective treatment option for human cases and no effective, legal (United States) options exist for cattle (Dr Keith Poulsen, WVDL, personal communication). As the application of modern molecular techniques becomes more commonplace, it is probable that diagnostic and surveillance efforts will place food animal species and production methods under greater scrutiny with respect to zoonotic enteric diseases. Increased awareness, rigor, and possibly limitations regarding antimicrobial use in food animals should not be surprising outcomes.

REFERENCES

1. Smith BP. Salmonellosis in ruminants. In: Smith BP, editor. Large animal internal medicine. 4th edition. St. Louis(MO): Mosby; 2009. p. 877–81.
2. Bopp CA, Brenner FW, Fields PI, et al. Escherichia, shigella, and salmonella. In: Murray PR, Baron EJ, Jorgensen JH, et al, editors. Manual of clinical microbiology, vol. 1, 8th edition. Washington, DC: ASM Press; 2003. p. 654–71.
3. Watthiau P, Boland C, Bertrand S. Methodologies for *Salmonella enterica* subsp. *Enterica* subtyping, gold standards and new methodologies. Appl Environ Microbiol 2011;77:7877–85.
4. Yachison CA, Yoshida C, Robertson J, et al. The validation and implications of using whole genome sequencing as a replacement for traditional serotyping for a national Salmonella reference laboratory. Front Microbiol 2017;8(1044):1–7.
5. Zhang S, Yin Y, Jones MB, et al. Salmonella serotype determination utilizing high throughput genome sequencing data. J Clin Microbiol 2015;53(5):1685–92.
6. Samuel G, Reeves P. Biosynthesis of O-antigens: genes and pathways involved in nucleotide sugar precursor synthesis and O-antigen assembly. Carbohydr Res 2003;338(23):2503–19.
7. Smith NH, Selander RK. Sequence invariance of the antigen-coding central region of the phase I flagellar filament (fliC) gene among strains of *Salmonella* typhimurium. J Bacteriol 1990;172:603–9.
8. Yoshida CE, Kruczkiewicz P, Laing CR, et al. The *Salmonella in silico* typing resource (SISTR): an open web-accessible tool for rapidly typing and subtyping draft *Salmonella* genome assemblies. PLoS One 2016;11(1):e0147101.
9. Peek SF, Cummings KJ, McGuirk SM, et al. Infectious diseases of the gastrointestinal tract. In: Peek SF, Divers TJ, editors. Diseases of dairy cattle. 3rd edition. St. Louis(MO): Elsevier; 2017.
10. United States Department of Agriculture (USDA). Salmonella, listeria and campylobacter on US dairy operations, 1996-2007. Fort Collins (CO): USDA-APHIS-VS-CEAH; 2007.
11. United States Department of Agriculture (USDA). E.coli O157:H7 and Salmonella status on dairy farms. Fort Collins (CO): USDA-APHIS-VS-CEAH; 1996.

12. Cummings KJ, Warnick LD, Alexander KA, et al. The incidence of salmonellosis among dairy herds in the Northeastern United States. J Dairy Sci 2009;92(8): 3766–74.

13. Fossler CP, Wells SJ, Kaneene JB, et al. Prevalence of *Salmonella* spp on conventional and organic dairy farms. J Am Vet Med Assoc 2004;225(4):567–73.

14. Morningstar-Shaw BR, Mackie TA, Barker DA, et al. Salmonella serotypes isolated from animals in the United States. Greensboro (NC): Proceedings 116th Annual Meeting US Animal Health Association; 2013. p. 397–407.

15. Valenzuela JR, Sethik AK, Aulik ND, et al. Antimicrobial resistance patterns of bovine Salmonella enterica isolates submitted to the Wisconsin Veterinary Diagnostic Laboratory: 2006-2015. J Dairy Sci 2017;100(2):1319–30.

16. Pecoraro HL, Thompson B, Duhamel GE. Histopathology case definition of naturally acquired *Salmonella enterica* serovar Dublin infection in young Holstein cattle in the northeastern United States. J Vet Diagn Invest 2017. https://doi.org/10.1177/1040638717712757.

17. Nielsen LR. Review of pathogenesis and diagnostic methods of immediate relevance for epidemiology and control of *Salmonella* Dublin in cattle. Vet Microbiol 2013;162(1):1–9.

18. Hardman PM, Wathes CM, Wray C. Transmission of salmonellae among calves penned individually. Vet Rec 1991;129(15):327–9.

19. Wathes CM, Zaidan WA, Pearson GR, et al. Aerosol infection of calves and mice with Salmonella typhimurium. Vet Rec 1988;123(23):590–4.

20. Mohler VL, Izzo MM, House JK. Salmonella in calves. Vet Clin North Am Food Anim Pract 2009;25(1):37–54.

21. Mohler VL, Heithof DM, Maham MJ, et al. Cross protective immunity conferred by a DNA adenine methylase deficient *Salmonella eneterica* serovar Typhimurium vaccine in calves challenged with *Salmonella* serovar Newport. Vaccine 2008; 26(14):1751–8.

22. Tsolis RM, Adams LG, Ficht TA, et al. Contribution of *Salmonella typhimurium* virulence factors to diarrheal disease in calves. Infect Immun 1999;67(9):4879–85.

23. Wray C, Davies R. Salmonella infections in cattle. In: Wray C, Wray W, editors. Salmonella in domestic animals. New York: CABI Publishing; 2000. p. 169–90.

24. De Jong H, Ekdahl MO. Salmonellosis in calves – the effect of dose rate and other factors on the transmission. N Z Vet J 1965;13(2):59–64.

25. Wotzka SY, Nguyen BD, Hardt WD. *Salmonella* Typhimurium diarrhea reveals basic principles of enteropathogen infection and disease-promoted DNA exchange. Cell Host Microbe 2017;21(4):443–54.

26. Stecher B. The roles of inflammation, nutrient availability and the commensal microbiota in enteric pathogen infection. Microbiol Spectr 2015;3(3). https://doi.org/10.1128/microbiolspec.MBP-0008-2014.

27. Muller AA, Dolowschiak T, Sellin ME, et al. An NK cell perforin response elicited via IL-18 controls mucosal inflammation kinetics during Salmonella gut infection. PLoS Pathog 2016;12(6):e1005723.

28. Waltman WD. Methods for the cultural isolation of Salmonella. In: Wray C, Wray A, editors. Salmonella in domestic animals. Wallingford (UK): CABI Publishing; 2000. p. 355–72.

29. Lombard JE, Beam AL, Nifong EM, et al. Comparison of individual, pooled, and composite fecal sampling methods for detection of Salmonella on U.S. dairy operations. J Food Prot 2012;75(9):1562–71.

30. Munoz N, Diaz-Osorio M, Moreno J, et al. Development and evaluation of a real time multiplex polymerase chain reaction procedure to clinically type prevalent *Salmonella enterica* serovars. J Mol Diagn 2010;12(2):220–5.
31. Lofstrom C, Hansen F, Hoorfar J. Validation of a 20h real time PCR method for screening of Salmonella in poultry fecal samples. Vet Microbiol 2010;144(3–4): 511–4.
32. Kasturi KN, Drgon T. Real time PCR method for detection of *Salmonella* spp. in environmental samples. Appl Environ Microbiol 2017;83(14) [pii:e00644–17].
33. Gokduman K, Avsaroglu MD, Cakiris A, et al. Recombinant plasmid based quantitative real time PCR analysis of *Salmonella enterica* serotypes and its application to milk samples. J Microbiol Methods 2016;122:50–8.
34. Peek SF, Hartmann FA, Thomas CB, et al. Isolation of Salmonella spp. from the environment of dairies without any clinical history of salmonellosis. J Am Vet Med Assoc 2004;225(4):574–7.
35. Fossler CP, Wells SJ, Kaneene JB, et al. Cattle and environmental sample level factors associated with the presence of *Salmonella* in a multi-state study of conventional and organic dairy farms. Prev Vet Med 2005;67(1):39–53.
36. Nilesen LR, Ersbell AK. Age stratified validation of an indirect *Salmonella* Dublin serum ELISA for individual diagnosis in cattle. J Vet Diagn Invest 2004;16(3): 205–11.
37. Robertsson JA. Humoral antibody responses to experimental and spontaneous *Salmonella* infections in cattle measured by ELISA. Zentralbl Veterinarmed B 1984;31:367–80.
38. Nilesen LR, Ersbell AK. Factors associated with variation in bulk tank milk *Salmonella* Dublin ELISA ODC% in dairy herds. Prev Vet Med 2005;68:165–79.
39. Warnick LD, Nielsen LR, Nielsen J, et al. Simulation model estimates of test accuracy and predictive values for the Danish *Salmonella* surveillance program in dairy herds. Prev Vet Med 2006;77:284–303.
40. McGuirk SM. Disease management of dairy calves and heifers. Vet Clin North Am Food Anim Pract 2008;24:139–54.
41. Warnick LD, Kanistanon K, McDonough PL, et al. Effect of previous antimicrobial treatment on fecal shedding of *Salmonella enterica* subsp. *Enterica* serogroup B in New York dairy herds with recent salmonellosis. Prev Vet Med 2003;56(4): 285–97.
42. Millner P, Ingram D, Mulbry W, et al. Pathogen reduction in minimally managed composting of bovine manure. Waste Manag 2014;34(11):1992–9.
43. Toth JD, Aceto HW, Rankin SC, et al. Survival characteristics of Salmonella enterica serovar Newport in the dairy farm environment. J Dairy Sci 2011;94(10): 5238–46.
44. Habing GG, Lombard JE, Kopral CE, et al. Farm level associations with the shedding of Salmonella and antimicrobial resistant Salmonella in US dairy cattle. Foodborne Pathog Dis 2012;9(9):815–21.
45. Bemis DA, Craig LE, Dunn JR. Salmonella transmission through splash exposure during a bovine necropsy. Foodborne Pathog Dis 2007;4(3):387–90.
46. Saklou NT, Burgess BA, Van Metre DC, et al. Comparison of disinfectant efficacy when using high-volume directed mist application of accelerated hydrogen peroxide and peroxymonosulfate disinfectants in a large animal hospital. Equine Vet J 2016;48(4):485–9.
47. Smith GW, Alley ML, Foster DM, et al. Passive immunity stimulated by vaccination of dry cows with a *Salmonella* bacterial extract. J Vet Intern Med 2014;28(5): 1602–5.

48. Hanson DL, Loneragan GH, Brown TR, et al. Evidence supporting vertical transmission of *Salmonella* in dairy cattle. Epidemiol Infect 2016;144(5):962–7.

49. Robertsson JA, Lindberg AA, Hoiseth S, et al. Salmonella Typhimurium infection in calves: protection and survival of virulent challenge bacteria after immunization with live or inactivated vaccines. Infect Immun 1983;41(2):742.

50. Smith BP, Habasha FG, Reina-Guierra M, et al. Immunization of calves against salmonellosis. Am J Vet Res 1980;41(12):1947–51.

51. Nielsen TD, Vesterbaek IL, Kudahl AB, et al. Effect of prevention of *Salmonella* Dublin exposure of calves during a one-year control programme in 84 Danish dairy herds. Prev Vet Med 2012;105:101–9.

52. Stockmarr A, Bodher R, Nielsen LR. Dynamic changes in antibody levels as an early warning of *Salmonella* Dublin in bovine dairy herds. J Dairy Sci 2013; 96(12):7558–64.

53. Nielsen TD, Kudahl AB, Ostergaard S, et al. Gross margin losses due to *Salmonella* Dublin infection in Danish dairy cattle herds estimated by simulation modelling. Prev Vet Med 2013;111:51–62.

54. Nielsen LR, Schukken YH, Grohn YT, et al. *Salmonella* Dublin infection in dairy cattle: risk factors for becoming a carrier. Prev Vet Med 2004;65:47–62.

55. Agren EC, Frossling J, Wahlstrom H, et al. A questionnaire study of associations between potential risk factors and salmonella status in Swedish dairy herds. Prev Vet Med 2017;143(1):21–9.

56. Nielsen LR, Doohoo I. Culling decisions of dairy farmers during a 3-year *Salmonella* control study. Prev Vet Med 2011;100(1):29–37.

57. Nilesen LR, van den Borne B, van Schalk G. *Salmonella* Dublin infection in young dairy calves: transmission parameters estimated from field data and an SIR model. Prev Vet Med 2007;79(1):46–58.

58. Cornell University Animal Health Diagnostic Center. NYSCHAP Recommendations for the control of Salmonella Dublin in dairy calf and heifer raising operations. Available at: https://ahdc.vet.cornell.edu/programs/NYSCHAP/docs/Calf_HeiferRaiserSDRecommendations_12_2012.pdf. Accessed 2017.

59. Smith GW, Smith F, Zuidhof S, et al. Characterization of the serologic response induced by vaccination of late gestation cows with a *Salmonella* Dublin vaccine. J Dairy Sci 2015;98(4):2529–32.

60. Cummings KJ, Warnick LD, Elton M, et al. The effect of clinical outbreaks of Salmonellosis on the prevalence of fecal shedding among dairy cattle in New York. Foodborne Pathog Dis 2010;7(7):815–23.

61. Karon AE, Archer JR, Sotir MJ, et al. Human multi-drug resistant *Salmonella* Newport infections, Wisconsin, 2003-2005. Emerg Infect Dis 2007;13:1777–80.

62. Mead PS, Slutsker L, Dietz V, et al. Food related illness and death in the United States. Emerg Infect Dis 1999;5(5):607–25.

63. Sanchez S, Hofacre CL, Lee MD, et al. Animal sources of salmonellosis in humans. J Am Vet Med Assoc 2002;221:492–7.

64. Dechet AM, Scallan E, Gensheimer K, et al. Outbreak of multi-drug-resistant *Salmonella enterica* serotype Typhimurium Definitive phage type 104 infection linked to commercial ground beef, northeastern United States, 2003-2004. Clin Infect Dis 2006;42(6):747–52.

65. Varma JK, Marcus R, Stenzel SA, et al. Highly resistant *Salmonella* Newport-MDRAmpC transmitted through the domestic US food supply: a FoodNet case–control study of sporadic *Salmonella* Newport infections, 2002-2003. J Infect Dis 2006;194:222–30.

66. Van Kessel JS, Sonnier J, Zhao S, et al. Antimicrobial resistance of Salmonella enterica isolates from bulk tank milk and milk filters in the United States. J Food Prot 2013;76:18–25.
67. Van Kessel JA, Karns JS, Lombard JE, et al. Prevalence of Salmonella enterica, Listeria monocytogenes and Escherichia coli virulence factors in bulk tank milk and in line filters from US dairies. J Food Prot 2011;74:759–68.
68. Karns JS, Van Kessel JS, McCluskey BJ, et al. Prevalence of Salmonella enterica in bulk tank milk from US dairies as determined by polymerase chain reaction. J Dairy Sci 2005;88(10):3475–9.
69. Ruzante JM, Lombard JE, Wagner B, et al. Factors associated with Salmonella presence in environmental samples and bulk tank milk from US dairies. Zoonoses Public Health 2010;57:e217–25.
70. Jayarao BM, Donalson SC, Straley BA, et al. A survey of foodborne pathogens in bulk tank milk and raw milk consumption among farm families in Pennsylvania. J Dairy Sci 2006;89(7):2451–8.
71. Cummings KJ, Perkins GA, Khatibzadeh SM, et al. Antimicrobial resistance trends among Salmonella isolates obtained from dairy cattle in the northeastern United States. Foodborne Pathog Dis 2013;10:353–61.
72. Ray KA, Warnick LD, Mitchell RM, et al. Prevalence of antimicrobial resistance among Salmonella on Midwest and northeast dairy farms. Prev Vet Med 2007; 79:204–23.
73. Fey PD, Safranek TJ, Rupp ME, et al. Ceftriaxone-resistant salmonella infection acquired by a child from cattle. N Engl J Med 2000;342:1242–9.
74. Edrington TS, Schultz CL, Bischoff KM, et al. Antimicrobial resistance and serotype prevalence of Salmonella isolated from dairy cattle in the southwestern United States. Microb Drug Resist 2004;10(1):51–6.
75. DeFrancesco KA, Cobbold RN, Rice DH, et al. Antimicrobial resistance of commensal Escherichia coli from dairy cattle associated with recent multi-resistant salmonellosis outbreaks. Vet Microbiol 2004;98(1):55–61.
76. Helke KL, McCrakin MA, Galloway AM, et al. Effects of antimicrobial use in agricultural animals on drug resistant foodborne salmonellosis in humans. A systematic literature review. Crit Rev Food Sci Nutr 2017;57:472–88.
77. Hohmann EL. Nontyphoidal salmonellosis. Clin Infect Dis 2001;322:263–9.
78. Alcaine SD, Sukhanand SS, Warnick LD, et al. Ceftiofur resistant Salmonella strains isolated from dairy farms represent multiple widely distributed subtypes that evolved by independent horizontal gene transfer. Antimicrob Agents Chemother 2005;49(10):4061–7.
79. Alexander KA, Warnick LD, Wiedmann M. Antimicrobial resistant Salmonella in dairy cattle in the United States. Vet Res Commun 2009;33:191–209.
80. Glenn LM, Lindsey RL, Frank JF, et al. Analysis of antimicrobial resistance genes detected in multi-drug resistant Salmonella enterica serovar Typhimurium isolated from food animals. Microb Drug Resist 2011;17:407–18.

Clostridial Abomasitis and Enteritis in Ruminants

Katharine M. Simpson, DVM, MS*, Robert J. Callan, DVM, MS, PhD,
David C. Van Metre, DVM

KEYWORDS

- *Clostridium perfringens* • *Clostridium difficile* • Abomasitis • Enteritis
- Enterotoxemia • Ruminant

KEY POINTS

- Clostridial abomasitis and enteritis are characterized by necrosis of the abomasal or intestinal mucosa caused by exotoxins produced by *Clostridium perfringens* or *Clostridium difficile* in the lumen of the gastrointestinal tract.
- *C perfringens* types A, B, C, D, and E can cause enteric disease in all species of domestic ruminants. The 5 genotypes are identified by the presence of the genes for the lethal exotoxins alpha, beta, epsilon, and iota.
- Multiplex polymerase chain reaction is used diagnostically to identify *C perfringens* genotypes from anaerobic culture of samples.
- Proliferation of *C perfringens* in the ruminant gastrointestinal tract is associated with a combination of increased availability of carbohydrate or protein, and alteration in gastrointestinal motility.
- Treatment of abomasitis and enteritis caused by *C perfringens* should focus on 6 goals: relief of abdominal distention, systemic fluid support, prevention of *C perfringens* proliferation, decreasing or preventing exotoxin production, restoration of normal gastrointestinal flora, and providing pain management as needed.

INTRODUCTION

Clostridial diseases affecting the gastrointestinal tract are common in ruminant livestock; however, their classification can be confusing because of the varied nomenclature of the disease conditions.[1–4] Described diseases have included hemorrhagic enterocolitis, enterotoxemia, pulpy kidney disease, overeating disease, braxy, bradsot, struck, lamb dysentery, enterotoxemic jaundice, yellow lamb disease, clostridial

Disclosure: The authors have nothing to disclose.
Livestock Medicine and Surgery, Department of Clinical Sciences, College of Veterinary Medicine and Biological Sciences, Colorado State University, 300 West Drake Road, Fort Collins, CO 80523-1678, USA
* Corresponding author.
E-mail address: katie.simpson@colostate.edu

abomasitis, and clostridial enteritis. Other than braxy (bradsot) of sheep, which is caused by *Clostridium septicum*, these diseases are all caused by different subtypes of *Clostridium perfringens*. *C perfringens* type A can also cause gangrenous mastitis and may be present in high numbers in spoiled milk.

Clinical disease is associated with rapid bacterial overgrowth within the gastrointestinal tract and subsequent exotoxin release. Although limited tissue invasion by *C perfringens* does occur, most local and systemic lesions result from the effects of potent exotoxins produced by certain genotypes of these bacteria. *C perfringens* is a large, gram-positive, anaerobic bacillus that exists ubiquitously in the environment and in the gastrointestinal tract of most mammals.[3,5–8] There are 5 defined types, or genotypes, of *C perfringens*: A, B, C, D, and E (**Table 1**). These genotypes are identified based on the lethal toxins that they produce: *C perfringens* alpha (CPA), *C perfringens* beta (CPB), epsilon (ETX), and *C perfringens* iota (CPI).[7–10] The alpha toxin gene (*plc*) is present on the chromosome of all *C perfringens* isolates.[7,8] All genotypes produce alpha toxin, although isolates differ significantly in the amount of alpha toxin produced.[11,12] The other lethal toxins, CPB (*cpb* gene), ETX (*etx* gene), and CPI (*iap/ibp* genes) are contained on transferrable plasmids.[7,8]

Two other toxins, enterotoxin (*C perfringens* enterotoxin [CPE], *cpe* gene) and the beta-2 toxin (CPB2, *cpb2* gene), are also carried on transferable plasmids in livestock isolates. Enterotoxin can be expressed by any of the subtypes if the plasmid containing this gene (*cpe*) is present, but it is not required for pathogenicity. Enterotoxin is not released by vegetative bacteria but only in sporulating *C perfringens* cells during lysis of the vegetative cell.[7] Thus, the toxin may not be present in intestinal contents of animals with *C perfringens* enteritis unless sporulation is occurring. The beta-2 toxin may be produced by type A as well as by some isolates of types B, C, and E.[13] Strains of *C perfringens* that carry the beta-2 toxin gene have been isolated from a variety of species of domestic animals, including horses, camelids, cattle, and swine.[13,14]

The genotype, and thus the specific subtype of *C perfringens*, can be determined by a multiplex polymerase chain reaction (mPCR) that detects the specific toxin genes carried by an individual isolate. Because the clinical and pathologic presentations of diseases caused by *C perfringens* types are not always distinct, anaerobic culture and polymerase chain reaction (PCR) genotyping of the isolates can be instrumental in determining the subtype involved and can help identify specific control measures. Each of the subtypes of *C perfringens* is associated with specific disease syndromes that are directly or indirectly related to the toxins they produce. The term enterotoxemia is often loosely used to describe enteric or systemic disease caused by any of the *C perfringens* toxinotypes. The term enterotoxemia refers to systemic disease caused by absorption of a toxin from the intestine. Clostridial abomasitis and enteritis does not require absorption of the toxins. The term enterotoxemia is best reserved for cases in

Table 1
Toxins, gene, genetic location, and toxin action expressed by different *Clostridium perfringens* toxinotypes (genotypes)

Toxin	*C perfringens* Type					Gene	Gene Location	Toxin Action
	A	B	C	D	E			
Alpha (CPA)	+	+	+	+	+	*plc*	Chromosome	Phospholipase
Beta (CPB)	−	+	+	−	−	*cpb*	Plasmid	Pore formation
Epsilon (ETX)	−	+	−	+	−	*etx*	Plasmid	Pore formation
Iota (CPI)	−	−	−	−	+	*lap/ibp*	Plasmid	Cytoskeleton disruption

which systemic disease is associated with absorption of bacterial exotoxins, including hemolytic diseases in lambs with *C perfringens* type A, and systemic disorders caused by the epsilon toxin of *C perfringens* types B and D. Some of the disease conditions described for *C perfringens* are listed in **Table 2**.

Table 2
Diseases caused by different subtypes of *Clostridium perfringens*

Organism	Disease	Notes
C perfringens type A	• Enterotoxemic jaundice (lambs) • Yellow lamb disease • Rare in cattle	• Nutritional factors may predispose to bacterial overgrowth • Depression, anemia, icterus, hemoglobinuria • Hemolysis caused by action of alpha toxin • Lambs die within 6–12 h
	• Abomasitis, enteritis (calves)[15]	• Abdominal tympany • Abomasal ulceration • Mucosal necrosis and hemorrhage • Dietary factors, milk quality, and storage may predispose to disease
	• Enteritis (swine)[16]	• Found in both diseased and normal pigs
C perfringens type B	• Lamb dysentery • Enterotoxemia (calves, foals)	• Rare in North America; more common in United Kingdom and Europe • Lambs up to 3 wk of age • Calves up to 10 d of age • Hemorrhagic enterocolitis with bloody diarrhea
C perfringens type C	• Hemorrhagic enterocolitis (calves, lambs, foals, swine)	• Calves up to 10 d of age • Trypsin inhibitors in colostrum/milk or other feeds (soy, sweet potatoes) may increase susceptibility by blocking degradation of beta toxin by trypsin • Hemorrhagic enterocolitis with bloody diarrhea • Immunize dam to provide lactogenic immunity to calf during critical first 10 d of life, when trypsin inhibitors are present in colostrum and milk
	• Struck (adult sheep)	• Acute fatal enterotoxemia of adult sheep • Organism in soil • Early spring • Colic, rigidity, sudden death • Rarely, diarrhea is observed • Abomasitis and enteritis
C perfringens type D	• Enterotoxemia • Pulpy kidney disease • Overeating disease	• Systemic distribution of epsilon toxin causes widespread endothelial damage and results in cerebral edema • Hyperglycemia and glucosuria occur caused by mobilization of hepatic glycogen • Primarily seen in lambs, less common in goat kids, and rare in calves • Lambs and goat kids 3–10 wk of age with heavy milking dams • Calves 1–4 mo of age • Predisposed by dietary conditions that promote high carbohydrate or protein bypass to the duodenum and secondary factors causing ileus • Vaccination of dams provides protective colostral antibodies in the neonates that last up to 8 mo
C perfringens type E	• Necrotic hemorrhagic enteritis (goats, calves)	• Outbreaks reported in adult goats • Otherwise rare in North America

Recent studies have suggested an association of hemorrhagic bowel syndrome (HBS) in cattle with *C perfringens* type A.[17–20] Although *C perfringens* is isolated from the intestinal tract and from lesions of animals with HBS, a causal link has not been established. It is possible that the heavy growth of *C perfringens* from animals with HBS is caused by an appropriate environment for growth that is associated with gastrointestinal (GI) hemorrhage and stasis. Studies trying to induce HBS by inoculation with *C perfringens* type A have not been able to reproduce the disease.[21]

CLOSTRIDIUM PERFRINGENS EXOTOXINS

The *C perfringens* exotoxins are all polypeptides that generally act by phospholipase damage to the plasma membrane or by forming pores or channels in the plasma membrane of host cells.[8] This process results in cellular membrane disruption and cell leakage of electrolytes or water. The alpha toxin gene is expressed from the chromosome of all *C perfringens* subtypes.[7,8] The genes encoding the other toxins are carried on large plasmids.[7,8] The enterotoxin gene can be either chromosomal or plasmid determined. In animal isolates, it is generally carried on a plasmid. However, it is chromosomally located on most (~70%) isolates from human cases of *C perfringens* food poisoning.[22] All of the toxins except CPE are secreted by vegetative bacteria. Enterotoxin is released after sporulation and bacterial cell lysis.[7,8,22]

Alpha Toxin

Alpha toxin is produced by all subtypes of *C perfringens*; however, the amount of toxin secreted varies by both isolate and type.[7] The alpha toxin gene (*plc*) is located on the bacterial chromosome. Alpha toxin is a phospholipase C sphingomyelinase (lecithinase) enzyme that binds to cell membranes and causes disruption of the lipid bilayer.[7,8,23] The toxin is hemolytic and dermonecrotic. Hydrolysis of lecithin by alpha -toxin produces diacylglycerol, which leads to stimulation of eukaryotic cell phospholipases and the arachidonic acid cascade.[8,23] This process can result in alterations in vascular permeability, platelet aggregation, and vasoconstriction. Alpha toxin has been shown to cause alterations in fluid transport within ileal and colonic loops in sheep.[24] Alpha toxin likely acts in concert with additional virulence factors, resulting in intestinal mucosal damage and, in particular, the *C perfringens* toxin perfringolysin (theta toxin) seems to work synergistically with alpha toxin in calves.[25,26]

Beta Toxin

Beta toxin is produced by type B and C strains of *C perfringens*. The beta toxin gene (*cpb*) is encoded on a large plasmid and codes for a small polypeptide protoxin. The protoxin is secreted from the vegetative bacteria and cleaved by proteases to produce the active toxin.[7] Beta toxin is classified as a pore-forming cytolysin, and is similar to other toxins, including *Staphylococcus aureus* alpha toxin. The channels formed by the beta toxin pores are selective for monovalent cations such as sodium and potassium.[27] Beta toxin is rapidly destroyed by trypsin.[3,7] Because of this, disease caused by types B and C tend to occur in young neonates less than 10 to 21 days of age because of the presence of trypsin inhibitors in colostrum and early milk. Disease may also occur later if bacterial or plant-derived trypsin inhibitors are present in the feed.

Epsilon Toxin

The epsilon toxin gene (*etx*) is carried by type B and D strains of *C perfringens*. The gene is encoded on a large plasmid.[7,8] The gene encodes a small polypeptide protoxin that is cleaved to the active toxin by intestinal proteases, including trypsin and chymo-trypsin.[28,29] C perfringens epsilon toxin is the third most potent bacterial toxin following botulinum toxin and tetanus toxins.[28] The toxin is lethal and dermonecrotic. Studies in lambs, goats, and calves show increased vascular permeability associated with exposure to epsilon toxin.[30–34] The toxin binds the plasma membrane of sensitive cells, including endothelial cells, and forms a complex with a particular membrane protein, resulting in altered membrane permeability by an unknown mechanism,[8,28,29] and this is the primary extent of disease observed in the intestine caused by epsilon toxin.

C perfringens epsilon toxin also results in systemic disorders in ruminant species (enterotoxemia). Toxin-induced damage to the intestinal mucosa allows absorption and systemic dissemination of the toxin. Disruption of endothelial cells causes vascular lesions and edema observed in the heart, lungs, and brain, resulting in peri-cardial effusion, pleural effusion, pulmonary edema, and perivascular cerebral edema.[28] Endothelial cell damage in the brain disrupts the blood-brain barrier, providing the toxin access to cerebral neurons and parenchymal cells. Epsilon toxin causes damage and necrosis to neurons, astrocytes, and oligodendrocytes, produc-ing the characteristic lesion of focal symmetric encephalomalacia.[29] Pore formation disrupts transmembrane K^+, Cl^-, Na^+, and Ca^{++} transport in affected cells. There is also an overexpression of the membrane channel protein aquaporin-4, resulting in a disruption of intracellular water balance. Sublethal intracerebroventricular injections of epsilon toxin into mice and rats produced neuronal degeneration in the cerebral cor-tex, hippocampus, striatum, and hypothalamus, resulting in permanent behavioral changes.[35] Dexamethasone was able to reduce the effects of epsilon toxin in these studies.

Iota Toxin

The iota toxin is a binary cytotoxin consisting of 2 subunits: Ia and Ib.[7,8,36] The genes coding for the toxin (iap and iab) are located on an extrachromosomal plasmid. Both subunits are required for toxicity. The Ib subunit constitutes the binding component and the Ia subunit is the enzymatic component. The Ib precursor protein is cleaved by trypsin and binds to the cell membrane, forming a heptameric complex. Ia subunits bind to this complex and enter the cell by receptor-mediated endocytosis. The Ib hep-tamer forms a pore within the endosome, allowing translocation of the Ia subunits to the cytoplasm. The Ia subunit has ADP-ribosylation activity resulting in the depolymer-ization of actin and inhibition of cell functions that are dependent on actin.

Enterotoxin

C perfringens enterotoxin is a primary toxin associated with food poisoning in humans, but its relationship to enteric disease in animals is not fully established. The CPE gene (cpe) can be located either on the bacterial chromosome or on an extrachromosomal plasmid.[7–9,22] The cpe gene is chromosomally determined in C perfringens isolates that cause food poisoning in humans. However, the cpe gene is plasmid determined in isolates from animals. The cpe gene is carried by less than 6% of C perfringens iso-lates. The enterotoxin gene is most commonly found in type A isolates but is also pre-sent in some type C, D, and E isolates.[22] Although the gene is expressed in A, C, and D isolates, it is silent in the type E isolates that have been identified. Enterotoxin is only expressed during the process of bacterial sporulation and then released when the vegetative C perfringens cells undergo lysis.[7,22] Expression is regulated at the tran-scriptional level. The toxin binds claudins in the cell membrane of enterocytes forming a large transmembrane pore complex that allows for calcium influx and cell death by either apoptosis or necrosis.[22] The CPE-claudin complex also causes destabilization of intercellular tight junctions and leakage between cells.

Beta-2 Toxin

The beta-2 toxin gene (cpb2) is located on an extrachromosomal plasmid and can be found in all subtypes of C perfringens. Although genetically distinct, the beta-2 toxin shows cytotoxic activity similar to that of C perfringens beta toxin (CPB; also designated beta-1 toxin).[8,37] The significance of the beta-2 toxin as related to disease caused by C perfringens has not been fully determined.[14,37–39] The toxin is likely a cofactor in the pathogenesis of abomasitis and enteritis when present but is not required for intestinal mucosal necrosis.

Novel Pore-forming Toxins

NetF toxin, a pore-forming toxin produced by a subset of C perfringens type A strains and related to the leukocidin/hemolysin superfamily, was recently associated with necrotizing enteritis in neonatal foals and with canine hemorrhagic gastroenteritis.[40,41] Similarly, NetB toxin (necrotic enteritis toxin B type) produced by some strains of C perfringens type A has been shown to be essential in causing necrotic enteritis in chickens.[42] These toxins form pores that result in disruption of the phospholipid membrane bilayer of cells and cause an ion influx that can lead to osmotic cell lysis.[43] Although it was previously thought that alpha toxin was the major toxin responsible for avian necrotic enteritis, Keyburn and colleagues[44] showed that alpha toxin null mutants were still virulent in an avian necrotic enteritis disease model. These novel toxins have not yet been shown to play a role in clostridial enteric diseases in ruminants.[45,46]

CLINICAL DISEASE

This article focuses on abomasitis and enteritis associated with C perfringens with clarification of the distinctions from true enterotoxemia. Enterotoxemia is a loosely used term for disease caused by C perfringens and is often used in reference to all clinical forms of C perfringens, including abomasitis and enteritis observed in cattle and other ruminants. This loose terminology can cause confusion when discussing the disease because it does not designate the specific genotype and clinical manifestations of C perfringens syndromes seen in cattle and other ruminants. The term enterotoxemia is best reserved for C perfringens diseases that include absorption and systemic spread of toxins with disorders in other organs beyond the intestinal tract. Clinical forms of the wide array of C perfringens disease syndromes are reviewed in **Table 2**.

Clostridial Abomasitis

All genotypes of C perfringens can cause abomasitis or enteritis in some or all domestic ruminant species. C perfringens type A is an increasingly common isolate associated with clostridial abomasitis in ruminants.[4,15,30,45,47–49] Type E has also been isolated in cases of abomasitis but seems to be rare.[47,49,50] Clostridial abomasitis has been reproduced experimentally by intraruminal inoculation of C perfringens type A in calves.[51] Clostridial abomasitis may be present by itself or combined with enteritis.

Type A abomasitis is most commonly observed in neonatal and juvenile animals but can also be observed in adult ruminants. C perfringens abomasitis is a sporadic disorder of neonatal to weanling calves, lambs, and kids.[15,45,47,49,52] The condition is common in both dairy and beef calves and seems to be less common in lambs and kid goats. Clinical signs include decreased nursing, lethargy, fluid distension of the abomasum, abdominal tympany, colic, and bruxism.[49] Animals generally have a normal temperature unless complications of systemic sepsis or peritonitis have developed, in which case their temperature can be decreased or increased. Mucous membranes may be pale with a prolonged capillary refill time indicating systemic shock. Hydration status is often normal in acute cases but dehydration can develop in animals that are not treated soon. Abdominal distension with a succussion splash is a predominant and consistent clinical sign (**Fig. 1**). The ability of *C perfringens* to produce gas contributes to gastric dilatation and intramural emphysema evident in affected animals. Abomasal tympany and the associated abdominal distension also causes respiratory difficulty because of pressure placed on the diaphragm. Abomasal distension can also result in hemodynamic effects that can lead to shock. The case fatality rate of clostridial abomasitis seems to be high when rapid treatment is not instituted (75%–100%).[15,45,47–49,51]

At necropsy, the abomasum is grossly distended and filled with hemorrhagic fluid and gas (**Fig. 2**A). Gross pathology is characterized by diffuse, hemorrhagic to necrotizing inflammation of the abomasal mucosa, frequently involving the deeper layers of the abomasal wall in severe or chronic cases (**Fig. 2**B). Abomasal ulceration (**Fig. 2**C) and perforation with peritonitis (**Fig. 2**D) may occur in a subset of affected animals. Intramural emphysema and edema of the abomasal wall may be present.

Other differential causes of abomasitis and abomasal tympany in ruminants include *Sarcina* spp,[47,53–55] *Salmonella*,[56–58] coccidiosis,[59] fungal infection,[60] immunosuppression, pica, trauma from coarse feed, trichobezoars, gastric ulcers, and

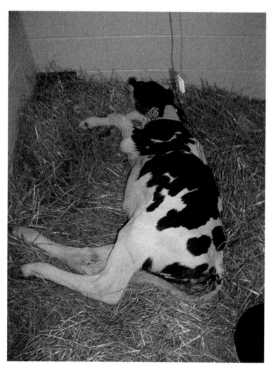

Fig. 1. A 3-week-old calf with abdominal distension caused by *C perfringens* type A abomasitis and enteritis.

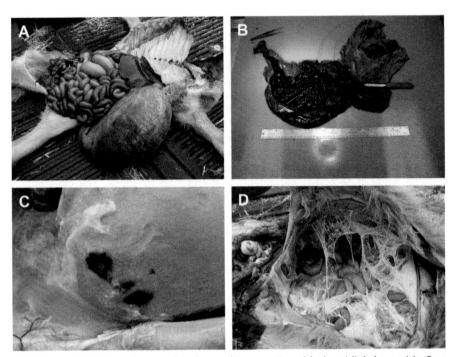

Fig. 2. Necropsy findings that may be observed in neonates with clostridial abomasitis. Common findings include grossly distended abomasum containing fluid and gas (*A*); diffuse, hemorrhagic to necrotizing inflammation of the abomasal mucosa (*B*); abomasal ulceration (*C*) with or without perforation resulting in fibrinous peritonitis (*D*).

vitamin or mineral deficiencies.[61] *Sarcina* spp are implicated as a cause of abomasitis and abomasal tympany in calves, sheep, and goats.[47,53–55] Abomasal coccidiosis is described in an 11-month-old female sheep with proliferative abomasitis.[59] *Salmonella typhimurium* DT104 was isolated from the abomasal wall of Midwestern veal calves with abomasitis.[56,57] *S typhimurium* was also isolated from an outbreak in ewes and lambs in which the primary clinical finding was abomasitis.[58] Copper deficiency has been associated with abomasitis and abomasal ulcers in beef calves.[61–63] However, Roeder and colleagues[51] showed that abomasitis can occur spontaneously and be induced experimentally in the absence of copper deficiency. Thus, although copper deficiency may act as a contributory factor for abomasitis and enteric disease of calves, it does not seem to be a requisite factor for either condition.

Clostridial Enteritis

Clostridial enteritis (inflammation of the small intestine) may be seen in concert with abomasitis or on its own. The condition is most commonly observed in young animals but may also occur in adult ruminants. Clostridial enteritis can be caused by all toxinotypes of *C perfringens*, although there are important differences. *C perfringens* type A is the most common cause of clostridial enteritis currently observed in ruminants in the United States, which may in part be caused by the routine use of clostridial C and D toxoids in ruminants in the United States resulting in antibodies to beta and epsilon toxins and providing effective protection against enteritis caused by *C perfringens* types B, C, and D. It may also be caused by geographic differences in the environmental and host distribution of toxinotypes B, C, D, and E.

Type A

Enteritis caused by *C perfringens* type A is observed in calves, lambs, and kid goats.[1,3,10,25,30,47,50,64,65] Enteritis is generally acute and develops over a period of hours. Appetite is significantly decreased. In most cases, diarrhea is not present in the acute stages. The animals generally have a normal temperature and may not show physical or clinicopathologic signs of sepsis or systemic inflammation unless the disease has progressed and generalized sepsis is present. At necropsy, the small intestine is hemorrhagic and distended with hemorrhagic contents (**Fig. 3**). The intestinal wall may be thickened with edema or, if intestinal distension is severe, may appear thin. Ultrasonography examination of affected patients often shows local or generalized areas of distended small intestine. The motility pattern of the affected segments is decreased, or seems to have a lack of coordinated progressive peristalsis. Gross pathology is characterized by segmental to diffuse, hemorrhagic or necrotizing inflammation of small intestinal mucosa. In some cases, mucosal damage can also affect the cecum or spiral colon.

    C perfringens type A is also associated with nonobstructive hemorrhagic enteritis in adult ruminants, particularly cattle. This condition in adult ruminants is poorly described in the literature. Type A hemorrhagic enteritis is less common in adults than in young animals. Clinical signs include acute onset of decreased appetite with right side or bilateral ventral abdominal distension (**Fig. 4**A). The animals may have a fever or be afebrile. Inflammatory changes to the complete blood count (CBC) are often absent but may be present because of translocation of enteric Gram-negative bacteria and secondary septicemia. Hemorrhagic diarrhea may not be apparent at the time of presentation (**Fig. 4**B) but may be apparent later in the course of the disease (**Fig. 4**D). Abdominal ultrasonography often reveals multiple loops of fluid-distended small intestine up to 5 cm in diameter (**Fig. 4**C). Intestinal motility is often decreased or lacks coordinated peristalsis. Scant feces may be noted upon rectal examination in early cases. The clinical signs are often difficult to discriminate from intestinal obstruction caused by intussusception, entrapment, or obstructing HBS. *C perfringens* type A can be cultured from affected small intestine and these

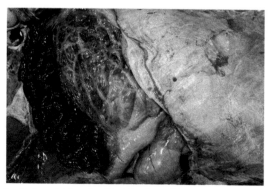

Fig. 3. Necropsy of a 3-day-old beef calf with *C perfringens* type A hemorrhagic enteritis. The cause was confirmed with anaerobic culture and mPCR genotyping.

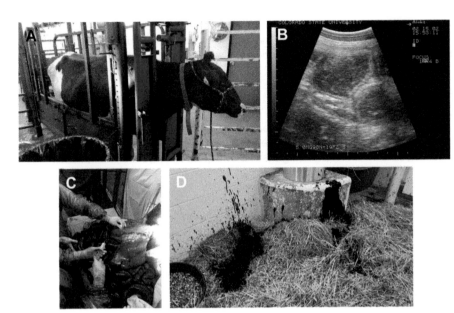

Fig. 4. Hemorrhagic *C perfringens* enteritis in an adult dairy cow. Note the right ventral abdominal distension caused by distension of the small intestine (*A*). Transabdominal ultrasonography shows dilated loops of small intestine up to 5 cm in diameter (*B*). A right flank exploratory laparotomy was performed and confirmed diffuse hemorrhagic enteritis (*C*). The cow received intraluminal procaine penicillin G in surgery. The following morning the cow had profuse hemorrhagic diarrhea (*D*), returned to eating, and recovered.

animals often respond to treatment directed toward intraluminal clostridial infection. At this time, it is unclear whether this is an enteritis condition distinct from HBS or part of a continuum of enteric disease caused by *C perfringens* type A that includes HBS.

Type A enterotoxemia of sheep (yellow lamb disease) is an apparently rare but highly fatal disorder that manifests as an acute hemolytic disease. Hemolysis is thought to be caused by either alpha toxin or perfringolysin (theta toxin) following absorption into the circulation secondary to damaged intestinal mucosa.

Type B
C perfringens type B causes acute hemorrhagic enterocolitis in neonatal ruminants. Type B enteritis is uncommon in North America but more common in the United Kingdom and Europe. In lambs, the condition is called lamb dysentery. Type B enteritis is also observed in calves and foals. The main contributing toxin is the beta toxin. The disease is restricted to young animals; generally, lambs less than 21 days of age and calves less than 10 days. The main factor responsible for this age restriction is the susceptibility of the beta toxin to destruction by trypsin (discussed further for *C perfringens* type C). Infection results in a severe acute hemorrhagic enterocolitis with high mortality similar to type C. Type C isolates also express epsilon toxin and can cause clinical signs of enterotoxemia because of systemic absorption and the action of the epsilon toxin.

Type C
Hemorrhagic enterocolitis caused by *C perfringens* type C is a commonly fatal disease that occurs in calves and lambs and is suspected to occur on rare occasions in

goats.[5,65,66] The hallmark of this disease is acute profuse hemorrhagic diarrhea. Neonates are most commonly affected, although disease losses in older calves and lambs can be significant. Intake of large quantities of soluble carbohydrate and/or protein is considered a risk factor for the development of type C enterotoxemia.[5,65] Neonates nursing heavily lactating dams seem to be at higher risk. Heavy grain feeding, foraging on grain crops, sudden access to high-quality forage, or overfeeding following a period of hunger are also considered risks.

The beta toxin is thought to be responsible for the acute necrohemorrhagic enterocolitis. The disease is generally restricted to neonatal ruminants because of the susceptibility of the beta toxin to proteolytic destruction by trypsin.[3,7] Beta toxin is active in young neonates because of the presence of trypsin inhibitors in colostrum and early postpartum milk. Trypsin inhibitors are present in milk for up to the first 10 to 21 days after parturition and place neonates that nurse postpartum dams at risk. The risk is less for neonates fed pooled milk, including milk from later lactation animals or milk replacer. Disease can occur in older ruminants if bacterial or plant-derived trypsin inhibitors are present in the feed.

Affected animals are acutely listless and reluctant to nurse. Ataxia, colic, bloody diarrhea, depression, and recumbency soon follow. Extensor rigidity and opisthotonus may be seen terminally, and death usually occurs within hours of the onset of signs. Severe hemorrhagic enterocolitis is the primary gross lesion at necropsy. This lesion tends to be most pronounced and is consistently found in the distal jejunum and ileum, although occasionally the entire small intestine or colon is involved.[5,67] Fibrin clots, casts of necrotic mucosa, and red-brown blood may be present within the intestinal lumen. An increased amount of clear, straw-colored, or serosanguinous fluid may be found within the peritoneal, pleural, and pericardial cavities.

Type D

Enteritis is not the predominant clinical feature of enteric infection with *C perfringens* type D. Clinical enteritis is rare in calves and lambs. Goats more consistently show clinical signs of GI dysfunction with type D infection, including gross and histologic lesions of enteritis.[33,68–71] In the peracute form of this disease, affected goats may be found dead or may have colic. Abdominal distension, vocalizing, dyspnea, tachypnea, and watery diarrhea containing fibrin, mucus, or strands of blood may occur. Recumbency, respiratory distress, and convulsions associated with true enterotoxemia usually follow, and death typically occurs within hours of the onset of signs.

C perfringens type D is responsible for true enterotoxemia in small ruminants of all ages.[5,65] Type D enterotoxemia in calves is rare.[72] Enteritis is not a consistent clinical finding with enterotoxemia except in goats. *C perfringens* type D is not considered to be a common inhabitant of the GI tract of normal ruminants, although it can be carried sporadically by healthy animals.[65] As with type C enterotoxemia, passage of soluble carbohydrates or protein into the small intestine is thought to induce rapid replication and elaboration of epsilon toxin from this organism.[66] Unlike beta toxin, however, epsilon toxin is activated by intestinal and pancreatic proteases.[5,7,8] Once absorbed into the bloodstream, epsilon toxin causes loss of endothelial integrity, increased capillary permeability, and edema formation in multiple tissues.[73] Epsilon toxin also causes damage and necrosis to neurons, astrocytes, and oligodendrocytes, producing the characteristic lesion of focal symmetric encephalomalacia and is responsible for the neurologic signs observed with this disease.[29]

Type D enterotoxemia in sheep is typically a peracute illness, with many cases simply being found dead. If a live ovine case is detected, neurologic signs predominate.

Lethargy and ataxia are evident early, with collapse, hyperesthesia, lateral recumbency, convulsive paddling, and opisthotonus following within hours. Diarrhea is inconsistently seen. Glucosuria is frequently present in sheep.[74]

At necropsy examination, the effusion is typically observed in the peritoneal, pleural, or pericardial spaces with variable volumes of straw-colored or red fluid that may contain fibrin clots. Petechial hemorrhages are often visible on the visceral surfaces. Pulmonary and mesenteric edema may be evident. Gross lesions of the intestinal tract are frequently absent in affected sheep. Dipstick analysis of urine collected from the bladder frequently reveals the presence of glucose in sheep. The renal cortex may be softened (hence the term pulpy kidney), although this is a nonspecific autolytic change seen on occasion in small ruminant cadavers. The classic pathologic lesion is focal symmetric encephalomalacia. Occasionally, no gross lesions are seen in ovine cases of type D enterotoxemia.[66]

Unlike sheep, goats affected by type D enterotoxemia more consistently show signs of GI dysfunction, and gross and histologic lesions are more consistently found in the GI tract.[33,68–71] In the peracute form of this disease, affected goats may be found dead or may have colic. Abdominal distension, vocalizing, dyspnea, tachypnea, and watery diarrhea containing fibrin, mucus, or strands of blood may occur. Recumbency, respiratory distress, and convulsions usually follow, and death typically occurs within hours of the onset of signs. Glucosuria is not consistently detected in goats with enterotoxemia.[69]

The clinical signs of the acute form of type D enterotoxemia in goats are similar to those of the peracute form, but the progression of the disease occurs over 2 to 4 days. Intermittent or protracted diarrhea, weight loss, and reduced milk production are evident in the chronic form of enterotoxemia in goats. In this form of the disease, clinical signs may persist for several days or occur intermittently over weeks or months. Chronic enterotoxemia may be difficult to diagnose unless prior peracute or acute cases are known to have occurred in the herd. GI parasitism, salmonellosis, Johne disease, and rumen acidosis are important differential diagnoses.

The most prominent gross postmortem lesion in goats with peracute or acute type D enterotoxemia is fibrinohemorrhagic colitis, which is usually most severe in the spiral colon.[33] Luminal casts of fibrin, blood, and mucus may be present, and a pseudomembrane may form in affected colonic segments. The colonic serosa may be hyperemic or edematous, with edema evident in the colonic mesentery and mesenteric lymph nodes. Pulmonary edema, fluid, and fibrin in the thoracic and abdominal cavities and pericardium, and scattered ecchymotic hemorrhages on serosal surfaces may be present. Occasionally caprine cases of peracute type D enterotoxemia show no gross lesions. Chronic cases may show scant body fat reserves and ulcerated colonic mucosa. Glucosuria is inconsistently found.[69]

Type E

Enteritis caused by C perfringens type E is rare but has been reported in goats, calves, and adult cattle.[50,75,76] Clinical signs range from mild diarrhea to severe hemorrhagic enteritis. Type E isolates are not considered to be a common cause of abomasitis or enteritis in cattle. However, their presence makes appropriate diagnostic differentiation important when evaluating cases of clostridial abomasitis or enteritis in ruminants.

PREDISPOSING FACTORS

The underlying factors that allow overgrowth and toxin expression of C perfringens in ruminants are considered multifactorial. Three key components seem to be involved in clostridial abomasitis and enteritis:

1. The presence of C perfringens within the GI tract
2. Sufficient carbohydrate or protein nutrients to support bacterial growth
3. Decreased GI motility that allows segmental overgrowth of the bacteria within the GI tract

C perfringens type A is ubiquitous in the livestock environment and is considered normal flora at low levels in the healthy ruminant.[7,8,45,47,77] Fecal shedding maintains persistence in the environment. Other toxinotypes are not found as consistently in the environment or from fecal samples of ruminants.

All forms of enteric disease caused by C perfringens seem to be associated with increased intake of feeds rich in soluble carbohydrate, protein, or both. Heavy grain feeding, foraging on grain crops, sudden access to high-quality forage, or overfeeding following a period of hunger are also considered risks. Consumption of large volumes of milk at individual feedings also seems to increase risk in nursing ruminants.

Clostridial abomasitis and enteritis in neonatal beef calves is associated with management practices that cause delays in regular nursing patterns (eg, calf separation at branding) or changes in environment that interrupt normal nursing patterns (eg, winter storms).[62] In dairy calves, poor milk hygiene, intermittent feeding of large volumes of milk, and milk replacers with higher carbohydrate or protein concentrations are thought to be contributory factors.

There are many factors that can decrease intestinal motility. Abomasal emptying in nursing calves can be delayed by feeding large volumes in single feedings, feeding with an esophageal tube, high caloric content, and high osmolality of the milk.[78] Enteric pathogens can alter intestinal motility, including rotavirus, coronavirus, cryptosporidia, and coccidia. Cases of C perfringens enteritis have been associated with concurrent coccidiosis in cattle and New World camelids.[79–81] Other factors, such as abomasal ulcers, coarse feed, foreign bodies, hairballs, and mineral deficiencies, may be associated with abomasal tympany and increase the risk of C perfringens overgrowth in the abomasum.[61]

CLINICAL PATHOLOGY

Because the pathogenesis of the disease is primarily an enterotoxemia, signs of systemic inflammation are often not observed. A CBC may show a neutrophilia without a left shift and normal fibrinogen, suggestive of a physiologic response or a stress response. An inflammatory leukogram is rarely seen unless there is sufficient mucosal compromise to allow for Gram-negative bacterial translocation and/or systemic endotoxin absorption. Most parameters on the serum chemistry are normal. The creatinine and/or blood urea nitrogen level may be increased if systemic shock has resulted in decreased renal perfusion. Sheep and sometimes goats with type D enterotoxemia may be hyperglycemic and glucosuric. Total protein level is usually not increased because systemic dehydration is often not present in peracute or acute cases. The serum chloride may be decreased because of intestinal ileus and delayed abomasal emptying, and metabolic alkalosis may be present in early cases. Metabolic acidosis and increased lactate levels are common in later stages of the disease.

DIAGNOSIS

Definitive diagnosis of C perfringens abomasitis or enteritis has challenges and must rely on clinical signs, gross and microscopic pathology, and appropriate microbiological tests to show the presence of the organism.[10] mPCR is currently used to categorize this diverse species into distinct types, or genotypes. Genotyping is based on detection of gene sequences for alpha, beta, beta-2, epsilon, and iota toxins and enterotoxin.[13,14,82,83] The presence of the gene for a particular toxin reflects the potential to produce that toxin. It is critical to note that expression of major lethal toxins is not consistent across clinical isolates within a particular genotype. Thus, the potential pathogenicity of isolates within each genotype is suspected to be variable.

Interpretation of positive culture results for *C perfringens* from the intestinal lumen of a ruminant is a complicated matter. *C perfringens* type A inhabits the intestine of normal animals and can overgrow in the gut lumen postmortem.[5,65] Thus, its isolation should be considered significant only from a fresh cadaver with compatible history, clinical signs, and lesions. The organism is easily grown in vitro; *C perfringens* type A grows rapidly in anaerobic culture and may overgrow other potential pathogens.[65] Although quantitative culture is considered helpful in discriminating normal flora from overgrowth, a recent study in veal calves showed no difference in bacterial counts between normal veal calves and veal calves with clostridial enteritis.[84] Diagnosis of clostridial abomasitis or enteritis therefore requires a combination of observations that may include:

- Observation of abdominal distension with colic.
- The presence of hemorrhagic abomasitis or enteritis (see **Figs. 2B** and **3**). Abomasitis or enteritis may additionally be suggested by ultrasonographic findings.
- Cytologic evidence of high numbers of gram-positive rods in abomasal or intestinal contents, feces, or on the mucosal surface of tissues (**Fig. 5**).
- Culture of *C perfringens* in high numbers from abomasal or intestinal contents, feces, or tissue samples.
- Demonstration of the presence of alpha, beta, or epsilon toxin by mouse neutralization test or enzyme-linked immunosorbent assay (ELISA). However, toxin assays for the lethal toxins are not readily available from commercial diagnostic laboratories in the United States. Toxin detection test kits are available from BioX in Belgium (http://www.biox.com).

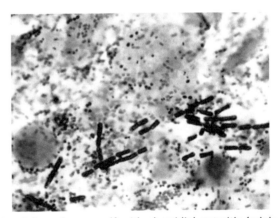

Fig. 5. Gram stain of feces from a calf with clostridial enteritis (original magnification, ×1000). Note the group of large Gram positive rods within the background of other bacterial flora. Cytologic evidence of high numbers of large Gram-positive rods in ingesta or feces is suggestive of, but not definitive for, clostridial abomasitis and/or enteritis. The presence of white blood cells, red blood cells, and sloughed mucosal epithelium indicates inflammation with mucosal necrosis and hemorrhage. In early cases of abomasitis or enteritis, changes in fecal flora may not initially be observed.

Recommended samples for diagnostic testing include[2,10]:

- Abomasal or intestinal contents or feces for cytologic evaluation.
- Impression smear of the mucosal surface of the affected GI tract for cytology including Gram stain.
- Intestinal contents, tissues, or feces for anaerobic culture and PCR identification of genotype. Samples should be collected antemortem and/or immediately post-mortem to avoid normal postmortem clostridial overgrowth.
- Abomasum, small intestine, and colon in 10% buffered formalin for histopathology.
- Brain in 10% formalin for histopathology if neurologic signs are observed and C perfringens type D (or B) is suspected.
- Intestinal contents, refrigerated or frozen for toxin detection.

TREATMENT

There is very limited information on the efficacy of treatment methods for abomasitis and enteritis caused by C perfringens. The following information is based on treatment protocols at the contributing authors' institution that seem to be effective in treating animals with clinical signs consistent with clostridial abomasitis or enteritis. Treatment of abomasal or enteric clostridial disease should focus on 6 goals:

1. Relief of abdominal distension, particularly if respiration is compromised because of abdominal pressure on the diaphragm.
2. Systemic and nutritional support with intravenous (IV) fluids if indicated.
3. Preventing ongoing bacterial proliferation.
4. Decreasing or preventing production of and neutralizing clostridial exotoxins.
5. Restore normal GI flora.
6. Pain management as needed.

The abdominal distension in cases of clostridial abomasitis and enteritis is caused by gas and fluid distension of the abomasum and/or small intestine. The gaseous distension is a result of a combination of ileus and bacterial gas production. In most cases, passage of an orogastric tube does not provide significant relief. If the distension is severe enough that it is compromising respiration, then percutaneous decompression of the abomasum can be performed. This decompression is best done with the animal in dorsal or left lateral recumbency (**Fig. 6**).[85] The area of tympany is localized and quickly clipped and prepared for an aseptic procedure. A percutaneous abomasocentesis can then be performed using a 16-gauge to 20-gauge, 38-mm (1.5-inch) needle inserted directly through the skin into the abomasum. An extension set can be attached to the needle. Allow the gas to freely escape while placing slight pressure on the abdomen. Fluid that drains from the needle can be collected for anaerobic culture, PCR typing, or toxin assays. Before removing the needle, antimicrobials and C perfringens type C and D antitoxin can be administered directly into the abomasum (these syringes should be prepared and ready before starting the abomasocentesis).

Systemic support generally involves administration of IV fluids. Because the animals typically have ileus and abdominal distension, oral fluids, including milk, are not indicated until the distension is resolved (generally 12–24 hours). IV fluids provide systemic support in treatment of the hypovolemic or maldistributive shock that is often observed in these patients. Some animals with clostridial enteritis do not show significant clinical dehydration, most likely because of the rapid effects of the toxins. Shock fluid rates are 80 mL/kg, and can be divided into one-quarter doses

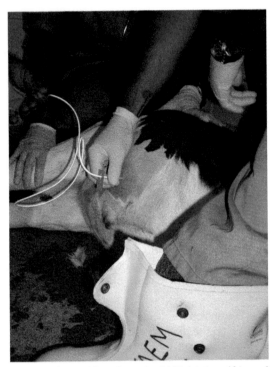

Fig. 6. Abomasocentesis performed in a 3-week-old Holstein calf in order to decompress a tightly distended abomasum. This procedure is best done with the calf in dorsal or left lateral recumbency. Following decompression, fluid samples can be obtained for culture and genotyping as well as cytology. Antibiotics and antitoxin can also be administered directly into the abomasum.

given to effect at intervals of 15 to 30 minutes. Once the shock has been addressed, the fluid rate can be decreased to a maintenance rate of 3 mL/kg/h. Dextrose (5%) can also be provided in the maintenance fluids, because milk is likely to be withheld for 12 to 24 hours. Many animals with clostridial enteritis show mild to moderate hypochloremic metabolic alkalosis caused by the intestinal ileus and delayed abomasal emptying. Thus, isotonic sodium chloride is a suitable initial fluid type to resolve the hypochloremic alkalosis if present. Animals in later stages of the disease may show metabolic acidosis and require the addition of sodium bicarbonate to fluids. IV fluids can be changed to a balanced electrolyte solution after resolution of the shock, or within the first 12 hours.

Antimicrobials are used to slow or stop clostridial proliferation in the GI tract. The challenge is that the bacteria reside within the lumen so antimicrobial treatment must be selected such that an appropriate antimicrobial is delivered to the lumen of the abomasum and small intestine. Many antimicrobials are effective against *C perfringens*. Penicillin is one of the most effective antibiotics at killing *C perfringens*; however, penicillin does not immediately kill the bacteria. During the initial phase, the bacteria may continue to produce and release lethal exotoxins.[86] Further, systemically administered penicillin is excreted via the renal system and is minimally excreted or secreted into the GI tract. Thus, oral procaine penicillin G (22,000 IU/kg, by mouth, every 24 hours for 3–5 days) may be recommended for treatment and has been used by the authors. Most *C perfringens* isolates are susceptible to oxytetracycline. Oxytetracycline is a bacteriostatic agent that inhibits protein synthesis. Oxytetracycline reduces *C perfringens* toxin production in vitro more rapidly than penicillin.[86] Systemically administered oxytetracycline is partially excreted through the liver and biliary system and enters the lumen of the GI tract through the common bile duct. Both oral penicillin and systemic or oral oxytetracycline, alone or in combination, have been found to be clinically effective in treating acute cases of clostridial enteritis at Colorado State University (authors' personal experience). Metronidazole, although effective against *C perfringens*, is a substituted benzimidazole and is illegal in all food animals including cattle, sheep, goats, and swine.

One study with a food safety focus has suggested that use of egg yolk antibody from hens immunized against *C perfringens* could significantly inhibit the growth and sporulation of *C perfringens* in vitro.[87] An oral product intended for calves that contains egg-derived antibodies from hens immunized against *C perfringens* types A, C, and D is commercially available (EPIC Calf Scour Formula, Tomlyn), but its use in treatment or prevention of clinical cases of *C perfringens* has not been described.

In addition to administering an appropriate antimicrobial, bacterial proliferation may be decreased by withholding milk feedings for a period of 12 to 24 hours. In cases in which medical treatment is successful, the calves generally want to nurse within 12 to 24 hours. It is critical that, after this time, milk feeding is reinstituted slowly in small volumes (500 mL [1 pint]) at more frequent intervals (every 4 to 6 hours). Overfeeding can result in a relapse of *C perfringens* overgrowth.

Attempts to restore normal GI flora may also be beneficial once oral intake resumes. Oral administration of fresh rumen fluid may help restore normal GI flora in affected animals. Alternatively, commercially available probiotics can be administered. Placement of an indwelling nasogastric tube greatly facilitates frequent administration of oral medications and transfaunation in patients that do not quickly regain nursing activity.

There is limited information on effective treatments for neutralizing *C perfringens* toxins. In the case of clostridial toxins that work directly on the GI mucosa, neutralization must occur within the GI lumen to be most effective. *C perfringens* type C and D antitoxin contains antibodies against the beta and epsilon toxins and may provide efficacy against enteritis caused by *C perfringens* types B, C, and D. Systemically administered antitoxin may not reach effective concentrations within the GI tract. However, it is highly effective at neutralizing systemically absorbed epsilon toxin (*C perfringens* types D and B) associated with neurologic signs of enterotoxemia. When treating enteric clostridiosis, the authors recommend a combination of both systemic and oral C and D antitoxin at the labeled amounts.

Di-tri-octahedral smectite (Bio-Sponge, Platinum Performance) has been shown to bind *C perfringens* alpha, beta, and beta-2 toxins, and enterotoxin.[88,89] Kaolin-pectin and bismuth subsalicylate have also been used to bind *C perfringens* toxins; however, there are limited data showing efficacy. Both kaolin-pectin and bismuth subsalicylate could have clinical benefit in treating the damaged mucosal epithelium. Kaolin in Kaopectate is a potent activator of the extrinsic clotting cascade and may help decrease intestinal blood loss in cases with hemorrhagic gastroenteritis. Use of proton pump inhibitors in an attempt to limit mucosal ulceration in clostridial abomasitis cases should likely be discouraged, because there is evidence that these are a risk factor for the development of some types of clostridial GI infections in humans.[90]

Pain management should be used on an as-needed basis in these cases. Nonsteroidal antiinflammatories should be used judiciously, because severe shock and decreased renal perfusion may be present. In addition, GI ulceration can occur from the primary disease process, and this could be exacerbated by use or overuse of nonsteroidal antiinflammatory drugs such as flunixin meglumine or meloxicam. A low dose of flunixin meglumine, as is used to treat the effects of Gram-negative sepsis (0.25 mg/kg IV every 6 hours or 0.3 mg/kg IV every 8 hours) may be preferable to using the labeled cattle dose (up to 2.2 mg/kg IV every 24 hours). Opioids are an alternative selection for pain control but can decrease GI motility and should therefore be used cautiously in cases of suspected clostridial gastroenteritis. However, use of butorphanol intramuscularly (0.02–0.1 mg/kg every 6–8 hours) or as a constant rate infusion (CRI) (13 µg/kg/h) in horses with anterior enteritis is reported to have minimal effects on GI motility.[91] As with all drugs used extralabel in food-producing species, the Food Animal Residue Avoidance Databank (www.farad.org) should be consulted for a meat and/or milk withdrawal time before the administration of any of these agents.

Early medical treatment of *C perfringens* type A abomasitis and enteritis cases can often have dramatic success (**Fig. 7**). Calves are often standing and eager to nurse within 12 to 24 hours when treatment is initiated early. It is important to initially limit milk intake to smaller frequent quantities and gradually return to a normal feeding over 5 to 10 days. Differentiation of *C perfringens* type A hemorrhagic enteritis in adult cattle may be difficult to distinguish from intestinal obstruction. In these cases, an exploratory laparotomy may be performed. Distended hemorrhagic small intestine without intraluminal obstruction is observed (see **Fig. 4**C). During surgery, intestinal samples can be obtained at surgery for bacterial culture, genotyping, and cytology if indicated. Treatment can be initiated intraoperatively with intraluminal injections of penicillin. In our experience, exploratory laparotomy in these cases has not seemed to be detrimental and greatly aids confirmation of a diagnosis and initial treatment.

PREVENTION
Vaccination

Vaccination is considered to be the cornerstone of preventive programs for clostridial diseases in livestock.[72,92] Conventional commercial *C perfringens* C and D or 7-way or

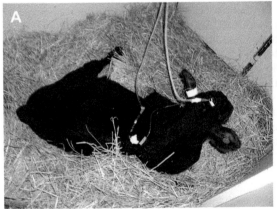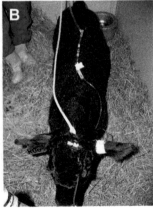

Fig. 7. Beef calf with suspected *C perfringens* abomasitis. The calf showed marked abdominal distension and abomasal tympany at presentation (*A*). The calf was treated medically and the abdominal distension resolved within 24 hours (*B*).

8-way toxoid vaccines are very effective at preventing disease caused by *C perfringens* types B, C, and D in young animals. Type B disease, however, is very rare in the United States. In the following review of the literature, summaries to facilitate evidence-based decisions are presented. It is critical to understand that the conclusions reached in these studies should be related to the specific vaccine products tested in each trial.

In sheep in North America, immunization against the major toxins of *C perfringens* types C and D is warranted. Tetanus is also considered an essential component of a flock immunization program.[93,94] In a 1962 study in sheep, Sterne and colleagues[95] showed that a multivalent, alum-adjuvanted, formalin-inactivated clostridial bacterin-toxoid administered to sheep in 2 doses induced titers deemed protective against the beta and epsilon toxins of *C perfringens*. In another study, antibody titers to epsilon toxin of *C perfringens* type D were induced in sheep immunized with a 2-dose series of a multivalent (8-way) clostridial vaccine.[96] Immunization of ewes 3 weeks before lambing has been shown to induce colostral antibody titers against epsilon toxin that were adequate to impart protection of lambs for up to 12 weeks of age.[97] In that study, adding a 2-dose immunization of the lambs at either days 1 and 21 of age or days 21 and 42 of age did not significantly change the titer of passively protected lambs. Immunization of lambs from vaccinated ewes (that do not have failure or suspected failure of passive transfer) with a *C perfringens* C and D and tetanus toxoid is recommended at 8 to 12 weeks of age and again 3 to 4 weeks later.[94] Feeder lambs (and ideally replacement ewe lambs) can also receive a booster before entering the feedlot or being placed on a high-grain ration.[94]

In goats, most enterotoxemia cases in North America seem to be caused by *C perfringens* type D.[66] Administration of multivalent ovine enterotoxemia vaccines twice annually to goats has been shown to be ineffective in protecting goats against fatal type D enterotoxemia.[70] Goats do respond, albeit variably, to the epsilon toxin component of *C perfringens* type D vaccines labeled for sheep.[68] The disparity in protection among the two species may reflect disparate mechanisms of disease. In sheep, most pathologic lesions seem to be the result of translocation of epsilon toxin from the gut to remote organs; for example, the brain. Circulating antitoxin antibodies against epsilon toxin seem to be critical in protecting sheep. In goats, however, the more localized disease process (enterocolitis) does not seem to be effectively or consistently curtailed by anti–epsilon toxin antibodies in the bloodstream.[33,68,69] However, in a 1998 study, immunization with an epsilon toxoid combined with Freund incomplete adjuvant did protect goats against intraduodenal challenge with purified epsilon toxin, whereas a commercial, aluminum hydroxide–adjuvanted product did not.[33] Existing *C perfringens* C and D toxoids may need to be administered to goats more than twice per year to confer adequate (albeit partial) protection.[70]

Administration of *C perfringens* type C and D to cattle has been shown to induce protective titers against both the beta toxin[98] and epsilon toxin[99] in recipients. Neonates and young, growing animals in stocker operations and feedlots are considered to be at higher risk for clostridial diseases relative to adults, but the risk seems to vary among herds.[72,92] For the former group, immunization of pregnant cows and heifers has been shown to produce antitoxin titers considered adequate for protection against type C and D infections in colostrum-fed calves.[99] Many ranchers immunize calves with multivalent clostridial vaccines before weaning, but, in many cases, repeat immunization of calves to provoke an anamnestic titer is not consistently performed during the preweaning period. Troxel and colleagues[99] determined that vaccination of colostrum-fed calves (from immunized dams) with a multivalent clostridial vaccine at 50 to 53 days of age and again at weaning at ~170 days produced titers to beta and epsilon toxin that were not considered protective for calves during the preweaning period. The investigators concluded that this 4-month gap between the first and second immunizations may not be optimal for herds in which clostridial diseases occur in preweaned calves, and alterations in management and/or vaccination schedule would be warranted in such cases. In another study, immunization of colostrum-fed calves (from immunized dams) at 3 weeks of age with a single-dose clostridial bacterin-toxoid did not significantly affect type C or D antitoxin titers over the first 4 months of life; however, significant differences in antitoxin titers among different vaccines were apparent.[100]

In a 2000 survey of feedlot operators, more than 90% of operators overseeing lots with a capacity more than 8000 head used at least 1 type of clostridial vaccine in their cattle.[101] In a prospective feedlot study involving nearly 19,000 animals, death losses were compared among calves immunized against clostridial diseases and those that were not.[102] Treated calves were administered a 7-way clostridial vaccine at arrival and 30 days later. Reduction in death loss in the vaccinated calves, weighed against purchase price and vaccine cost, provided an additional net profit of more than $10 per vaccinate.[102] More recently, DeGroot and colleagues[103] found no detectable effect of booster vaccination with a multivalent clostridial vaccine on sudden death syndrome mortality in feedlot cattle.

Although the former study has sometimes been used as justification for use of clostridial vaccines in feedlot calves,[92] additional research has investigated the potential detrimental effects of this use. Because ownership is not always retained for groups of cattle moving from ranch to feedlot, the immunization history of incoming cattle at a feedlot is not always known. As a result, some animals may receive multiple (predicted as many as 6) clostridial vaccinations before marketing, potentially compounding problems with injection site reactions in carcasses.[104] When administered subcutaneously twice to feedlot calves, a 7-way clostridial vaccine induced significant reduction in feed intake after the second immunization and larger injection site lesions than did a C perfringens type C and D toxoid.[104]

C perfringens type C and D toxoid vaccines are not designed to specifically stimulate an immune response against alpha toxin. Thus, these vaccines are generally not considered to be effective at preventing abomasitis or enteritis caused by type A strains. One commercial type A toxoid vaccine is available (Clostridium Perfringens Type A Toxoid, Elanco) and has been shown to be safe and stimulate an antibody response against alpha toxin. However, because of the difficulty in developing a satisfactory experimental challenge model, efficacy has not yet been shown in order to have a preventive label. Autogenous C perfringens type A vaccines can also be used. The efficacy of these vaccines for C perfringens is still not established. A recent study has shown that although formaldehyde inactivated alpha toxin vaccines stimulated antibody production similar to native alpha toxin vaccines, only antibodies produced from the native toxin vaccines provided protection in an intestinal loop assay.[105] Recombinant vaccines may offer advantages compared with conventional toxoid vaccines in the future.[106]

C perfringens vaccination strategies based on species, age, and animal use are provided in **Table 3**.

Feeding and Environmental Management

Presentation of excessive amounts of starch, sugar, or soluble protein into the stomach and/or intestines is considered pivotal in the development of these diseases; thus, all potential influences on this crucial event must be considered when formulating a preventive plan. Evaluation of ration net energy, fiber content and forage length, bunk space, animal hierarchy within a pen, feeding frequency, the rate and magnitude of changes in ration between successive production groups, and feed mixing practices is essential to identify and correct problems with carbohydrate overload and/or so-called slug feeding. For pasture-fed animals, turnout onto a new, particularly lush pasture should be very gradual (eg, day 1, 15 minutes of grazing; day 2, 30 minutes; day 3, 1 hour; day 4, 2 hours; and so forth).

Prevention of enterotoxemia in nursing animals requires consideration of environmental or management factors that may trigger changes in milk composition or volume for lactating dams. Intermittent provision of high-energy supplements to range animals may trigger changes in milk production. Similarly, management practices that cause prolonged interruption of suckling (eg, cow processing for pregnancy examination) must be made time-efficient in order to limit engorgement of the udder and subsequent ingestion by the neonate of a larger-than-normal milk meal. Sudden and severe changes in weather may cause dams and their offspring to seek shelter or remain recumbent for prolonged periods of time; provision of multiple locales for shelter and bedding, or simply encouraging dams to eat by providing hay (weather permitting) may encourage more frequent nursing than if the animals were left to "sit the storm out."

In dairy calves, variable or improper mixing of milk replacers may increase the incidence of clostridial GI disease. Milk replacers should be mixed at the appropriate concentration and temperature. Some milk replacers are prone to settling out and can result in variable concentrations between what is fed from the start to the finish of a single batch. Milk replacers high in protein and carbohydrate may also promote clostridial overgrowth in the GI tract.

Clostridium difficile

Clostridium difficile is another potential cause of enteritis, but the relationship between *C difficile* infection (CDI) and GI disease in ruminants is unclear because the bacterium may be present in the feces of clinically normal animals. A high prevalence of *C difficile* shedding has been described in otherwise healthy young calves; in one study, 14.9% of calves without clinical disease were shedding the organism.[108] In otherwise healthy veal calves, CDI has been reported to be as high as 51%.[109] *C difficile* shedding has also been detected in dairy cows,[110] feedlot cattle,[111] sheep,[112] and goats.[113]

Hammitt and colleagues[114] found *C difficile* and its toxins (toxin A and toxin B) in 25.3% and 22.9%, respectively, of calves with diarrhea. Diarrheic calves were twice as likely to be culture positive compared with those without diarrhea.[114] Nondiarrheic calves, however, more commonly had toxin-positive stools.[114] This team of researchers concluded that these findings lent credence to the idea that CDI may manifest as diarrhea in young cattle.[114]

C difficile–associated diarrhea (CDAD) was also suspected in a neonatal elk calf, based on finding a toxigenic *C difficile* fecal isolate in the absence of other more common enteropathogens.[115] Similarly, the authors have tentatively diagnosed 3 alpaca crias with CDAD based on fecal ELISAs positive for *C difficile* toxins A and/or B, in combination with exclusion of other common infectious causes of camelid diarrhea and a history of prior antimicrobial administration (authors' personal experience). It is possible that CDAD in livestock occurs more frequently than reported, but it remains underdiagnosed because attempted identification of *C difficile* and its toxins is not routinely performed in most diarrheic ruminants.

Table 3
Summary of current best-practice *Clostridium perfringens* toxoid vaccine recommendations for disease prevention, based on review of the literature

Species and Age Group	Type of Vaccine	Timing and Frequency of Vaccination	Reasoning and Type of Immunity Induced
Bred heifers and adult cows, both beef and dairy	• *C perfringens* type C and D, or 7-way or 8-way vaccines	• Initial immunization followed by booster 3–4 wk later • Second dose (and additional boosters) 2–3 wk before calving[107]	• Provides immunity against the beta and epsilon toxins in calves via colostral transfer • Enteric immunity from anti–beta toxin colostral antibody during the first 2 wk of life is critical in preventing disease from types B and C, because trypsin inhibitors in colostrum prevent denaturation of beta toxin • Systemic immunity from anti–epsilon toxin antibodies are effective at neutralizing systemically absorbed epsilon toxin and preventing neurologic signs from type D ± type B infections
	• *C perfringens* type A	• Initial immunization followed by booster in 2–4 wk, then: • Yearly 2–4 wk before calving	• *C perfringens* C and D toxoid vaccines are not designed to specifically stimulate an immune response against alpha toxin and usually are not considered effective at preventing abomasitis or enteritis caused by type A • May be particularly important in farms with a history of type A outbreaks in calves • Might also be useful in adult cows on dairies with a history of HBS
Feedlot cattle	• *C perfringens* types C and D, 7-way or 8-way vaccines	• At arrival and 30 d later, or: • Initial immunization and booster 3–4 wk apart before arrival	• Potential reduction in death loss • 7-way vaccines may induce decreased feed intake and larger injection-site lesions after booster compared with C and D vaccines
Beef and dairy calves (particularly from herds with previous *C perfringens* type C or D outbreaks)	• *C perfringens* types C and D, or 7-way or 8-way vaccines	• 3–6 mo of age • Initial immunization followed by booster 3–4 wk later	• In cattle, classic type D disease most commonly observed in older, weaned animals on high-concentrate feed • Maternal antibodies may have decreased to nonprotective levels by this age

Adult sheep	• C perfringens types C and D, or 7-way or 8-way vaccines	• Initial series of 2 doses 3–4 wk apart, then yearly boosters[94]	• Provides immunity against beta and epsilon toxins
Bred ewes	• C perfringens types C and D, or 7-way or 8-way vaccines	• Yearly booster 3–4 wk before lambing	• Provides immunity in lambs against epsilon toxin for up to 12 wk
Lambs from vaccinated dams	• C perfringens types C and D	• 8–12 wk of age and booster 3–4 wk later	• Feeder lambs and replacement ewe lambs should receive boosters again before feedlot entry or being placed on high-grain diet
Lambs from unvaccinated dams or with suspected FPT	• C perfringens types C and D	• 1–3 wk of age • Booster twice: 3–4 wk and 6–8 wk later[94]	• Feeder lambs and replacement ewe lambs should receive boosters again before feedlot entry or being placed on high-grain diet
Adult goats and kids	• C perfringens types C and D, or 7-way or 8-way vaccines	• >2 immunizations per year • 3 immunizations per year, with initial booster dose 3–4 wk later	• May still only provide partial protection • Type D disease most common in goats, and is not prevented by 2 doses of multivalent ovine enterotoxemia vaccines • This may in part be caused by minimal antibody excretion into GI tract in localized enterocolitis in goats vs systemic antibody protection needed in sheep because of effects of absorbed epsilon toxin
Bred does	• C perfringens types C and D, or 7-way or 8-way vaccines	• One of the yearly boosters given 3–4 wk before kidding	—

Abbreviation: FPT, failure of passive transfer.

SUMMARY

Clostridial abomasitis and enteritis remain common clinical diseases in livestock, particularly in young ruminants. *C perfringens* types A, B, C, and D are the most common causes, although enteritis caused by *C difficile* is also reported. Commercial *C perfringens* C and D vaccines are effective at preventing disease caused by type B, C, and D strains but do not provide adequate protection for type A strains. When clinical cases are identified early, treatment can be successful if provided promptly.

REFERENCES

1. Lebrun M, Mainil JG, Linden A. Cattle enterotoxaemia and *Clostridium perfringens*: description, diagnosis and prophylaxis. Vet Rec 2010;167(1):13–22.
2. Uzal FA, Songer JG. Diagnosis of *Clostridium perfringens* intestinal infections in sheep and goats. J Vet Diagn Invest 2008;20(3):253–65.
3. Songer JG. Clostridial enteric diseases of domestic animals. Clin Microbiol Rev 1996;9(2):216–34.
4. Lewis CJ. Control of important clostridial diseases of sheep. Vet Clin North Am Food Anim Pract 2011;27(1):121–6.
5. Borriello SP, Carman RJ, editors. Clostridia in gastrointestinal disease. Boca Raton (FL): CRC Press; 1992. p. 195–221.
6. Vance HN. A survey of the alimentary tract of cattle for *Clostridium perfringens*. Can J Comp Med Vet Sci 1967;31(10):260–4.
7. Rood JI. Virulence genes of *Clostridium perfringens*. Annu Rev Microbiol 1998; 52:333–60.
8. Petit L, Gibert M, Popoff MR. *Clostridium perfringens*: toxinotype and genotype. Trends Microbiol 1999;7(3):104–10.
9. Stiles BG, Barth G, Barth H, et al. *Clostridium perfringens* epsilon toxin: a malevolent molecule for animals and man? Toxins (Basel) 2013;5(11):2138–60.
10. Deprez P. *Clostridium perfringens* infections - a diagnostic challenge. Vet Rec 2015;177(15):388–9.
11. Hofshagen M, Stenwig H. Toxin production by *Clostridium perfringens* isolated from broiler chickens and capercaillies (*Tetrao urogallus*) with and without necrotizing enteritis. Avian Dis 1992;36(4):837–43.
12. Katayama S, Matsushita O, Minami J, et al. Comparison of the alpha-toxin genes of *Clostridium perfringens* type A and C strains: evidence for extragenic regulation of transcription. Infect Immun 1993;61(2):457–63.
13. Bueschel DM, Jost BH, Billington SJ, et al. Prevalence of cpb2, encoding beta2 toxin, in *Clostridium perfringens* field isolates: correlation of genotype with phenotype. Vet Microbiol 2003;94(2):121–9.
14. Garmory HS, Chanter N, French NP, et al. Occurrence of *Clostridium perfringens* beta2-toxin amongst animals, determined using genotyping and subtyping PCR assays. Epidemiol Infect 2000;124(1):61–7.
15. Songer JG, Miskimins DW. Clostridial abomasitis in calves: case report and review of the literature. Anaerobe 2005;11(5):290–4.
16. Songer JG, Uzal FA. Clostridial enteric infections in pigs. J Vet Diagn Invest 2005;17(6):528–36.
17. Dennison AC, Van Metre DC, Morley PS, et al. Comparison of the odds of isolation, genotypes, and in vivo production of major toxins by *Clostridium perfringens* obtained from the gastrointestinal tract of dairy cows with hemorrhagic bowel syndrome or left-displaced abomasum. J Am Vet Med Assoc 2005; 227(1):132–8.

18. Dennison AC, VanMetre DC, Callan RJ, et al. Hemorrhagic bowel syndrome in dairy cattle: 22 cases (1997-2000). J Am Vet Med Assoc 2002;221(5):686–9.
19. Ceci L, Paradies P, Sasanelli M, et al. Haemorrhagic bowel syndrome in dairy cattle: possible role of *Clostridium perfringens* type A in the disease complex. J Vet Med A Physiol Pathol Clin Med 2006;53(10):518–23.
20. Abutarbush SM, Radostits OM. Jejunal hemorrhage syndrome in dairy and beef cattle: 11 cases (2001 to 2003). Can Vet J 2005;46(8):711–5.
21. Ewoldt JM, Anderson DE. Determination of the effect of single abomasal or jejunal inoculation of *Clostridium perfringens* type A in dairy cows. Can Vet J 2005;46(9):821–4.
22. Freedman JC, Shrestha A, McClane BA. *Clostridium perfringens* enterotoxin: action, genetics, and translational applications. Toxins (Basel) 2016;8(3) [pii:E73].
23. Sakurai J, Nagahama M, Oda M. *Clostridium perfringens* alpha-toxin: characterization and mode of action. J Biochem 2004;136(5):569–74.
24. Fernandez Miyakawa ME, Uzal FA. Morphologic and physiologic changes induced by *Clostridium perfringens* type A alpha toxin in the intestine of sheep. Am J Vet Res 2005;66(2):251–5.
25. Goossens E, Valgaeren BR, Pardon B, et al. Rethinking the role of alpha toxin in *Clostridium perfringens*-associated enteric diseases: a review on bovine necro-haemorrhagic enteritis. Vet Res 2017;48(1):9.
26. Verherstraeten S, Goossens E, Valgaeren B, et al. The synergistic necrohemorrhagic action of *Clostridium perfringens* perfringolysin and alpha toxin in the bovine intestine and against bovine endothelial cells. Vet Res 2013;44:45.
27. Tweten RK. *Clostridium perfringens* beta toxin and *Clostridium septicum* alpha toxin: their mechanisms and possible role in pathogenesis. Vet Microbiol 2001; 82(1):1–9.
28. Alves GG, Machado de Avila RA, Chavez-Olortegui CD, et al. *Clostridium perfringens* epsilon toxin: the third most potent bacterial toxin known. Anaerobe 2014;30:102–7.
29. Freedman JC, McClane BA, Uzal FA. New insights into *Clostridium perfringens* epsilon toxin activation and action on the brain during enterotoxemia. Anaerobe 2016;41:27–31.
30. Greco G, Madio A, Buonavoglia D, et al. *Clostridium perfringens* toxin-types in lambs and kids affected with gastroenteric pathologies in Italy. Vet J 2005; 170(3):346–50.
31. Finnie JW. Pathogenesis of brain damage produced in sheep by *Clostridium perfringens* type D epsilon toxin: a review. Aust Vet J 2003;81(4):219–21.
32. Uzal FA, Kelly WR, Morris WE, et al. Effects of intravenous injection of *Clostridium perfringens* type D epsilon toxin in calves. J Comp Pathol 2002; 126(1):71–5.
33. Uzal FA, Kelly WR. Experimental *Clostridium perfringens* type D enterotoxemia in goats. Vet Pathol 1998;35(2):132–40.
34. Uzal FA, Kelly WR. Effects of the intravenous administration of *Clostridium perfringens* type D epsilon toxin on young goats and lambs. J Comp Pathol 1997; 116(1):63–71.
35. Morris WE, Goldstein J, Redondo LM, et al. *Clostridium perfringens* epsilon toxin induces permanent neuronal degeneration and behavioral changes. Toxicon 2017;130:19–28.
36. Barth H, Aktories K, Popoff MR, et al. Binary bacterial toxins: biochemistry, biology, and applications of common *Clostridium* and *Bacillus* proteins. Microbiol Mol Biol Rev 2004;68(3):373–402. Table of contents.

37. Schotte U, Truyen U, Neubauer H. Significance of beta 2-toxigenic *Clostridium perfringens* infections in animals and their predisposing factors–a review. J Vet Med B Infect Dis Vet Public Health 2004;51(10):423–6.

38. Gkiourtzidis K, Frey J, Bourtzi-Hatzopoulou E, et al. PCR detection and prevalence of alpha-, beta-, beta 2-, epsilon-, iota- and enterotoxin genes in *Clostridium perfringens* isolated from lambs with clostridial dysentery. Vet Microbiol 2001;82(1):39–43.

39. Manteca C, Daube G, Jauniaux T, et al. A role for the *Clostridium perfringens* beta2 toxin in bovine enterotoxaemia? Vet Microbiol 2002;86(3):191–202.

40. Mehdizadeh I, Parreira V, Prescott J, et al. 2015 ACVIM proceedings: a novel pore-forming toxin in type A *Clostridium perfringens* associated with fatal canine hemorrhagic gastroenteritis and neonatal foal necrotizing enterocolitis. J Vet Intern Med 2015;29:1205.

41. Gohari IM, Parreira VR, Timoney JF, et al. NetF-positive *Clostridium perfringens* in neonatal foal necrotising enteritis in Kentucky. Vet Rec 2016;178(9):216.

42. Keyburn AL, Boyce JD, Vaz P, et al. NetB, a new toxin that is associated with avian necrotic enteritis caused by *Clostridium perfringens*. PLoS Pathog 2008; 4(2):e26.

43. Keyburn AL, Yan XX, Bannam TL, et al. Association between avian necrotic enteritis and *Clostridium perfringens* strains expressing NetB toxin. Vet Res 2010; 41(2):21.

44. Keyburn AL, Sheedy SA, Ford ME, et al. Alpha-toxin of *Clostridium perfringens* is not an essential virulence factor in necrotic enteritis in chickens. Infect Immun 2006;74(11):6496–500.

45. Schlegel BJ, Nowell VJ, Parreira VR, et al. Toxin-associated and other genes in *Clostridium perfringens* type A isolates from bovine clostridial abomasitis (BCA) and jejunal hemorrhage syndrome (JHS). Can J Vet Res 2012;76(4):248–54.

46. Valgaeren B, Pardon B, Goossens E, et al. lesion development in a new intestinal loop model indicates the involvement of a shared *Clostridium perfringens* virulence factor in haemorrhagic enteritis in calves. J Comp Pathol 2013; 149(1):103–12.

47. Van Kruiningen HJ, Nyaoke CA, Sidor IF, et al. Clostridial abomasal disease in Connecticut dairy calves. Can Vet J 2009;50(8):857–60.

48. Manteca C, Jauniaux T, Daube G, et al. Isolation of *Clostridium perfringens* from three calves with hemorrhagic abomasitis. Revue de Médecine Vétérinaire 2001;152:637–9.

49. Roeder BL, Chengappa MM, Nagaraja TG, et al. Isolation of *Clostridium perfringens* from neonatal calves with ruminal and abomasal tympany, abomasitis, and abomasal ulceration. J Am Vet Med Assoc 1987;190(12):1550–5.

50. Songer JG, Miskimmins DW. *Clostridium perfringens* type E enteritis in calves: two cases and a brief review of the literature. Anaerobe 2004;10(4):239–42.

51. Roeder BL, Chengappa MM, Nagaraja TG, et al. Experimental induction of abdominal tympany, abomasitis, and abomasal ulceration by intraruminal inoculation of *Clostridium perfringens* type A in neonatal calves. Am J Vet Res 1988; 49(2):201–7.

52. Russell WC. Type A enterotoxemia in captive wild goats. J Am Vet Med Assoc 1970;157(5):643–6.

53. Leite Filho RV, Bianchi MV, Fredo G, et al. Emphysematous abomasitis in a lamb by bacteria of the *Sarcina* genus in Southern Brazil. Ciência Rural 2016;46(2): 300–3.

54. Edwards GT, Woodger NG, Barlow AM, et al. *Sarcina*-like bacteria associated with bloat in young lambs and calves. Vet Rec 2008;163(13):391–3.

55. DeBey BM, Blanchard PC, Durfee PT. Abomasal bloat associated with *Sarcina*-like bacteria in goat kids. J Am Vet Med Assoc 1996;209(8):1468–9.

56. Carlson SA, Stoffregen WC, Bolin SR. Abomasitis associated with multiple antibiotic resistant *Salmonella enterica* serotype Typhimurium phagetype DT104. Vet Microbiol 2002;85(3):233–40.

57. Carlson SA, Meyerholz DK, Stabel TJ, et al. Secretion of a putative cytotoxin in multiple antibiotic resistant *Salmonella enterica* serotype Typhimurium phagetype DT104. Microb Pathog 2001;31(4):201–4.

58. Hunter AG, Mathieson AO, Scott JA, et al. An outbreak of S typhimurium in sheep and its consequences. Vet Rec 1976;98(7):126–30.

59. Maratea KA, Miller MA. Abomasal coccidiosis associated with proliferative abomasitis in a sheep. J Vet Diagn Invest 2007;19(1):118–21.

60. Morin M, Lariviere S, Lallier R. Pathological and microbiological observations made on spontaneous cases of acute neonatal calf diarrhea. Can J Comp Med 1976;40(3):228–40.

61. Marshall TS. Abomasal ulceration and tympany of calves. Vet Clin North Am Food Anim Pract 2009;25(1):209–20, viii.

62. Lilley CW, Hamar DW, Gerlach M, et al. Linking copper deficiency with abomasal ulcers in beef calves. Vet Med 1985;(80):85–8.

63. Mills KW, Johnson JL, Jensen RL, et al. Laboratory findings associated with abomasal ulcers/tympany in range calves. J Vet Diagn Invest 1990;2(3):208–12.

64. Goossens E, Verherstraeten S, Timbermont L, et al. *Clostridium perfringens* strains from bovine enterotoxemia cases are not superior in in vitro production of alpha toxin, perfringolysin O and proteolytic enzymes. BMC Vet Res 2014; 10:32.

65. Niilo L. *Clostridium perfringens* in animal disease: a review of current knowledge. Can Vet J 1980;21(5):141–8.

66. Guss SB. Enterotoxemia. Paper presented at: symposium on health and disease of sheep and goats, American Association of Sheep and Goat Practitioners. Salt Lake City, 1979.

67. Niilo L. *Clostridium perfringens* type C enterotoxemia. Can Vet J 1988;29(8): 658–64.

68. Uzal FA, Kelly WR. Enterotoxaemia in goats. Vet Res Commun 1996;20(6): 481–92.

69. Blackwell TE, Butler DG, Prescott JF, et al. Differences in signs and lesions in sheep and goats with enterotoxemia induced by intraduodenal infusion of *Clostridium perfringens* type D. Am J Vet Res 1991;52(7):1147–52.

70. Blackwell TE, Butler DG. Clinical signs, treatment, and postmortem lesions in dairy goats with enterotoxemia: 13 cases (1979-1982). J Am Vet Med Assoc 1992;200(2):214–7.

71. Blackwell TE. Enteritis and diarrhea. Vet Clin North Am Large Anim Pract 1983; 5(3):557–70.

72. Songer JG. Clostridial vaccines. In: Smith BP, editor. Large animal internal medicine. 3rd edition. St Louis (MO): Mosby; 2002. p. 1430–2.

73. Gardner DE. Pathology of *Clostridium welchii* type D enterotoxaemia. II. Structural and ultrastructural alterations in the tissues of lambs and mice. J Comp Pathol 1973;83(4):509–24.

74. Bullen JJ, Battey I. Enterotoxaemia of sheep. Vet Rec 1957;69:1268–76.

75. Kim HY, Byun JW, Roh IS, et al. First isolation of *Clostridium perfringens* type E from a goat with diarrhea. Anaerobe 2013;22:141–3.

76. Redondo LM, Farber M, Venzano A, et al. Sudden death syndrome in adult cows associated with *Clostridium perfringens* type E. Anaerobe 2013;20:1–4.

77. Fohler S, Klein G, Hoedemaker M, et al. Diversity of *Clostridium perfringens* toxin-genotypes from dairy farms. BMC Microbiol 2016;16(1):199.

78. Burgstaller J, Wittek T, Smith GW. Invited review: abomasal emptying in calves and its potential influence on gastrointestinal disease. J Dairy Sci 2017;100(1): 17–35.

79. Rosadio R, Londone P, Perez D, et al. *Eimeria macusaniensis* associated lesions in neonate alpacas dying from enterotoxemia. Vet Parasitol 2010;168(1–2): 116–20.

80. Rojas M, Manchego A, Rocha CB, et al. Outbreak of diarrhea among preweaning alpacas (*Vicugna pacos*) in the southern Peruvian highland. J Infect Dev Ctries 2016;10(3):269–74.

81. Kirino Y, Tanida M, Hasunuma H, et al. Increase of *Clostridium perfringens* in association with *Eimeria* in haemorrhagic enteritis in Japanese beef cattle. Vet Rec 2015;177(8):202.

82. Meer RR, Songer JG. Multiplex polymerase chain reaction assay for genotyping *Clostridium perfringens*. Am J Vet Res 1997;58(7):702–5.

83. Daube G, Simon P, Limbourg B, et al. Hybridization of 2,659 *Clostridium perfringens* isolates with gene probes for seven toxins (alpha, beta, epsilon, iota, theta, mu, and enterotoxin) and for sialidase. Am J Vet Res 1996;57(4):496–501.

84. Valgaeren BR, Pardon B, Verherstraeten S, et al. Intestinal clostridial counts have no diagnostic value in the diagnosis of enterotoxaemia in veal calves. Vet Rec 2013;172(9):237.

85. Kümper H. A new treatment for abomasal bloat in calves. Bovine Practitioner 1995;(29):80–2.

86. Stevens DL, Maier KA, Mitten JE. Effect of antibiotics on toxin production and viability of *Clostridium perfringens*. Antimicrob Agents Chemother 1987;31(2): 213–8.

87. Song MS, Kim CJ, Cho WI, et al. Growth inhibition of *Clostridium perfringens* vegetative cells and spores using chicken immunoglobulin Y. J Food Saf 2009;29(4):511–20.

88. Weese JS, Cote NM, de Gannes RV. Evaluation of in vitro properties of di-tri-octahedral smectite on clostridial toxins and growth. Equine Vet J 2003;35(7): 638–41.

89. Lawler JB, Hassel DM, Magnuson RJ, et al. Adsorptive effects of di-tri-octahedral smectite on *Clostridium perfringens* alpha, beta, and beta-2 exotoxins and equine colostral antibodies. Am J Vet Res 2008;69(2):233–9.

90. Furuya-Kanamori L, Stone JC, Clark J, et al. Comorbidities, exposure to medications, and the risk of community-acquired *Clostridium difficile* infection: a systematic review and meta-analysis. Infect Control Hosp Epidemiol 2015;36(2): 132–41.

91. Javsicas LH. Duodenitis-proximal jejunitis. In: Reed SM, Bayly WM, Sellon DC, editors. Equine internal medicine. 3rd edition. St Louis (MO): Saunders; 2010. p. 848–9.

92. Radostits OM, Gay CC, Blood DC, et al. Veterinary medicine. London: WB Saunders; 2000.

93. System NAHM. Reference of 1996 US sheep health management practices. In: USDA: APHIS:VS, ed. Fort Collins (CO): 1996.

94. Krueder AJ, Plummer PJ. Ovine and caprine vaccination programs. In: Smith BP, editor. Large animal internal medicine. 5th edition. St. Louis (MO): Elsevier; 2015. p. 1461–2.

95. Sterne M, Batty I, Thomson A. Immunization of sheep with multi-component clostridial vaccines. Vet Rec 1962;74:909–13.

96. Kerry JB, Craig GR. Field studies in sheep with multicomponent clostridial vaccines. Vet Rec 1979;105(24):551–4.

97. de la Rosa C, Hogue DE, Thonney ML. Vaccination schedules to raise antibody concentrations against epsilon-toxin of *Clostridium perfringens* in ewes and their triplet lambs. J Anim Sci 1997;75(9):2328–34.

98. Kennedy KK, Norris SJ, Beckenhauer WH, et al. Antitoxin response in cattle vaccinated with *Clostridium perfringens* type C toxoid. Vet Med Small Anim Clin 1977;72(7):1213–5.

99. Troxel TR, Burke GL, Wallace WT, et al. Clostridial vaccination efficacy on stimulating and maintaining an immune response in beef cows and calves. J Anim Sci 1997;75(1):19–25.

100. Troxel TR, Gadberry MS, Wallace WT, et al. Clostridial antibody response from injection-site lesions in beef cattle, long-term response to single or multiple doses, and response in newborn beef calves. J Anim Sci 2001;79(10): 2558–64.

101. NAHMS. Part II: Baseline reference of feedlot health and management, 1999. In: USDA: APHIS:VS, editor. Fort Collins (CO): National Animal Health Monitoring System; 2000.

102. Knott GKL, Erwin BG, Classick LG. Benefits of a clostridial vaccination program in feedlot cattle. Vet Med 1985;80:95–7.

103. De Groot B, Dewey CE, Griffin DD, et al. Effect of booster vaccination with a multivalent clostridial bacterin-toxoid on sudden death syndrome mortality rate among feedlot cattle. J Am Vet Med Assoc 1997;211(6):749–53.

104. Stokka GL, Edwards AJ, Spire MF, et al. Inflammatory response to clostridial vaccines in feedlot cattle. J Am Vet Med Assoc 1994;204(3):415–9.

105. Goossens E, Verherstraeten S, Valgaeren BR, et al. Toxin-neutralizing antibodies protect against *Clostridium perfringens*-induced necrosis in an intestinal loop model for bovine necrohemorrhagic enteritis. BMC Vet Res 2016;12(1):101.

106. Ferreira MR, Moreira GM, Cunha CE, et al. Recombinant alpha, beta, and epsilon toxins of *Clostridium perfringens*: production strategies and applications as veterinary vaccines. Toxins (Basel) 2016;8(11) [pii:E340].

107. Songer JG. Clostridial vaccines. In: Smith BP, editor. Large animal internal medicine. 5th edition. St. Louis (MO): Elsevier; 2015. p. 1488–90.

108. Rodriguez-Palacios A, Stampfli HR, Duffield T, et al. *Clostridium difficile* PCR ribotypes in calves, Canada. Emerg Infect Dis 2006;12(11):1730–6.

109. Costa MC, Stampfli HR, Arroyo LG, et al. Epidemiology of *Clostridium difficile* on a veal farm: prevalence, molecular characterization and tetracycline resistance. Vet Microbiol 2011;152(3–4):379–84.

110. Bandelj P, Blagus R, Briski F, et al. Identification of risk factors influencing *Clostridium difficile* prevalence in middle-size dairy farms. Vet Res 2016;47:41.

111. Costa MC, Reid-Smith R, Gow S, et al. Prevalence and molecular characterization of *Clostridium difficile* isolated from feedlot beef cattle upon arrival and midfeeding period. BMC Vet Res 2012;8:38.

112. Koene MG, Mevius D, Wagenaar JA, et al. *Clostridium difficile* in Dutch animals: their presence, characteristics and similarities with human isolates. Clin Microbiol Infect 2012;18(8):778–84.

113. Avbersek J, Pirs T, Pate M, et al. *Clostridium difficile* in goats and sheep in Slovenia: characterisation of strains and evidence of age-related shedding. Anaerobe 2014;28:163–7.
114. Hammitt MC, Bueschel DA, Kee AK, et al. A possible role for *Clostridium difficile* in the etiology of calf enteritis. Vet Microbiol 2008;127(3–4):343–52.
115. Arroyo LG, Rousseau JD, Staempfli HR, et al. Suspected *Clostridium difficile*-associated hemorrhagic diarrhea in a 1-week-old elk calf. Can Vet J 2005; 46(12):1130–1.

Gastrointestinal Nematodes, Diagnosis and Control

 CrossMark

Thomas M. Craig, DVM, PhD, DACVM

KEYWORDS

- Ostertagia • Cooperia • Haemonchus • Anthelmintic resistance

KEY POINTS

- Gastrointestinal nematode infection is completely different depending on the species and age of ruminant and the environment. The disease, control measures, and drugs used must be focused on different ages and environments.
- Infection and disease are not synonymous. We try to prevent disease and ensure the animal's immune system is stimulated, not overwhelmed.
- Different drugs should be used against the parasites most likely affected by the specific drug and administered how and when it will accomplish the best sustainable control.
- Nematode larvae undergo hypobiosis in their hosts to evade unfavorable environmental conditions for their offspring and the immunologic response of the host, then emerge to ensure the survival of the species.

Gastrointestinal parasites of ruminants may adversely affect their hosts either clinically or economically; differentiating them is important to the veterinarian and producer. Clinical diseases are manifest as abnormal signs in dermal, gastrointestinal, or cardiovascular systems and are common in small ruminants. Economic disease is the level of parasitism that causes a less than genetic potential rate of gain, feed conversion, development, reproduction, or less than optimum production of milk or meat, as seen in cattle. Most losses in ruminants are economic, not as morbidity or mortality. Understanding the interactions of parasitism, nutrition, and livestock management is the key to understanding losses. Parasitism is not the most important cause of economic loss in the livestock industry but has the potential of being so with increased stocking rates and limited nutritional intake.

Disclosure Statement: Dr T.M. Craig provides service for, and has done research and consultation with, several pharmaceutical companies. He owns no stock nor has any monetary affiliation with any.
Department of Veterinary Pathobiology, Texas A&M University, Raymond Stotzer Parkway, College Station, TX 77843-4467, USA
E-mail address: tcraig@cvm.tamu.edu

The life cycles of the gastrointestinal nematode parasites of ruminants in temperate areas are direct. Climate determines which parasites will be present in a given geographic region and weather determines when livestock will acquire the infection. The class of livestock and the management of the stock will, to a large extent, determine the magnitude of the infection acquired. The nutritional status of the livestock may determine how adversely the individual animal will be affected by the parasites it acquires.

Because of the way each class of ruminants is managed, the likelihood of parasitic disease varies tremendously among them. Therefore, the parasites of ruminants will be approached as a herd/class problem rather than as a problem in an individual animal. The herd/class problem is a component of individual problems. Control programs for individual host species are addressed, but the anthelmintics used and relative importance of the species of parasites targeted may change over time; however, the general approaches to parasite control will remain more or less constant.

Parasitic gastroenteritis is a term used for the disease complex of nematodes affecting ruminants. Usually 1 or 2 species are more important than others in a given host and situation. The genera most often associated with this complex are *Haemonchus, Ostertagia, Teladorsagia,* and *Trichostrongylus* in the abomasum; *Trichostrongylus, Cooperia,* and *Nematodirus* in the small intestine; and *Oesophagostomum* in the large intestine. The eggs of these genera are thin shelled, segmented, and cannot be readily differentiated with the exception of *Nematodirus,* which has a distinctive large football-shaped egg. The eggs are commonly referred to as trichostrongyle type and are easily differentiated from whipworm or tapeworm eggs in feces.

The general life cycle is the eggs are passed in feces, and in the pasture L_1 larvae hatch in a few days. The larvae feed on bacteria in the feces and develop to the infective stage, which retains the cuticle as a protective sheath for the L_3 in the environment. The L_3 larvae do not feed; they are aquatic and are able to go where a film of moisture exists on surface of soil, underground, or on vegetation. These larvae go where the moisture is and if that is on the vegetation, the larvae are ingested during grazing. The worms complete development to adults in the gastrointestinal tract in approximately 3 weeks.

TRANSMISSION

In the pasture, larval development is temperature and moisture dependent. Larvae are more active at higher temperatures. Optimal development occurs near 100% relative humidity and 22 to 26°C (72–79°F) in 7 days; longer in cold weather. The development is fast in summer but life expectancy is short. Development is slow during the winter, but survival is lengthy. Larvae survive only a month in humid tropics. Larvae may survive in low temperatures on pasture up to 1 year but usually 2 to 6 months. The larvae are susceptible to high temperatures, excess moisture, desiccation, and UV light. During adverse weather conditions, larvae survive by moving into the soil or being entrapped in the dung pat. Another strategy for survival is by remaining within the host as arrested larvae (hypobiosis).

Each species of parasite has its own optimum requirements, minimum and maximum, for development and survival. Because of these differences, certain species of parasites will be important in various geographic regions and at different times of the year, that is, *Haemonchus* is a warm season parasite; *Ostertagia* a winter parasite in Texas but a summer parasite in Michigan. It is possible to have transmission of parasites at virtually any time of the year in mild climates if there is sufficient moisture. However, various species of parasites tend to follow a pattern of transmission which is seasonally based. *Cool season parasites*: *Ostertagia*, *Teladorsagia*, *Cooperia oncophora*, *Oesophagostomum*, *Trichostrongylus axei*, and *Trichostrongylus colubriformis*. *Warm season parasites*: *Bunostomum*, *Haemonchus*, *Cooperia punctata*, and *Cooperia pectinata*. Genera such as *Nematodirus*, *Trichuris* and *Toxocara* do not appear to be as seasonal as other parasites. Transmission of larvae requires at least 2 inches of rainfall during a month, and for cool season transmission mean monthly mean temperatures of 40 to 68°F (4–20°C) or warm season 60 to 95°F (15.5–35.0°C).

DISEASE

Disease is seldom due to just one species but rather to the cumulative effects of a mixed Infection. Outbreaks, however, due to a predominance of a single species of parasite are common.

The economic loss associated with this disease is usually associated with a failure to gain weight or produce milk at an optimum rate. Occasionally disease is manifested by death or severe weight loss. However, the primary loss is decreased production. Nutritional interactions are important with this complex, as an excess of high-quality intake may obscure the presence of parasites or nutritional failures may be blamed on the presence of parasites.

The effects of gastric parasitism are those of anorexia, hypertrophy of mucosa, reduced primary digestion, decreased hydrochloric acid and pepsin production, dyspepsia, loss of plasma protein, and blood loss. Intestinal parasitism is manifest as lowered absorption and transport due to water and electrolyte loss with increased peristalsis, loss of plasma protein, and malabsorption. The malabsorption is due to rapid turnover of epithelial cells. Immature epithelial cells lack enzymes needed for digestion, thus reducing transportation of vitamins, amino acids, and carbohydrates. Diarrhea also occurs due to fermentation of carbohydrates in the gut. Nonabsorbed protein is broken down into indoles and amines that contribute to the foul smell of diarrheic stools. Diarrhea is also due to increased peristalsis, which is due in turn to mechanical irritation and "solvent drag" of transportation of water and other materials of malabsorption. In addition, immunologic events, such as histamine release, cause separation of tight junctions between epithelial cells, which allows further release of protein and fluid.

IMMUNITY

Acquired immunity may be manifest as a retardation or inhibition of development of larval nematodes (hypobiosis), but is usually seen as a reduction in establishment of infection with smaller worms and suppressed egg production. Immunity is not a 100% reduction in worm numbers but protection from disease. Most animals in a herd will manifest some level of immunity. Some species of nematodes provoke an early strong resistance to infection, others require repeated exposure. Genetic selection of animals in a herd with resistance to worms may become more important over time with the increase in the failure of anthelmintics.[1,2]

The periparturient relaxation of resistance occurs at parturition and early lactation. As prolactin levels rise, arrested larvae are no longer inhibited, and there is little or no resistance against new infection. Pastures become seeded with large numbers of eggs at this time such that susceptible animals (the young) will come in contact with many larvae when they begin to graze. Some animals rather than ridding themselves of parasites become resilient or tolerant of the infection. Individual animals may have a heavy parasite burden but are able to thrive despite the presence of worms, manifested as less weight loss, increased erythrocyte production, or increased fecundity.

Certain breeds and individuals within breeds have increased resistance to or resilience from the effects of gastrointestinal parasitism. Resistance may be innate but is probably more often acquired resistance. Young animals are not able to manifest resistance for the first several months of life. Resistance to worms may or may not be associated with other phenotypic characteristics. There are many genes involved in this process that may be limited to specific parasites.

CATTLE NEMATODES

Most infections in cattle are a combination of several parasitic species but a few stand out as being more economically important than others. The most important nematode parasite of cattle in temperate regions of the world is *Ostertagia ostertagi*. The parasite is pathogenic and may cause severe clinical disease and, even when encountered in comparatively low numbers, it causes anorexia and an inability to efficiently convert forage into milk or meat. The economic importance of this parasite was not fully appreciated until the availability of anthelmintics that were extremely effective against this parasite. The primary economic effects of these anthelmintics are those of increased milk production[3–5] and the increased growth rate in calves.[6,7] Not only do the cows produce more milk, there is evidence they breed back more rapidly following calving. To be certain, not all trials replicated these findings, as there is considerable variability among herd genetics, geographic localities, and years.[8,9]

The most common genus encountered in younger cattle is *Cooperia*, and from the standpoint of egg numbers is often the dominant worm present. However, when compared with *Ostertagia* or *Haemonchus,* it is of lesser clinical significance. The genus has become more important in recent years, as it has changed from a worm that was controlled by anthelmintics to a genus that is often resistant to macrocyclic lactones.[10] Other genera that are locally important include *Trichostrongylus, Bunostomum, Oesophagostomum,* and *Nematodirus*. At this time, control programs for adult cattle directed toward *Ostertagia* are likely to aid in the control of other species, but in younger animals the environment, time of year, history, and source of cattle or worms must be considered to prevent disease caused by gastrointestinal nematodes.

SMALL RUMINANT NEMATODES

In North America, fewer nematodes are associated with disease, but the economic impact is far greater than in cattle. Two species stand out where sheep, goats, camelids, deer, or exotics are raised: *Haemonchus contortus* and *Trichostrongylus colubriformis. Haemonchus* kills by exsanguination and *Trichostrongylus* causes ill thrift and diarrhea. In cooler moist regions *Teladorsagia circumcincta* may be an important pathogen causing weight loss and diarrhea. To be certain, in some geographic areas, other species may be important but in general they have disappeared from North America largely due to our attempts to control parasites. Many populations of *Haemonchus* and *Trichostrongylus* have become resistant to all extant anthelmintics,[11] and our attempts to control them have led to the virtual extermination of other species.

The selection for anthelmintic-resistant worms by small ruminant producers should be an important lesson for cattle veterinarians and efforts to control parasitic disease rather than the "kill 'um all" approach. Anthelminthic resistance to important cattle nematodes is limited or widespread depending primarily on the movement of cattle. Importing resistant worms in apparently healthy livestock occurs and moving older cattle that have not been exposed to specific parasites can result in severe disease in animals normally resistant to that worm species.

IMPORTANT GASTROINTESTINAL NEMATODE PARASITES
Ostertagia

Ostertagia ostertagi is the most important species of nematode throughout most of the temperate world and may even cause clinical disease in adult cattle. The strategies directed toward the control of parasitic gastroenteritis are based on *Ostertagia,* but the timing must be different geographically. For instance, *Ostertagia* is transmitted in the northern United States and Canada during the summer and autumn, and during the winter and spring in the southern United States and is absent from south Texas, Florida, and lower altitudes in Mexico. The disease ostertagiosis is due to abomasal damage caused by maturing worms emerging from the abomasal glands.

Two disease patterns are recognized. Type I disease occurs during the grazing period, which is seasonal: summer/autumn (North) or autumn/winter (South). The disease is caused by the emergence of immature worms from the gastric glands 10 to 14 days after the ingestion of infective larvae. Type II is seen months following pasture exposure during the spring (North) or autumn (South) and is caused by the simultaneous emergence of arrested larvae that were acquired over an extended period during the grazing season. Larvae remain hypobiotic (usually several months) within the gastric glands until a stimulus triggers the resumption of their development.

Several factors have been implicated in the emergence of hypobiotic worms, but the climate selection for the geographic region appears to be most important for *Ostertagia.* Simultaneous emergence of thousands of maturing worms from the gastric glands causes marked structural and physiologic changes within the abomasum. The abomasum becomes edematous with hypertrophy of gastric mucosa. Specialized cells of the gastric glands degenerate or are replaced by cuboidal mucus-secreting cells resulting in lowered production of HCl and pepsinogen. The normal abomasal pH is 2 to 3, when pH levels rise to 4.5 there is little activity in the conversion of pepsinogen into pepsin, and by the time the pH level reaches 6.0, pepsinogen is not activated, with diarrhea a common sign. At a pH of 7.0, there is diarrhea, sloughing of mucosa, and bacterial invasion of the stomach wall. There is hyperplasia of cuboidal cells; the cells lining the gastric glands become incompletely fused and leak plasma protein and pepsinogen, sloughing the superficial epithelium with bacterial proliferation.

Other Ostertaginae, such as *Teladorsagia circumcincta* in sheep and goats and other species of small ruminants, can cause a similar disease especially when the animals are also infected by small intestinal *Trichostrongylus* as well. The disease manifestations are similar to that of *Ostertagia* in cattle in that the inflammatory response to the parasite is damaging to the host.[12,13] Treating to remove hypobiotic larvae and/or the use of anthelmintics, which have residual effect so that incoming larvae are destroyed before they can establish, is the basis of *Ostertagia* control. Winter treatment in the north and summer treatment in the south may accomplish this. Beef cows and their single suckled calves are the primary thrust of the basic program. *Ostertagia ostertagi* is a common parasite of cattle, but they must be infected before they develop acquired immunity to prevent disease.[14–16] Disease prevention means that not only does the animal look healthy but it also produces to its genetic potential when provided adequate nutrition. In some regions, weather conditions and management are such that cattle do not get sufficient exposure to *Ostertagia* to stimulate resistance in every year, so we may have more disease in older cattle than expected if the level of exposure were more consistent.

Reports of *Ostertagia* populations resistant to formerly effective anthelmintics are rare but have been seen[17]; however, the increased use of these drugs is a cause for concern. Resistance (immunity) to parasite infection appears to be primarily acquired, but has a strong genetic component. Therefore, species or breeds that evolved with their parasites have a greater chance of responding to those specific parasites. In the case of *Ostertagia,* Zebu cattle, in general, are unable or delayed in mounting an effective protective immune response. The immunity expressed is protection from disease not infection. More or less regular exposure is necessary to maintain resistance. However, exposure in almost all geographic regions is not constant but comes in waves, and the interval between waves may allow waning of resistance. Cattle must be exposed to *Ostertagia* over time to stimulate a protective immune response. The worms also have the capacity to reduce the immune competence of the host.[18] If cattle are not exposed or only minimally so they remain susceptible, this may explain the high incidence of adult ostertagiosis in cattle raised in arid areas compared with those in higher rainfall areas.

Haemonchus

Haemonchus placei is generally recognized as being the cattle parasite, and *H contortus* is in small ruminants. However, both species can be found in the other hosts with comingled species, such as white-tailed deer having either or both species. Whatever the species name, it is a genus that is able to exploit opportunities by having a wide host range, tremendous fecundity, and the ability to rapidly adapt to anthelmintics. *Haemonchus* is a warm season parasite and undergoes hypobiosis during the winter or prolonged dry season. Cattle generally become immune to disease caused by *Haemonchus* more readily than goats or sheep, but calves are fully susceptible to the parasite.

Haemonchus, the largest worm in the abomasum, is an avid bloodsucker. The females are 2.5 to 3.0 cm in length, with a barber-pole or candy-cane appearance of the white, egg-filled uterus, wrapped around the blood-filled intestine, they produce 5 to 6000 eggs per day. Pastures grazed by large numbers of susceptible calves have billions of infective larvae in them and become killing grounds. Anemia with packed cell volumes occasionally in the single digits and hypoproteinemia with intermandibular edema (bottle jaw) are the primary signs of disease.

Reports of *Haemonchus* resistant to macrolide and benzimidazole anthelmintics in stocker calves in North America are a cause for concern.[19,20] The resistance was first seen in calves that originated from many farms and were held on common small pastures to complete the weaning process. These calves were vaccinated and administered an anthelmintic at this time. They were then placed on a warm season perennial pasture laden with larvae that survived the winter or the calves were carrying worms that escaped the anthelmintic. After a period of grazing, the numbers of infective larvae in the pasture rapidly escalated due to the susceptibility of the calves and the fecundity of the worms. Disease is seen later in the grazing season if weather conditions are favorable for the transmission of the parasite. However, if the calves are grazed on a cool season annual pasture even if a few worms survive the anthelmintic the exposure level never becomes sufficient to cause clinical disease.

Trichostrongylus

Trichostrongylus axei occurs in the abomasum of cattle and small ruminants and the stomach of horses and swine. *Trichostrongylus* are small worms, the adults only 5.5 to 8.0 mm in length, with an easily seen excretory notch. There are approximately 12 eggs (end to end) in the female and the male spicules are variable in size and shape.

For the most part *T axei* is considered a nonpathogen that occupies space usually used by *Ostertagia*. However, it can cause a disease similar to that caused by *Ostertagia* and suppresses the immune system.[18]

Trichostrongylus colubriformis, often called the black scour worm or bankrupt worm, is found in the small intestine of sheep, goats, llamas, and exotic ruminants, and may cause anorexia, abdominal pain, diarrhea, and progressive weakness. Infected animals require twice the feed to gain comparable weights. Infection in young lambs has been associated with osteodystrophy due to interference with calcium, phosphorous, and vitamin A absorption from the intestine. It is seen as a winter/spring disease in southern North America but can survive summers in pastures. In winter, rainfall areas, or in the northern United States, the *T colubriformis* and *T circumcincta* complex can be the most economically important parasites of small ruminants.

Cooperia

Cooperia spp inhabit the small intestine and are associated with anorexia, villous atrophy, and diarrhea when there are large numbers of parasites present. As a result, there will be lowered weight gains. However, when they are present, there are usually also abomasal helminths and the combination of worms is more debilitating than each species contributes in its own right. As effective treatment of *Ostertagia* has become more widely practiced, *Cooperia* has become more common and perhaps its importance should be reassessed. Under feedlot conditions during a 60-day trial, 460-lb calves infected with *Cooperia punctata* gained one-quarter pound per day less than noninfected calves.[21]

From the time of first release, macrocyclic lactone anthelmintics have not been as effective against *Cooperia* as with other genera. This tolerance has evolved into anthelmintic resistance.[10,17,22,23] As calves mature, *Cooperia* disappear, apparently due to acquired immunity, and by the time calves are 12 to 18 months old it is unusual to find high levels of infection except in cattle never before exposed to the local species. Because macrocyclic lactone anthelmintics are not as effective against this genus in light stockers or dairy calves, other anthelmintics are preferable.

Nematodirus

Nematodirus adults are 10 to 25 mm in length and they are very slender worms, which are coiled in a springlike fashion. They are commonly called the twisted wireworm. They possess a cephalic vesicle and the tail of the female is blunt with a small hairlike spine on the end. The male has very long slender spicules. The genus is characterized by large football-shaped eggs (140–180 × 75–90 μm) containing 8 cells, which do not hatch until the L3 has developed within the egg. The parasite is seen in dry or frigid climates where other genera die due to desiccation. The apparent prevalence of *Nematodirus* is increasing in cattle as more ranchers use avermectins and milbemycins for treatment. These drugs are effective against abomasal parasites but are less effective against *Nematodirus* and *Cooperia*. Control by treating only the young to lower pasture contamination for the next year and using an anthelmintic other than a macrocyclic lactone may be preferred.

Bunostomum

The hookworm *Bunostomum phlebotomum* is a large 3-cm robust white worm capable of causing anemia in calves. In areas in which anthelmintics are widely used, the parasite has disappeared, but should be considered a cause of anemia in other areas. Infection can occur both by ingestion or skin penetration, and may be a problem in young calves housed in moist environments, especially in the tropics.

Calves establish rapid immunity to reinfection. The prepatent period is 1 to 2 months and hypobiosis is a strategy for avoiding prolonged dry conditions.

Strongyloides

Strongyloides papillosus is a parasite of the young and is usually the first parasite egg passed by young calves. It is shared with other ruminant species. The parasite has both free-living and parasitic generations. Only females are parasitic, with eggs that are 50 to 60 $\times$ 30 µm, thin shelled, and larvated when passed in the feces. The eggs rapidly hatch and either develop into free-living adult worms or infective L3 larvae. Transmammary, skin penetration, or oral routes may transmit the L3. The L3 in cow's milk goes directly to the small intestine. However, L3s transmitted from the environment to naïve hosts undergo a skin/mucous membrane to tracheal migration, where they are coughed up, swallowed, and become adult females in the small intestine. When L3s are transmitted to resistant hosts, they undergo a skin/mucous membrane, aortic migration where larvae remain in hypobiosis until the cow gives birth and the larvae are activated and go to the mammary glands. Free-living adult worms live in moist environments, with high levels of organic material (ie, soiled bedding, especially sawdust saturated with urine and feces).

There is usually no disease associated; with the infection, occasionally loose feces are seen. However, rapid death due to cardiac arrhythmias in calves housed on sawdust due has been reported.[24] The sudden cardiac death syndrome is a ventricular fibrillation preceded by sinus tachycardia and has been associated with the presence of adult worms in the duodenum.[25] *Strongyloides* may become problem with poor sanitation manifested as dermatitis. Sanitation is vital to control and many modern anthelmintics are effective against the worms in the intestine.

Toxocara (Neoascaris)

Toxocara vitulorum are large robust worms up to 30 cm long with 3 large prominent lips. The eggs, 75 to 95 $\times$ 60 to 75 µm, are dark, subglobular, and single celled with a thick-pitted shell and are usually passed only by calves. The adults live in the small intestine of cattle, and buffalo in southern Europe, Asia, and South America and have been a reported in bison in North America.[26] *Toxocara* are observed in calves in Florida, where fenbendazole at 5 mg/kg was only 85% effective.[27] The life cycle is direct, the thick-shelled eggs are unsegmented when passed in feces of calves and requires 3 weeks to become infective. When the egg is ingested by a cow, the larva hatches and undergoes somatic migration remaining in the tissues until parturition. Transmammary transmission for up to 3 weeks following parturition is the only proven method of transmission. The worms develop in the intestine of the calf and there is a prepatent period of 1 month. The diagnosis is the recovery of roughly pitted clear ascarid-type eggs, which are spherical, or observing expelled adult worms in calf feces. The signs associated with infection include diarrhea, emaciation, obstruction, and death. There are usually no clinical signs, and calves undergo spontaneous cure when 3 to 5 months of age. Treatment with most broad-spectrum anthelmintics at effective dosages should be effective.

Oesophagostomum

Oesophagostomum radiatum adults live in the in large intestine, primarily the caecum of cattle. The larvae may be found from pylorus to anus in the gut mucosa. The adults are 1-cm to 2-cm robust worms whose anterior end is bent in a spiral with inflations or vesicles. The buccal cavity is large and leaf crowns are present. The eggs are 70 to 90 $\times$ 34 to 45 µm, and thin shelled and segmented when passed. Before modern anthelmintics, *Oesophagostomum* was a most important parasite during cool, wet seasons. The parasite is commercially important due to loss of intestine for human consumption (eg, sausage casing).

There is evidence of transmission in North American cattle feed lots, apparently due to a skin penetration. As with other intestinal nematodes, the life cycle is direct but transmission can be through either ingestion or skin penetration by infective L3 larvae. Once in the gut, larvae penetrate intestinal wall into mucosa, and molt to L4, which emerge in 7 to 10 days in a susceptible host. However, nodules surrounding larvae are formed in hypersensitive hosts. The larvae may remain within the nodule for up to 1 year. The prepatent period is variable, lasting 45 days to 5 months.

When larvae leave the gut wall, diarrhea may occur in heavily infected calves. In nodules containing *O radiatum,* there is a lymphocytic, eosinophilic infiltration with fibroblasts. The nodules may become as large as 1 to 2 cm in diameter, often filled with greenish purulent material that may calcify. The nodules formed in sensitized animals are larger and more likely to contain purulent exudate. The diagnosis is by postmortem examination identifying the worms or nodules. There may be emaciation; and a fibrous reaction interferes with normal gut motility or an ulcerative colitis. Broad-spectrum anthelmintics appear to be effective against most populations of this parasite but resistance has been reported[28] and should be expected elsewhere. Cattle become resistant to infection and apparently larvae trapped in the nodules are not exposed to anthelmintics. If some are able to emerge, they can contaminate an environment, such as a feedlot, with numerous larvae that infect naïve animals by skin penetration.

Trichuris

Whipworms infect ruminants. The adult worms are 3.5 to 8.0 cm with a very long threadlike anterior end and a short thick posterior end. The long anterior end contains the characteristic stichosome esophagus. The eggs are approximately 75×35 μm, brownish, barrel shaped, and have bipolar plugs. The eggs are single celled when passed. They live in the caecum and upper colon of cattle, *Trichuris discolors* and *Trichuris globulosa* are the most common species in cattle and, apparently, they are very similar. The life cycle is direct by the ingestion of infective eggs from the environment. It requires approximately 10 days to develop to the infective stage, but the egg can survive for several years. The prepatent period is 7 to 9 weeks. Finding the eggs by fecal flotation is diagnostic. In cattle, *Trichuris* are usually not pathogenic even when present in large numbers. However, in small ruminants and camels, disease is seen. Treatment is usually not required; however, benzimidazoles should be effective especially if administered in feed over several days.

DIAGNOSIS OF GASTROINTESTINAL NEMATODES

How do we know that cattle have problems with gastrointestinal nematodes? If cattle lose weight, become anemic, or have diarrhea or other clinical signs, we can certainly put parasitism on the list and look for eggs produced by adult worms. Eggs are found, so that is the problem. Maybe, how many eggs? Which host? What time of year? Answering those questions will increase the chances of ruling in or out parasites. Fecal egg counts in small ruminants can be highly suggestive, with counts greater than 1000 eggs per gram (EPG) in the spring and 2000 EPG in the late summer or autumn associated with disease or soon will be. With numbers that high in calves, we may see clinical signs.

Adult cows with counts greater than 20 EPG are probably not grazing enough to meet all their needs and therefore produce less milk so their calves are not growing as well as those nursing cows with lower egg counts. Doing egg counts for individual animals may give an idea if the counts for the herd are high or low, but there is a great deal of variation among the individual animals. Generally speaking, 20% of the herd will have 80% of the worms and if those animals are identified and administered anthelmintics the numbers of larvae in pastures would be decreased and there will be almost no selection for anthelmintic resistance. However, that is not a practical way for selection of whom to treat unless they are showing clinical signs.

The egg counts are low in adult cattle because *Ostertagia* produce few eggs and most of the damage occurs while the worms are larvae not adults. The high egg counts for *Cooperia* and *Haemonchus* in calves are because resistance to these worms has not yet occurred and they are fecund worms whose adults are doing the damage. Anemia or diarrhea is more likely seen with those worms. The eggs of the worms cannot be consistently differentiated, but with high egg counts the young should be treated and then the effectiveness of the anthelmintic determined at the property by comparing individual fecal egg counts at the time of treatment and 2 weeks later using a minimum of 10 to 12 animals from which samples are obtained.

In calves, a McMasters test in increments of 25 to 50 EPG is a practical approach, but in older cattle, a Wisconsin double-centrifugation with sensitivity of 1 egg per gram is more likely to give useful results. Other tests, such as serum pepsinogen, may be extremely helpful in determining the damage done to the abomasum by *Ostertagia* or possibly *Trichostrongylus,* but is not a specific test. Essentially, there are no good tests that will tell you if adult cattle will benefit from anthelmintics except controlled studies that use body weight of the cow and/or the calf or by observing how many hours the individual cows spend grazing. Cattle herds in arid areas may not benefit economically from a parasite control program, but the calves from these herds will be at greater risk than others if they move. The time of year, the geographic location, and the management of the cattle should determine if or when the cattle will benefit from treatment and the approach used will give different results depending on weather.

CONTROL PROGRAMS FOR GASTROINTESTINAL NEMATODES OF CATTLE

Approaches designed to lessen the chances of acquiring a large number of worms should be the goal of any control program. The program must address the species, environment, nutrition, management, and time of year. When dairy or background calves leave a barn/stable or dry lot and enter a pasture, parasitic gastroenteritis infection is a major concern. In climates in which calves are stabled or kept in dry lots, introduction to pasture and parasites can be overwhelming. The first 4 months on pasture is extremely dangerous for dairy calves, whereas beef calves do not usually show signs of disease until after weaning. In both groups, the more dangerous parasites encountered in most areas are *Ostertagia, Cooperia* spp, and *Haemonchus,* which affects calves the same as sheep or goats, with severe anemia the most obvious clinical sign. Even calves that are clinically normal may benefit from removal of gastrointestinal parasites while remaining on pasture or going to the feedlot.[6,29]

With single suckled beef calves, the transition is easier and the provision of high-quality feed (milk) ensures that the suckling calf will probably not show signs of disease. Suckling calves, 3 months or older, may benefit by deworming. After weaning, deworming calves becomes essential.[30] Remember they were getting high-quality food from mommy who is no longer there. Parasitic gastroenteritis may be a greater problem when stocker calves are imported from arid areas. They have not been exposed to worms at the levels to which the local cattle have begun to develop resistance, and we see disease in the imports. *Ostertagia, Cooperia*, and *Haemonchus* are problems in stockers and replacement calves.

With calves either suckling or early weaned, a benzimidazole is the drug of choice if the parasites have not already been selected for resistance to this class of drug. To be certain, there is no long-term residual effect, but this is probably the best class of drug for calves at this time. Treat the replacement calves at the time of vaccination, weaning, and then before breeding.

Yearling heifers may benefit by the use of a macrocyclic lactone as she becomes resistant to *Cooperia*. The first calf heifer is still growing and will give birth and have to suckle her calf. This animal will benefit the most from the use of a macrocyclic lactone with residual activity.

The selection as to when and what to use to deworm adult beef cattle should be determined as to when the hypobiotic *Ostertagia* are likely to be in the abomasum and if there are also other parasites the drugs may control, such as flukes or flies (grubs), ticks, or mites. You know when the breeding season is and should have an idea when there are arrested larvae in your geographic area. The host's hormonal state may interfere with acquired immunity. Normally, males are more susceptible to parasitic worms, except at parturition and early lactation when females are at greatest risk. Benzimidazoles may kill arrested larvae, which may be sufficient if the cattle are not being continually exposed to high pasture levels of nematodes. With macrocyclic lactones, cattle should benefit not only from the removal of worms at the time of treatment, but the residual effects that kill incoming larvae for 3 to 6 weeks or longer, depending on the drug and carrier. However, the approach that is quite effective in adult cattle may cause problems in calves. The widespread use of the macrocyclic lactones with their residual effects in calves has been the driving force for anthelmintic resistance in cattle. *Cooperia* spp are resistant to macrocyclic lactones throughout North America, and resistance to both benzimidazoles and macrocyclic lactones by *Haemonchus* is a real concern.

In general, adult cattle will probably benefit from a spring deworming using a macrocyclic lactone. In the south, *Ostertagia* will be transmitted throughout the fall, winter, and early spring. The worms acquired during the later period will be in arrested development, and the warm season worms will become active in the pastures. In the north, the arrested larvae acquired last year will be emerging if they were not removed at the end of the previous grazing season. If the cows were treated last fall, then waiting until they have grazed a few weeks will let them harvest the overwintering larvae before they contribute to a new generation of worms. This strategic approach will lessen the exposure the cattle will have later. What about production units, which are not considered north or south? Limited information from such areas indicates that there are *Ostertagia* with both winter arrest and summer arrest in the same herd of cattle. The studies were done some years ago and with the movement of livestock, changes in climate, and widespread use of anthelmintics, the pattern of arrest may not be accurate in all places. We do know if cattle acquired arrested *Ostertagia* larvae from northern pastures and moved into a southern environment, the larvae emerged in the spring and vice versa, which indicates that over time, the worm was able to adapt to the new environment or died out. So, it appears that a spring deworming should benefit cattle on pasture in high-rainfall areas.

There are so many different management programs that no one parasite control program will work on all farms or ranches. We need to think, "How does the parasite survive here?" to control it. Anthelmintic resistance will become more widespread in cattle with the movement of cattle carrying resistant worms from one farm to another. It may take 2 or 3 years for the resistance to become apparent on a property, but once established, it is there for the foreseeable future. Anthelmintics with a long residual effect are a mechanism for selecting resistant worms if the products are not 100% effective.

Leaving some cattle untreated, at least in theory, will provide the refugia necessary to preserve the effectiveness of the anthelmintics. The idea of refugia is that the offspring of worms in the untreated animals will mate with the offspring of the worms that demonstrated their resistance by surviving. The larvae then acquired from the pasture will be a combination of resistant and susceptible larvae, and the drugs will continue to be somewhat effective for a longer time. Bulls and cows through their third calving should be treated, but not treating all the older cows is probably the best source of a refugia. If other species can be used as a model, the teenage cow's immune system is slowing down and she probably also should be treated. Refugia has been used by small ruminant producers by using either fecal egg counts or evaluating the level of anemia determined by comparing ocular mucous membrane color with a FAMCHA chart. The chart (FAffa MAlan CHArt named for an acronym of the developer), compares ocular mucous membrane color with the level of anemia. It is used to specifically identify animals in a flock that should be administered an anthelmintic.[31] However, young animals (younger than 12–15 months) are the hosts for most of the *Cooperia* spp that are largely resistant to macrocyclic lactones. Therefore, if a herd of adult beef cattle was treated with a macrocyclic lactone and their calves with a benzimidazole, they would serve as the refugia for worms treated by the other family of anthelmintic.

How should anthelmintics be administered: as pour-on, oral, or injectable? The pour-on products in adult cattle should cover the important worms and control ecto parasites as well. However, there are some problems. The drugs must be administered to the skin of the cow, not her hair or the air. Also, some products have an effective anthelmintic listed on the label but have different carriers and apparently are not equal in effectiveness.[32] Pour-on drugs should not be administered to calves, as they are ineffective against *Cooperia* and possibly *Haemonchus,* which may enhance anthelmintic resistance. Benzimidazoles are administered orally and it is important to give a dose appropriate for the size of the individual animal or to the largest animals in a group to ensure an adequate dose is administered, as underdosing selects for resistant worms. The injectables, except for levamisole, have a residual effect that varies with the drug and carrier. The residual effect is positive in that incoming larvae will be killed for weeks to months, but as they are metabolized from the body, they act as a sorting gate by allowing only worms with genes for resistance to enter and mate with similar worms, resulting in resistant offspring.

Never inject the prolonged macrocyclic lactone into growing calves or small ruminants unless the pasture they are in is temporary and other calves will not follow until the next year and they are going to a feedlot. The calves are administered a drug based on body weight, and within 1 to 2 months their body weight has increased enough that the level of drug in their tissues is definitely an underdose, which selects for resistance. Too much deworming will result in worms that cannot be killed by any of the available anthelmintics or combinations thereof, and the cattle's immune system may not have had experience with important worms.

GRAZING MANAGEMENT

With the availability of inexpensive, safe, and effective dewormers, most of the control of parasitic disease has relied on the use of drugs rather than management. With high-intensity grazing systems and the selection of cattle for maximum production of meat or milk, this approach has generally served well. However, if lessons can be learned from small ruminants, the sustained use of these drugs will require some level of management in the selection of which animals to treat and when to treat them. Without exception, the disease caused by parasitic nematodes is a numbers game. When a host has a few parasites, there is no disease, but it is an opportunity to stimulate a protective immune response. With greater numbers, the opportunities for disease increase as the numbers rise. Therefore, young animals whose immune systems have not matured or encountered parasites are at greatest risk of disease.

To lessen the chances of disease, the most logical approach is to lessen exposure to infective larvae. Pastures can become parasite-safe by producing hay or cropping. An abandoned pasture is not a source of useful forage, because as vegetation matures, it becomes less palatable and is of lower nutritional quality; therefore, alternate species grazing or making hay/silage is preferred. The intervals of rest from grazing by a specific host species may be as short as 1 month in a warm, wet summer, but takes months in cool, humid climates for the larval population to dissipate. Husbandry practices to prevent disease include improved nutrition, which may lessen the amount of grazing close to the fecal pat. Separate age groups, as replacement dairy heifers or stocker calves are most susceptible when they are exposed to large numbers of parasites, especially by following animals that are only slightly older. Most hosts develop acquired resistance if not overwhelmed by parasites, and they obtain sufficient dietary protein. Management offers a substantially cheaper and more effective means for controlling helminths than drugs alone.[33] Most clinical helminthiasis occurs in young naïve hosts or those on marginal rations. Anthelmintics will not lead to increased weight gain unless adequate rations are consumed.

There is no system ideal for control of parasites unless the pasture is rested 1.5 to 12 months, depending on the time of year, but rotational grazing is better for animal nutrition and pasture quality. What does resting a pasture mean? You cannot simply abandon a pasture for 6 months in high-rainfall areas and expect eatable forage to be present. Resting a pasture means that the "at-risk" animals are not constantly occupying the pasture or with only short intervals without grazing. Grazing pastures with animals that have developed a level of immunity may harvest larval nematodes, resulting in safer pastures than occurs following abandonment. Pastures, especially improved pastures, must be managed. Fifty percent of the infective larvae occur within 1 inch of the ground. The use of temporary pastures or hay meadows after harvest is a parasite clean pasture. Overstocking varies with the year and available forage, and competition for food also results in more parasite exposure.

Short-duration, high-density grazing systems have become popular in that more livestock can be maintained on less land. There are many animals on limited area of forage, and the livestock are moved frequently (hours to days), and pastures are rested for 2 to 4 weeks (like growing and mowing a lawn). This approach is parasite heaven, but also produces maximum high-quality forage production per acre. The reason that this system is so favorable for parasites is that the time span required to produce high-quality forages is similar to the time required for the development from egg to infective larvae, and translation of the larvae onto the forage. Also, in high-density systems, the livestock do very little selective grazing and consume forage they may normally avoid, such as the rank grass surrounding a fecal pat, because there is no choice and the forages available are a monoculture or only a limited number of plant species. Raising replacement heifers on permanent pastures not used by similar calves the preceding year is a wise way of avoiding overwintering larvae. Older cattle can act as biological vacuum sweepers harvesting the larvae of which only a small percentage will become reproducing adults. Moving spring-born replacement calves at the midpoint of the grazing season is another way of avoiding heavy exposure to infective larvae.

This movement at the time of anthelmintic administration will not only remove the adult worms in the calves but has given the calves a level of exposure that may stimulate immunity. Having calves rotationally graze in front of cows or other resistant hosts allows the pasture to be used and lowers the risk of infection.

No single strategy of management will suffice for all herds, even in a given region. A few practices can be advantageous in most circumstances, but not all. One practice that is widely used is that after deworming, move to a clean pasture. The idea is that animals that have been freed of infection will not immediately encounter a new worm population to replace the one just removed. This is true, and when animals enter an annual pasture that is replanted each year is a very sound approach. If, however, the worms have not all been removed and the animals are to remain in the new pasture, it is an effective method of establishing resistant worms onto the new pasture. The reason for this, is that the only worms not removed by the anthelmintic used at the time of moving will be produce eggs in the new environment and the larvae produced from these eggs will have only other resistant worms to mate with when they mature.

REFERENCES

1. Gasbarre LC, Leighton EA, Sonstegard T. Role of the bovine immune system and genome in resistance to gastrointestinal nematodes. Vet Parasitol 2001;98:51–64.
2. Saddiqi HA, Jabbar A, Sarwar M, et al. Small ruminant resistance against gastro-intestinal nematodes: a case of *Haemonchus contortus*. Parasitol Res 2011;109: 1483–500.
3. Gross SJ, Ryan WG, Ploeger HW. Anthelmintic treatment of dairy cows and its effect on milk production. Vet Rec 1999;144:581–7.
4. McBeath DG, Dean SP, Preston NK. The effect of a preparturient fenbendazole treatment on lactation in yield in dairy cows. Vet Rec 1979;105:507–9.
5. Walsh TA, Tournis PJ, Morton JM. The effect of Ivermectin treatment of late pregnant dairy cows in Southwest Victoria on subsequent milk production and reproductive performance. Aust Vet J 1995;72:201–7.
6. Forbes AB, Huckle CA, Gibb MJ, et al. Evaluation of the effects of nematode parasitism on grazing behavior, herbage intake and growth in young grazing cattle. Vet Parasitol 2000;90:111–8.
7. Stomberg BE, Vatthauer RJ, Schlotthauer JC, et al. Production responses following strategic parasite control in a beef cow/calf herd. Vet Parasitol 1997; 68:315–22.
8. Reinemeyer CR. The effects of anthelmintic treatment of beef cows on parasito-logic and performance parameters. Compendium of Continuing Education 1992;14:678–86.
9. Zajac AM, Hansen JW, Whitten WD, et al. The effect of parasite control on fertility in beef heifers. Vet Parasitol 1991;40:281–91.
10. Coles GC, Watson CL, Anziani OS. Ivermectin-resistant *Cooperia* in cattle. Vet Rec 2001;148:283–4.
11. Fleming AS, Craig T, Kaplan RM, et al. Anthelmintic resistance of gastrointestinal parasites in small ruminants. J Vet Intern Med 2006;20:435–44.
12. Grossner AG, Venturina VM, Shaw DJ, et al. Relationship between susceptibility of Blackface sheep to *Teladorsaiga circumcincta* infection and inflammatory mucosal T cell response. Vet Res 2012;43:26–37.
13. Simpson HV, Przemeck SMC, Scott I, et al. Pathophysiology in *Teladorsaiga (Ostertagia) circumcincta*-infected sheep selected for high fleece weight. Vet Parasitol 2009;163:73–80.

14. Forbes AB, Rice BJ. Patterns of parasitic nematode infection and immunity in dairy heifers treated with ivermectin in a sustained-release bolus formulation either at turnout or in the middle of the grazing season. Vet Rec 2000;147:295–7.

15. Ploeger HW, Kloosterman A, Borgsteede FHM, et al. Effect of naturally occurring nematode infection in first and second grazing season on the growth performance of second year cattle. Vet Parasitol 1990;36:57–70.

16. Williams JC, Loyacano AF. Internal parasites of cattle in Louisiana and other southern states. Experiment Station Research Information. Louisiana State University; 2001. p. 1–20.

17. Edmonds MD, Johnson EG, Edmonds JD. Anthelmintic resistance of *Ostertagia ostertagi* and *Cooperia oncophora* to macrocyclic lactones in cattle from the western United States. Vet Parasitol 2010;170:224–9.

18. Snyder TG, Williams JC, Karnes PA, et al. Immunosuppression of lymphocyte blastogenesis in cattle infected with *Ostertagia ostertagi* and/or *Trichostrongylus axei*. Vet Immunol Immunpathol 1986;11:251–64.

19. Gasbarre LC, Smith LL, Pilitt PA. Identification of cattle nematodes resistant to multiple classes of anthelmintics in a commercial cattle population in the US. Proc Am Assoc Vet Parasitol 2005;50:46.

20. Gasbarre LC. Anthelmintic resistance in cattle nematodes in the US. Vet Parasitol 2014;204:3–11.

21. Stromberg BE, Gasbarre LC, Waite A, et al. *Cooperia punctata*: effect on cattle productivity? Vet Parasitol 2012;183:284–91.

22. Anziani OS, Suarez V, Guglielmone AA, et al. Resistance to benzimidazole and macrocyclic lactone anthelmintics in cattle nematodes in Argentina. Vet Parasitol 2004;122:303–6.

23. Familton AS, Mason P, Coles GC. Anthelmintic resistant *Cooperia* in New Zealand cattle. Vet Rec 2001;149:719–20.

24. Taira N, Ura S. Sudden death in calves associated with *Strongyloides papillosus* infection. Vet Parasitol 1991;39:313–9.

25. Nakamura Y, Ooba C, Hirose H. Recovery from arrhythmias in lambs infected with *Strongyloides papillosus* following worm elimination. J Helminthol 1998;72:43–6.

26. Woodbury MR, Copeland S, Wagner B, et al. *Toxocara vitulorum* in a bison (*Bison bison*) herd from western Canada. Can Vet J 2012;53:791–4.

27. Davila G, Irsik M, Griner EC. *Toxocara vitulorum* in beef calves in North Central Florida. Vet Parasitol 2010;168:261–3.

28. Condi GK, Soutello RG, Amarante AFT. Moxidectin-resistant nematodes in cattle in Brazil. Vet Parasitol 2009;161:213–7.

29. MacGregor DS, Yoder DR, Rew RS. Impact of doramectin treatment at the time of feedlot entry on the productivity of yearling steers with natural nematode infections. Am J Vet Res 2001;62:622–4.

30. Enteracasso CM, Parkins JJ, Armour J, et al. Production, parasitological and carcass evaluation studies in steers exposed to trichostrongyle infection and treated with a morantel bolus or fenbendazole in two consecutive grazing seasons. Res Vet Sci 1986;36:57–70.

31. vanWyk JA, Stenson MO, van der Merwe JS, et al. Anthelmintic resistance in South Africa; surveys indicate an extremely serious situation in sheep and goat farming. Onderstepoort J Vet Res 1999;66:273–84.

32. Yazwinski TA, Tucker CA, Hornsby JA, et al. Field trial evaluation of several commercial ivermectin pour-on products in cattle. Arkansas Cattle Business 2004;20:44–6.

33. Hoste H, Torres-Acosta JF. Non chemical control of helminths in ruminants: adapting solutions for changing worms in a changing world. Vet Parasitol 2013;180:144–54.

Coccidiosis in Large and Small Ruminants

Sarah Tammy Nicole Keeton, PhD, MS[a],*, Christine B. Navarre, DVM, MS[b]

KEYWORDS

- Coccidia • Coccidiosis • Diarrhea • Ruminants • Cattle • Sheep • Goats
- Ionophores

KEY POINTS

- Coccidiosis is an important parasitic disease of ruminant livestock caused by the protozoan parasite of the genus *Eimeria*.
- Calves between 6 and 12 months of age and lambs and kids between 1 and 6 months of age are most susceptible.
- Subclinical disease is characterized by poor growth.
- Clinical disease is most commonly characterized by diarrhea.
- Control of coccidiosis is based on sound management, the use of preventive medications, and treatment of clinical cases as necessary.

INTRODUCTION: NATURE OF THE PROBLEM

Coccidiosis is a parasitic disease of vertebrate animals, including domestic ruminants.[1] It is economically significant, with losses from both clinical and subclinical disease.

Coccidiosis is caused by the protozoan parasite of the genus *Eimeria*. *Eimeria* are host specific, meaning that an *Eimeria* species that infect goats does not infect sheep or cattle and vice versa. Certain species of *Eimeria* are nonpathogenic and do not cause disease. The pathogenic species and sites of infection are listed in **Table 1**. Mixed infections with multiple pathogenic and nonpathogenic species is common.

LIFE CYCLE

Proper treatment and control of coccidiosis requires an understanding of the complex life cycle and transmission of *Eimeria* spp (**Fig. 1**). The life cycle can be divided into

Disclosure: The authors have nothing to disclose.
[a] Department of Veterinary Clinical Sciences, School of Veterinary Medicine, Louisiana State University, Skip Bertman Drive, Baton Rouge, LA 70803, USA; [b] LSU AgCenter, School of Animal Sciences, Louisiana State University, 111 Dalrymple Bldg, 110 LSU Union Square, Baton Rouge, LA 70803-0106, USA
* Corresponding author. 909 Durnin Drive, Denham Springs, LA 70726.
E-mail address: Sorlik1@lsu.edu

Table 1
Pathogenic species of *Eimeria* and site of infestation in cattle, sheep, and goats

	Species of *Eimeria*	Site of Infestation
Cattle	*Eimeria zuernii*	Small and large intestine
	Eimeria bovis	Small and large intestine
	Eimeria alabamensis	Small and large intestine
Sheep	*Eimeria ovinoidalis*	Cecum and colon
	Eimeria crandalis	Small and large intestine
Goats	*Eimeria arloingi*	Small intestine
	Eimeria christenseni	Small intestine
	Eimeria ninakohlyakimovae	Small and large intestine

Data from Taylor MA, Coop RL, Wall RL. Veterinary parasitology. Fourth edition. Chichester (United Kingdom): Wiley Blackwell; 2016; and Chartier C, Paraud C. Coccidiosis due to *Eimeria* in sheep and goats, a review. Small Ruminant Res 2012;103(1):84–92.

2 phases: an exogenous phase (free living in the environment) and an endogenous phase (parasitic phase within host). The life cycle takes between 2 and 4 weeks to complete depending on the species of *Eimeria* and environmental conditions.[2]

In the exogenous phase of sporogony, unsporulated oocysts are excreted in feces and undergo sporulation under ideal environmental conditions of oxygen,

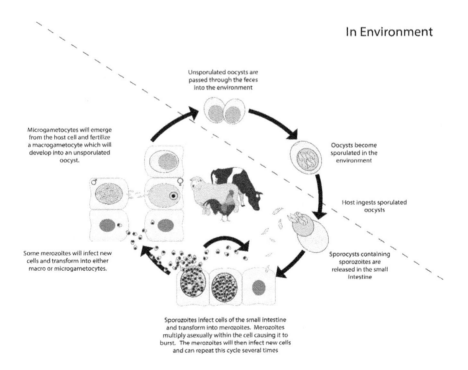

In Environment

Unsporulated oocysts are passed through the feces into the environment

Microgametocytes will emerge from the host cell and fertilize a macrogametocyte which will develop into an unsporulated oocyst.

Oocysts become sporulated in the environment

Host ingests sporulated oocysts

Some merozoites will infect new cells and transform into either macro or microgametocytes.

Sporocysts containing sporozoites are released in the small intestine

Sporozoites infect cells of the small intestine and transform into merozoites. Merozoites multiply asexually within the cell causing it to burst. The merozoites will then infect new cells and can repeat this cycle several times

In Host

Fig. 1. *Eimeria* life cycle. (*From* Javier Garza, PhD, USDA-NIFA Fellow, Parasite Immunology, Division of Animal and Nutritional Sciences, West Virginia University, with permission.)

moderate temperatures, and high moisture. Sporulation takes 1 to 4 days if environmental conditions are ideal but can take several weeks in less favorable conditions.[3]

The endogenous phase begins with the animal ingesting sporulated oocysts. Once ingested, the oocysts undergo excystation, in which the sporozoites are released and subsequently invade the intestinal cells. The sporozoites then transform into schizonts and multiply asexually to generate merozoites (merogony). Merozoites may then penetrate additional intestinal epithelial cells and multiply further or progress to macrogametes or microgametes. During the sexual phase (gametogony), microgametes (sperm) fertilize macrogametes (ova), producing oocysts. When the oocysts are mature, they rupture the host cell, are released into the lumen of the intestine, and are passed in the feces as unsporulated oocysts.[4–7] The damage to the gut caused by this phase is what contributes most to the clinical signs.

EPIDEMIOLOGY

Coccidia are highly prolific because each sporulated oocyst has the potential to produce 23 million oocysts during the endogenous phase after just 21 days.[6] This ability leads to high levels of environmental contamination. Sporulated oocysts are resistant in the environment and can survive for weeks to months, especially in favorable conditions of moderate heat and moisture.[7]

Buildup of high levels of contamination are most common in areas where animals congregate or are crowded and feces are more concentrated in the environment. Feedlots, drylots, and barns are common types of housing associated with coccidiosis. It can also be a problem in heavily stocked pastures, especially around watering and feeding areas.

Healthy ruminants are generally immune to disease by 1 year of age but serve as a reservoir to younger animals. The magnitude of infection, clinical signs, and oocyte shedding are affected by the species of *Eimeria* involved, level of environmental exposure, and animal immunity. Age, other stressors (weaning, weather, transportation, other diseases, and so forth), nutrition, and genetic susceptibility all contribute to animal immunity and susceptibility to coccidiosis.[7,8]

HISTORY AND PHYSICAL EXAMINATION

Calves are most susceptible to infection between 6 and 12 months of age. Lambs and kids are susceptible from 1 and 6 months of age, but most clinical disease is seen in lambs and kids between 4 and 8 weeks of age.[9,10]

There are subclinical and clinical forms coccidiosis. Subclinical infection can cause depressed appetite as well as decreased feed efficiency from gut damage, which leads to poor growth rates and weight gains.[10,11]

The following clinical signs may be associated with clinical coccidiosis:

- Diarrhea
- Anorexia
- Depression
- Weakness
- Abdominal pain
- Dehydration
- Pale mucous membranes
- Acute weight loss
- Straining to defecate and subsequent rectal prolapse

Diarrhea is the most common clinical sign, and it may be bloody or mucoid. The severity of disease varies from self-limiting, in which animals recover without treatment, to severe cases, in which animals quickly succumb to the infection and die.[8,12]

Speed and degree of recovery depend on the severity of infection and area of the gut involved. Animals that recover from more severe infection may become chronic so-called poor-doers because of permanent scarring of the gut.

Nervous coccidiosis is a condition that occurs in calves after heavy infections with *Eimeria zuernii*. Clinical signs include muscle tremors, convulsions, nystagmus, and other central nervous system signs. Animals may fall to the ground, show neurologic signs, then recover and have periods of normality. Mortality associated with nervous coccidiosis can be 80% to 90%. The pathophysiology of this condition is not known.[7,13]

DIAGNOSIS

A tentative ante mortem diagnosis of clinical coccidiosis is usually based on flock/herd history and clinical signs along with observation of coccidia oocysts in feces. A definitive diagnosis is complicated by the difficulty in interpreting results of fecal examination for oocytes. Quantitative fecal analysis by sugar or salt flotation techniques that give results in oocysts per gram of feces are superior to nonquantitative tests. Low numbers of oocytes are commonly shed in normal animals. Counts of 5000 oocysts per gram or higher in combination with a typical clinical picture are highly suggestive of coccidiosis. Speciation of the oocysts is important because high numbers of nonpathogenic species in animals with other diarrheal diseases is possible. It is also possible to have clinical signs develop in the early stages of the disease when fecal shedding is low or in animals that are in the chronic stages of the disease and have intestinal scarring. Fecal examinations on multiple animals during a suspected outbreak and over time in the herd or flock are helpful in interpreting results[7,10,14–17]

Necropsy may also help confirm coccidiosis in a herd or flock. Intestinal hemorrhage and white/gray patches or lines on the mucosa on gross examination are suspicious of coccidiosis. Histopathology can help confirm the diagnosis.

PHARMACOLOGIC TREATMENT OPTIONS

Prevention of coccidiosis is superior to treatment because subclinical production losses and potential permanent damage unresponsive to treatment are costly and have animal welfare implications. Some exposure to the organism is necessary to develop immunity, but it should be limited. Minimizing stress and other diseases, and optimizing nutrition are important, as is minimizing environmental contamination. Prevention of overcrowding, feeding off the ground, and sanitation of feeding and watering equipment are important. Exposure to sunlight and desiccation are effective means of decreasing of oocysts in the environment.

Where environmental control is not adequate, the use of anticoccidial drugs can be helpful for both treatment and prevention. Anticoccidial drugs work by impeding the growth and reproduction of coccidian parasites. They have little impact on existing infection but should help limit both subclinical and clinical disease and environmental contamination.

There are several anticoccidial drugs available for treatment and prevention of coccidiosis in ruminants (**Table 2**). Species and class approval varies and extralabel use should only be undertaken following the Animal Medicinal Drug Use Clarification Act (AMDUCA) in the United States. These agents may also be restricted in organic

Table 2
Anticoccidial agents for use in treatment and prevention of coccidiosis in cattle (C), sheep (S), and goats (G). Consult product label for specific class restriction within species and withdrawal times

Agent	Treatment	Prevention	Comments
Amprolium[a] (Corid)	10/mg/kg BW for 5 d (C) 25–40 mg/kg BW for 5 d (S, G, ELDU)	5 mg/kg BW for 21 d (C) 50 mg/kg BW for 21 d (S, ELDU)	Available in multiple forms: • 9.6% oral solution • 20% soluble powder • 1.25% or 2.5% crumbles/pellets
Decoquinate (Deccox)		0.5 mg/kg BW for at least 28 d (C, S, G)	Feed additive For prepartum use in sheep and goats • 1 kg of 13% premix in 22 kg of trace mineralized salt
Lasalocid (Bovatec)		1 mg/kg BW continuously (C, S) G = ELDU)	Feed additive For prepartum use in sheep and goats • 1 kg of 6% premix in 22 kg of trace mineralized salt
Monensin (Rumensin)		20 g/ton of feed (G) (S = ELDU) Cattle doses vary by class-see specific labels	Feed additive May be best choice for goats
Sulfaquinoxaline	10–20 mg/kg BW for 3–7 d (C) (S, G = ELDU)		As a 0.015% solution in water

Abbreviations: BW, body weight; ELDU, extralabel drug use.
[a] Amprolium is a thiamine analog and can cause polioencephalomalacia, especially at high doses.
Data from Refs.[15–17]

and natural programs. Anticoccidial agents used in other species, such as poultry, may be toxic to ruminants.[15]

The most commonly used anticoccidial drugs from those listed in **Table 2** are the ionophores (decoquinate, lasalocid, and monensin). They are feed additives classified as antibiotics. By altering the rumen bacteria, they also improve feed efficiency and control bloat and acidosis.[18] Sulfa drugs are commonly used to treat coccidiosis in many species but the exact mechanism is not known. Their clinical effectiveness may be more related to control of secondary bacterial enteritis than to a direct effect on coccidia. Sulfaquinoxaline is the only sulfa drug approved for control of coccidiosis and only in cattle.

When using anticoccidial drugs for prevention or treatment of weaned young stock, all animals in the group should be medicated. Resistance to coccidiostats can occur, and is common in poultry.[7] To minimize this potential, longer-term preventive uses should be limited to high risk-situations. Although resistance is possible, evidence that it occurs in ruminant *Eimeria* spp is mostly circumstantial at this time. Treatment success of clinical coccidiosis is frequently unrewarding, and no drug has ever been documented to be highly efficacious for treatment.[19] Once clinical signs appear, damage to the intestines has already occurred. What seems to be lack of efficacy of a treatment (continued diarrhea), is most likely caused by a damaged gut.[20] Use of drugs such as amprolium and sulfas for treatment may help prevent worsening of clinical signs by limiting reinfection in animals that cannot be removed from a contaminated environment and for which addition of ionophores to feed is impractical.

As mentioned before, the degree of oocyst shedding is affected by many factors, including initial dose, stage of the infections, age of the animal, and individual susceptibility. Therefore, using oocyst counts to determine drug efficacy/resistance in 1 or a small number of animals is difficult. The use of products not approved for food animal species, such as ponazuril (Marquis), for clinical cases that seem to be refractory to approved treatments is not recommended. It is unlikely to be any more clinically effective once clinical signs appear, and the meat withdrawal time is more than 120 days (contact FARAD.org for exact withdrawal times).[21] Use of ponazuril for convenience (1 dose compared with multiple doses of approved products) is illegal under AMDUCA.

Coccidiosis prevention is usually reserved for calves after weaning, when they are most susceptible, and in drylot or crowded condition. If problems occur in nursing calves, an anticoccidial drugs in creep feed may be necessary. Because lambs and kids are most at risk while still on the dam, coccidiostats can be provided to the dams for 30 days before lambing/kidding to reduce environmental contamination. An added benefit to the use of ionophores prepartum in sheep and goats is a potential decrease in the incidence pregnancy toxemia.[16]

NONPHARMACOLOGIC TREATMENT OPTIONS

Coccidiosis vaccines are commercially available for poultry. Despite ongoing research, a commercially available product in ruminants has not been developed.

Sericea lespedeza, a leguminous plant containing condensed tannins with antiparasitic properties, has been shown to be successful in preventing and controlling coccidiosis and gastrointestinal nematode infections in lambs. In a study conducted by the Louisiana State University Agricultural Center, sericea lespedeza was fed to experimentally infected lambs to evaluate efficacy. The increase, peak, and decline of fecal egg counts observed in the control lambs indicated a typical patent infection. The comparatively unchanged fecal egg count in the treatment lambs indicated that sericea lespedeza effectively controlled infection compared with the control lambs.[21] In addition, fecal egg count remained lower than in control lambs, which is in agreement with other reports of reduced fecal egg count in sericea lespedeza–fed animals.[21–23] Under the conditions of this study, sericea lespedeza effectively controlled *Eimeria* spp infection, as well as reducing nematode infections. The use of this plant could be beneficial in weaning management to control coccidiosis.[24]

SUMMARY

Coccidiosis is an important parasitic disease of ruminant livestock. Control of coccidiosis in cattle, sheep, and goats is based on sound management, the use of preventive medications, and treatment of clinical cases as necessary.

REFERENCES

1. Taylor MA, Coop RL, Wall RL. Veterinary parasitology. 4th edition. Ames (IA): Wiley Blackwell; 2016.
2. Soulsby EJL. Helminths, arthropods and protozoa of domesticated animals. 7th edition. London: Baillière Tindall; 1982.

3. Coccidiosis in Lambs. Farm health online – animal health and welfare knowledge hub. Available at: http://www.farmhealthonline.com/disease-management/sheep-diseases/coccidiosis-in-lambs/. Accessed May 18, 2017.

4. Chartier C, Paraud C. Coccidiosis due to *Eimeria* in sheep and goats, a review. Small Rumin Res 2012;103(1):84–92.

5. Foreyt WJ. Coccidiosis and cryptosporidiosis in sheep and goats. Vet Clin North Am Food Anim Pract 1990;6(3):655–70.

6. Dendrickson J. Coccidia lifecycle | prevention and treatment of coccidiosis. Corid. Available at: http://www.corid.com/Coccidia.html. Accessed May 18, 2017.

7. Jolley WR, Bardsley KD. Ruminant coccidiosis. Vet Clin North Am Food Anim Pract 2006;22(3):613–21.

8. Coffey L. Coccidiosis: symptoms, prevention, and treatment in sheep, goats, and calves. NCAT ATTRA Sustainable Agriculture. Available at: https://attra.ncat.org/attra-pub/viewhtml.php?id=483. Accessed May 1, 2017.

9. Coccidiosis in beef cattle - frequently asked questions. Alberta agriculture and forestry. Available at: http://www1.agric.gov.ab.ca/$department/deptdocs.nsf/all/faq8011. 2015. Accessed May 18, 2017.

10. Schoenian S. Coccidiosis: deadly scourge of lambs and kids. Maryland small ruminant page. Available at: http://www.sheepandgoat.com/coccidiosis. 2016. Accessed May 18, 2017.

11. Coccidiosis. Calfology. Available at: http://calfology.com/library/wiki/coccidiosis. Accessed May 18, 2017.

12. Richards C Step DL, Giedt EJ. Coccidiosis treatment and prevention in cattle. Division of Agricultural Science and Natural Resources Oklahoma State University. Available at: http://pods.dasnr.okstate.edu/docushare/dsweb/Get/Document-2677/VTMD-9129web-2015.pdf. Accessed May 16, 2017.

13. White P. Coccidiosis. American highland cattle association. Available at: https://www.highlandcattleusa.org/content/management/Coccidiosis.pdf. Accessed May 20, 2017.

14. Leite-Browning ML Coccidiosis in goats and prevention. Alabama cooperative extension system. Available at: http://www.aces.edu/pubs/docs/U/UNP-0109/UNP-0109.pdf. 2009. Accessed May 18, 2017.

15. Smith BP. Large animal internal medicine. St Louis (MO): Mosby; 2002.

16. Pugh DG, Navarre CB. Internal parasite control strategies. Vet Clin North Am Food Anim Pract 2001;2(3):231–44.

17. Pugh DG, Baird AN. Sheep and goat medicine. Maryland Heights (MO): Elsevier Saunders; 2012.

18. Hersom M, Thrift T. Application of ionophores in cattle diets. Every day information source Institute of Food and Agricultural Sciences, University of Florida 2015. Available at: http://edis.ifas.ufl.edu/pdffiles/AN/AN28500.pdf. Accessed June 18, 2017.

19. Constable, PD. Overview of coccidiosis. In: Merck Veterinary Manual. 2016. Available at: www.merckvetmanual.com/digestive-system/coccidiosis/overview-of-coccidiosis. Accessed June 7, 2017.

20. Howard JL. Current veterinary therapy 3: food animal practice. Philadelphia: WB Saunders; 1995.

21. Gibbons P, Love D, Craig T, et al. Efficacy of treatment of elevated coccidial oocyst counts in goats using amprolium versus ponazuril. Vet Parasitol 2016; 218:1–4.

22. Keeton STN. Integrated methods for controlling gastrointestinal nematode infections in ewes and lambs [dissertation]. Baton Rouge (LA): Louisiana State University and Agricultural and Mechanical College; 2016.
23. Lange KC, Olcott DD, Miller JE, et al. Effect of sericea lespedeza (*Lespedeza cuneata*) fed as hay, on natural and experimental *Haemonchus contortus* infections in lambs. Vet Parasitol 2006;141(3–4):273–8.
24. Burke JM, Miller JM, Mosjidis JA, et al. Grazing sericea lespedeza for control of gastrointestinal nematodes in lambs. Vet Parasitol 2012;186(3–4):507–12.

Paratuberculosis in Cattle

Marie-Eve Fecteau, DVM

KEYWORDS

- Johne disease • *Mycobacterium avium* ssp *paratuberculosis* • Ruminants • Herd
- Pathogenesis • Diagnosis • Control • Vaccination

KEY POINTS

- Paratuberculosis, or Johne disease, is caused by *Mycobacterium avium* ssp *paratuberculosis* (MAP), which has a long incubation period leading to delayed fecal shedding and a delayed humoral response in infected animals.
- Although the classic signs of Johne disease in cattle include diarrhea and weight loss, most infected cattle are in the subclinical phase of the disease and appear healthy; however, they have decreased milk production and reduced fertility when compared with uninfected herd mates.
- Subclinically, infected cattle can shed large amounts of MAP in their feces, contaminating the environment and infecting the replacement stock.
- Control of the disease relies on preventing infection of the susceptible animals in the herd, testing and culling the infected animals, and increasing resistance to MAP.

INTRODUCTION

Paratuberculosis is a chronic, granulomatous infection of the intestinal tract of cattle and other domestic and wild ruminants caused by *Mycobacterium avium* ssp *paratuberculosis* (MAP). The organism is an acid-fast, gram-positive, facultative intracellular pathogen that requires iron for growth and has the ability the survive within macrophages.[1] The organism is extremely resistant and, in ideal conditions, can survive for up to a year in the environment.[2] MAP has also been shown to survive pasteurization.[3,4] Because of MAP's long incubation period (between 2 and 7 years), most infected cattle (around 95%) are considered to be in the subclinical stages of the disease, with less than 5% of infected cattle displaying clinical signs of illness.[5] The term *Johne disease* typically refers to the clinical syndrome of diarrhea and weight loss that results from advanced MAP infection.

PREVALENCE OF PARATUBERCULOSIS IN CATTLE

Paratuberculosis is widely distributed throughout the world in many ruminant species. Many studies have been conducted in the United States as well as in other countries to

Disclosure Statement: The author has nothing to disclose.
Department of Clinical Studies–New Bolton Center, School of Veterinary Medicine, University of Pennsylvania, 382 West Street Road, Kennett Square, PA 19348, USA
E-mail address: mfecteau@vet.upenn.edu

estimate MAP prevalence in cattle. Fecal cultures and antibody-detection methods have been the most common diagnostic methods used for determination of prevalence.[6] Estimates of MAP prevalence are complicated by several factors, including the low sensitivity of the diagnostic tests available for subclinical animals, and that cattle in the clinical phase of the disease are usually culled before a final diagnosis of MAP infection is made. In the United States, at least 68% of dairy herds have MAP-infected cattle, with a much lower prevalence (less than 10%) among beef herds.[7,8] The most recent estimates of within-herd prevalence among a sample of 106 US dairy herds were reported to range from 0% to 27.3%, with a mean of 5.5%.[9] High within-herd prevalence is usually associated with higher MAP fecal shedding among positive animals, MAP fecal shedding at a younger age, shorter incubation period, and higher numbers of animals in the clinical phase of the disease.[6] It has also been proposed that the number of advanced clinical cases found in a herd can be used as a proxy for the determination of within-herd prevalence, in that for every cow with advanced Johne disease, it is likely that 15 to 25 others in the herd are infected.[10]

TRANSMISSION OF PARATUBERCULOSIS IN CATTLE
Routes of Transmission

Most new infections occur via the fecal-oral route, although other routes are possible. Calves born to seropositive dams were shown to be 6.6 times more likely to be seropositive compared with calves born to seronegative dams.[11] A meta-analysis estimated that 9% of fetuses born from subclinically infected dams and 39% born from clinically affected dams were infected in utero.[12] These findings indicate that the likelihood of fetal infection depends on the severity of the dam's infection. As the infection status of the dam represents a major risk factor for the newborn calf, it is not advised to keep a clinical cow within the herd in the hopes of obtaining the calf before culling, as the cow will continue to shed MAP organisms into the environment while the calf has a good chance to be infected.

MAP has been isolated from uterine flush fluids of infected cattle, and MAP organisms have been shown to adhere to embryos in vitro.[13] Therefore, an embryo obtained from an infected cow could result in an infected fetus; however, oocytes and embryos processed according to current embryo transfer recommendations are unlikely to result in infected calves.[14] Semen from infected bulls can be infected with MAP, even subclinically infected bulls.[15] However, semen from bulls kept in commercial bull studs is considered to have a very low risk of transmission, as these animals are rigorously tested for MAP. Herd sires (dairy and beef) should, therefore, be tested annually to ensure their negative status.

Most infections with MAP occur in the early neonatal period and are often associated with the calf sucking the manure-contaminated teat and udder when ingesting colostrum.[16] Multiple-use maternity pens can serve as focal points to spread the infection to the neonates. MAP may be passed through the colostrum and milk of cattle in the later stages of infection.[17,18] It has been demonstrated that colostrum from known infected cows is a much greater risk to spread MAP to calves compared with colostrum from known negative dams.[19] The practice of feeding pooled colostrum or waste milk may help spreading the infection from infected adults to many calves in the herd and should be discouraged. It is also important to note that MAP can survive pasteurization temperatures, therefore, colostrum and milk from known infected cows should not be used.[20]

Because beef calves nurse their dams from birth to several months of age, there may be more opportunity for transmission via MAP-positive colostrum and milk as well as through the exposure to adult cattle that may potentially be shedding MAP. With dairy calves, physical separation to calf hutches or, better yet, to another property, such as a commercial heifer-raising facility, reduces the risk of MAP transmission to the replacement stock.

Susceptibility to Infection

It is widely accepted that resistance to MAP infection increases with age.[21–23] The mechanism for increased susceptibility of young calves has not been determined with certainty; but possible explanations may include (1) the openness of the newborn calf's gut that allows him to absorb immunoglobulins in colostrum could represent a permissive barrier for MAP organisms and (2) the calf's immune system is immature when compared with that of an adult cow.[24]

Age-related resistance to infection can, however, be overcome by the pressure of infection. Replacement stock and adult cattle that are exposed to MAP-contaminated forages, water, and extremely contaminated environments could get infected with MAP. For example, the practice of offering feed refusals from adult cattle to younger heifers has been shown to be a significant risk factor to spread MAP.[25] Additionally, dairy herds using an intensive grazing system (also known as a leader-follower system) may have an increased risk of transmission to the replacement stock due to the continuous low-level exposure to MAP organisms in the pasture.[26] As noted earlier, unless massive and repeated doses of MAP are consumed, this is likely to be a relatively low risk for adult cows but could represent an important risk to younger replacement stock. One could also argue that cattle that become infected later in age may not start shedding MAP and develop clinical signs of Johne disease before they leave the herd for other unrelated reasons.

Susceptibility to infection with MAP can also be genetically influenced. It was suggested that certain breeds of cattle (Guernsey, Jersey, and *Bos indicus* breeds) and certain family lines may have a genetic predisposition to becoming infected with MAP.[27–30] Based on numerous published studies, the heritability of paratuberculosis in dairy cattle is estimated to be approximately 9% to 12%.[31] Several factors contribute to the variation in reported heritability estimates, including the level of MAP exposure in a given herd, the accuracy of the diagnostic tests and samples used, herd management, and sample size.[32] The nucleotide-binding oligomerization domain containing 2 gene, a well-characterized gene that contributes to the predisposition to Crohn disease in humans,[33,34] was also shown to have a significant association with MAP infection status in Brahman X Angus crossbred and Holstein-Friesian populations.[35,36] Other candidate genes have been associated with susceptibility to MAP infection in cattle, though few candidate genes or markers have been validated between studies.[37–40] In a recent study looking at the identification of loci associated with susceptibility to MAP tissue infection in cattle, the investigators concluded that many positional candidate genes are involved in signal transduction, have immunologic functions, or have putative functional relevance in MAP entry into host cells.[32] More specifically, the study supported 2 previously identified single nucleotide polymorphisms within a quantitative trait loci (QTL) on BTA16 and identified 16 new QTL, including 2 found in the US Pacific Northwest and the Northeast, associated with MAP tissue infection.[32] Genotyping assays targeting those specific genes may be useful in the future to allow producers to select cattle that are less susceptible to the disease.

Introduction into the Herd

In a herd with no previous history of Johne disease, the introduction of the infection is most likely to occur through the purchase of infected animals. Because of the long incubation period, an infected cow could show no clinical signs of Johne disease, and may test negative on both serologic and fecal culture tests. The carrier animal could then be purchased, brought into the herd, and later serve as a source of infection when she begins shedding the organism. Other breaks in biosecurity, such as farm equipment, boots, and clothing contaminated with feces, could all, in theory, serve as ways of transmission of MAP into a new herd. However, the most important way of introducing MAP into a susceptible herd remains by the addition of subclinically infected animals.

PATHOGENESIS AND STAGES OF *MYCOBACTERIUM AVIUM* SUBSPECIES *PARATUBERCULOSIS* INFECTION
Entry of the Organism

Early studies suggested that 10^3 bacilli were infectious and that with a concentration of 10^6 to 10^8 MAP colony forming units (CFU) per gram of feces, only a few milligrams of manure ingested by a young calf would be infectious.[41–43] Experimental studies have shown that 1.5×10^6 CFU per dose given orally at days 21 and 22 of age reliably induced infection in multiple tissues, yet at a low level.[44] Higher doses at younger ages resulted in greater tissue infection.[44] Following oral ingestion, most evidence points to the ileum as the main portal of entry. More specifically, the M cells are thought to have a major role in the uptake of MAP from the intestinal lumen.[45] The MAP organisms are taken up by the M cells and released on the submucosal side of the intestinal epithelium where they will be captured by macrophages. The time required for intestinal translocation from the mucosa to the adjacent lymph nodes may be as short as 1 hour.[46]

From this point on, whether an animal becomes infected with MAP depends on its immune response. If the macrophages are successful at killing the phagocytosed MAP, the host has a chance of fighting and clearing MAP. But because MAP organisms have the ability to survive within macrophages, most likely by preventing maturation and acidification of the phagocytic vacuole,[47] the animal may become infected and start the long incubation period that is typical of MAP infections.

Stage I: Silent Infection

Once infection occurs, the organism proliferates slowly in the jejunal and ileal mucosa and spreads to the regional lymph nodes over time.[48] This silent infection phase (also known as the eclipse phase) usually lasts for a minimum of 2 years and possibly for 10 years or more. In herds with a high prevalence of Johne disease, cattle in stage I may proceed to stage II or even stage III by 1 year of age. From this, it is inferred that the rate of progression of paratuberculosis is dose dependent and also depends on the age at infection.

Stage I–infected cattle show no outward clinical signs of infection, and there is no appreciable effect on growth or production. Cattle in this phase of infection have no detectable serum antibodies to MAP and may shed MAP in their feces but at a level less than the levels of detection using current methods, including culture and polymerase chain reaction (PCR), hence, the name eclipse phase. At postmortem examination, the organisms in the tissues may not be visible on microscopic examination but may be detectable by culture of multiple intestinal tissues,[44,49] suggesting that widespread dissemination occurs early in the disease development.

Stage II: The Infection Progresses

Cattle enter this disease stage with higher concentrations of MAP in their intestinal tissues. Although these animals still do not manifest weight loss or diarrhea, they have histologic changes consistent with the intestinal granulomatous inflammatory response characteristic of paratuberculosis. Cattle in stage II may have an altered immune response with an increased gamma interferon response by sensitized T cells to specific mitogens and/or an increased antibody response to MAP.[50] Animals in stage II may shed MAP in their manure, contaminating the environment and serving as sources of infection to other animals on the farm.

The rate of disease progression through stage II is highly variable and is most likely influenced by a wide range of factors that may include the age at the initial exposure to MAP, the dose of MAP at the initial exposure, the frequency of re-exposure over time, genetic factors of both the host and the organism, environmental factors, nutritional factors, production effects, and a variety of stressors. In addition to the progression of the intestinal infection, dissemination of MAP organisms to other organs, such as the uterus and mammary gland, may now occur.[17,18,51]

Although these animals still do not show signs of Johne disease, studies have shown that subclinically infected cattle have a reduced milk production and reduced reproductive efficiency when compared with uninfected animals.[52-54] Those differences, however, may be mild enough that they may not be detectable to the producer or veterinarian.

Stage III: Clinical Disease Begins

Animals at this stage have gradual weight loss and loose manure despite a normal appetite. The vital signs, heart rate, respiratory rate, and temperature are normal. Milk production and reproductive efficiency are affected.[10] Nearly all animals at stage III are positive for MAP organisms on fecal culture or fecal PCR and have increased antibodies detectable by the enzyme-linked immunosorbent assay (ELISA) test or the agar gel immunodiffusion (AGID) test.[24]

At this stage, the MAP population within the intestinal mucosal cells is very high.[10] The normal absorptive capacity of the bowel is abrogated, resulting in weight loss associated with a protein-losing enteropathy.[24] The proliferation of reactive lymphocytes, epithelioid macrophages, and giant cells results in infused blunted villi with decreased absorptive capacity.[24] The infection becomes disseminated with MAP detectable in several extraintestinal sites. These cows are at a higher risk of transmitting the organism in utero and have a higher frequency of MAP isolated from the milk.[17,18,51] Cattle in stage III shed high concentrations of MAP in their feces, contaminating the environment.[10]

Stage IV: Advanced Clinical Disease

Animals in the advanced stages of the disease are weak, emaciated, and usually have chronic, profuse diarrhea.[10] The feces do not have blood or mucus, and the cows do not exhibit tenesmus. Intermandibular edema or bottle jaw is characteristic of this phase of the disease secondary to the hypoproteinemia. Animals can progress quickly from stage II to stage IV, sometimes within a few weeks; but a more gradual progression is more typical. Animals in stage IV shed massive amounts of MAP in their feces and have a high antibody response on ELISA. Once the diarrhea is profuse and hypoproteinemia occurs, the animal's condition deteriorates rapidly, often in a matter of days. Most animals are sent to slaughter for salvage at this point. Otherwise, death occurs as a result of dehydration and cachexia.

DIAGNOSIS OF PARATUBERCULOSIS IN CATTLE

Several diagnostic methods are available for the detection of MAP infection in cattle, and each have their relative merits and applications. They are classically divided into 2 categories: (1) immune-based tests that detect the animal's immune response to MAP and (2) organism detection tests that detect MAP organisms or MAP bacterial DNA.

Immune-Based Tests

The most commonly applied immune tests are those that detect antibodies in serum or milk. These tests include the complement fixation test, AGID, and ELISA. ELISA is the most specific and sensitive of the commercially available tests.[55]

The main advantages of ELISA are that many samples can be processed at the same time, the rapid turnaround time, and relatively lower cost, when compared with culture. If run on milk, ELISA can be incorporated to routine Dairy Herd Improvement Association testing, adding convenience of sampling to its advantages. The main disadvantage of any antibody detection method is related to the biology of the organism and its long incubation period and, consequently, the delay in the development of antibodies to MAP following infection.[56] As a result, the sensitivity of milk or serum ELISA in subclinical animals is low (around 15%) but much higher (around 90%) in clinically affected cattle.[57] Overall, the sensitivity of serum ELISA is estimated at 30% when compared with necropsy.[58] The specificity of milk or serum ELISA is high (around 98% to 100%).[57] It is highly recommended to interpret ELISA results quantitatively (ie, based on ELISA optical density or sample to positive [S/P] ratios) rather than qualitatively (ie, positive/negative), as the former has a better correlation with the likelihood of infection and level of fecal shedding.[59,60]

Organism-Detection Tests

Diagnostic tests that aim at detecting MAP include bacterial culture of fecal or tissue samples and detection of MAP DNA in fecal or tissue samples by PCR. Tissue culture or PCR is mostly used in research settings and will not be discussed here, focusing rather on fecal culture and PCR.

Advantages of organism-detection tests over antibody detection methods include (1) earlier detection in subclinically infected animals as fecal shedding typically precedes antibody detection; (2) definitive identification of MAP (or MAP DNA) in a herd at the time of testing; and (3) quantification of the MAP fecal shedding within an individual. Both culture and PCR can be applied to individual, pooled, and environmental samples. The main disadvantages of culture are related to the relatively higher cost per sample and the slow turnaround process (up to 8 weeks for liquid culture systems and up to 16 weeks for solid media). PCR has a much faster turnaround time than culture but is also more expensive when compared with ELISA. PCR allows for quantitative estimation of fecal shedding and has been shown to correlate well with fecal culture results.[61] A positive culture result confirms the presence of viable MAP, and allows strain differentiation. Detection of MAP by PCR does not confirm the presence of viable organisms and does not permit strain differentiation. In herds that are heavily infected with MAP, culture and PCR results should also be interpreted carefully, as low-positive results could represent pass-through of MAP organisms consumed by the animals, rather than active shedding.[26,62] The sensitivity of culture is estimated to be around 60% when compared with necropsy, with a specificity greater than 99%.[58] Sensitivity and specificity of PCR are similar to that of culture.[63,64]

Testing Strategies

The diagnosis of infection in cattle depends in part on whether diagnostic efforts are aimed at detecting infection in an individual animal or a herd. A consensus statement regarding testing recommendations for US cattle was published in 2006.[58] The main purpose of the report was to provide simple, practical, and cost-effective recommendations for cattle herds. Those recommendations were summarized and adapted by Collins[60] in a 2011 review article on the diagnosis of paratuberculosis. Another consensus statement on paratuberculosis issued by the American College of Veterinary Internal Medicine and published in 2012 covered diagnostic test recommendations for various testing purposes.[62] **Table 1** is a summary of the testing recommendations for various purposes encountered in dairy and beef cattle production, adapted from the previously mentioned recommendations.[58,60,62] In **Table 1**, a separate mention is given to seed stock herds (dairy and beef herds that produce cattle for sale as breeding stock), as MAP-infected cattle are not considered suitable for breeding stock and should, therefore, be held to more rigorous testing.[60]

Diagnostic Testing in a Known-Infected Herd

In a known-positive herd, the main goal is to decrease the environmental MAP load and, therefore, decrease the risk of exposure to susceptible animals. The determination of individual cow's MAP infection status will facilitate cow and calf management around calving (ie, segregation of calving areas, colostrum management) and culling of high-positive cows. In commercial herds with high prevalence (>5%), individual ELISA on milk or serum is recommended, keeping in mind to interpret results quantitatively, based on S/P ratios. In low-prevalence herds (<5%), organism detection tests

Table 1			
Recommended diagnostic tests for dairy and beef cattle by testing purpose			
Testing Purpose	**Commercial[a] Dairy Cattle**	**Commercial[a] Beef Cattle**	**All Seed Stock[b]**
Control program in high prevalence (>5%) herds	ELISA (milk or serum)	ELISA (serum)	Fecal culture or PCR on individual animals
Control program in low prevalence (<5%) herd	Pooled or individual fecal culture or PCR	Pooled or individual fecal culture or PCR	Fecal culture or PCR on individual animals
Surveillance[c]	Environmental or pool fecal culture	Confirmatory testing of clinical suspects	NR[e]
Eradication[d]	Pooled fecal culture or pooled fecal PCR	Pooled fecal culture or pooled fecal PCR	Fecal culture or PCR on individual animals
Confirm a clinical diagnosis in herds with no prior confirmed MAP	Necropsy, fecal culture, or PCR on affected animals	Necropsy, fecal culture, or PCR on affected animals	Culture or PCR and histopathology on biopsy or necropsy-collected tissues
Confirm a clinical diagnosis in MAP-positive herd	ELISA, fecal culture, or PCR	ELISA, fecal culture, or PCR	Culture or PCR and histopathology on biopsy or necropsy-collected tissues

Abbreviation: NR, not recommended

[a] Commercial indicates dairy and beef herds that do not produce cattle for sale as breeding stock.

[b] Seed stock indicates dairy and beef herds that produce cattle for sale as breeding stock.

[c] Surveillance = estimation of biological burden.

[d] Eradication = eliminate MAP from the herd.

[e] Seed stock should either be classified as test-negative or work toward this goal.

Adapted from Collins MT. Diagnosis of paratuberculosis. Vet Clin Food Anim 2011;27(3):582; with permission.

(culture or PCR) on pooled or individual fecal samples is recommended based on the low predictive value of ELISA positive in those herds.[60]

Diagnostic testing to determine herd Mycobacterium avium subspecies paratuberculosis status (surveillance)

A producer or practitioner may elect to determine the MAP status of a given herd as part of, or outside the boundaries of, a voluntary Johne disease control program. Specific guidelines have been put in place for participation in the US Voluntary Bovine Johne's Disease Control Program, the Canadian Voluntary Johne's Disease Prevention and Control Program, and control programs at other governing bodies. The reader should defer to those guidelines for more specifics on what the programs entail in the respective countries. Commonly used strategies aiming at determining the MAP status of a herd often include environmental testing, testing of pooled fecal samples via culture or PCR, testing of individual animals via fecal culture/PCR or ELISA, and bulk tank milk ELISA testing. Individual animal testing can be done on each animal in the herd (very expensive), a random statistical subset of animals, or from specifically targeted animals based on age or suspicion of diseases.

Environmental testing: Composite environmental manure samples can serve as an excellent proxy to detect herd infection. In one study, composite environmental manure samples from 64 herds known to be infected with MAP detected 50 (78%) of the 64 herds.[65] Refinement of the environmental manure sampling to include composite or pooled manure samples from high cow traffic areas, manure storage areas, and manure from pens/lots representing all cow groups has further increased diagnostic sensitivity to detect herd infection.[66,67]

Fecal pooling: As expected, the sensitivity of pooled fecal cultures strongly depends on the pool size and the shedding level of the cows included in the pool. An evaluation of pooled fecal samples (1:5) in a range of infected dairy herds detected at least 88% of samples that contained at least one animal with moderate to high shedding.[67] Optimal pool size depends on both prevalence and herd size. Samples size can vary from 3 samples per pool for a 500-cow herd with low prevalence to 5 samples per pool for a 1000-cow herd with high prevalence.[68]

Diagnostic testing for eradication

The choice of test is dictated by herd prevalence and by how quickly and aggressively producers want to eradicate MAP from their herd. In general, the fastest approaches are also the most expensive to the producer. For example, whole-herd individual fecal culture or PCR followed by culling of positive animals has a better chance of quickly eradicating MAP from a seed stock herd but may be costly, whereas a less expensive (and less aggressive) approach might involve pooled fecal culture or PCR or serum/milk ELISA.

Diagnostic testing for individual animals

Diagnostic testing for individual animals that is aimed at confirming a clinical diagnosis (or suspicion) of Johne disease is summarized in **Table 1**. Diagnostic testing of an individual or group of animals that are not showing signs of Johne disease (prepurchase screening) is difficult, especially in animals that are less than 36 months of age, as most of those animals are still in the incubation phase and are not shedding MAP at detectable levels or producing antibodies to MAP yet. A producer would be better advised to acquire information on the Johne disease status of the herd of origin and buy cattle only from certified negative herds or, better yet, never purchase cattle from outside sources.

CONTROL OF PARATUBERCULOSIS IN CATTLE

Testing for MAP is of very little value if there are little to no efforts made at pursuing management changes within the herd or poor commitment to act on the test results. Johne disease can be successfully controlled with the implementation of long-term management strategies.

For negative herds, the goal is to remain MAP free. For that, herds need to be run in a closed fashion without the introduction of animals from other herds or participation to auctions or shows where there is a potential for contact with infected animals and herds must grow from within.

For infected herds, the goal is to work toward reducing the prevalence of MAP infection within the herd. The 3 cornerstones are to (1) prevent new infections, (2) manage infected cattle appropriately, and (3) improve resistance to MAP.

Prevent New Infections

It is widely accepted that most new infections occur during the neonatal period and that most infections occur via the fecal-oral route. Therefore, management strategies that are aimed at decreasing MAP exposure to the young replacement stock are likely to have the most impact.

- *Calving area*: Identify MAP-positive cows and use separate calving areas than for MAP-negative cows; use individual calving pens and maintain clean pens; and separate calves from cows immediately after birth. The main goal is to decrease fecal exposure to the newborn calf.
- *Colostrum management*: Only feed colostrum from MAP-negative cows; bank MAP-free colostrum; do not pool colostrum; and heat-treat colostrum.
- *Calf rearing*: Same as for the calving area, the goal here is to decrease fecal exposure to the replacement stock. Raise calves away from adult cattle (different farm or geographic location, calf hutches, and so forth); feed milk replacer or pasteurized milk; prevent contamination of feed and water with manure from the adult herd; do not feed manger sweepings or share the pasture/water source with the adult herd.
- *Chemoprophylaxis*: Prophylactic administration of an antimicrobial agent to neonatal calves during the period of high susceptibility and high exposure may represent an additional approach to preventing or controlling MAP infection. Gallium, a trivalent semimetal that shares many similarities with ferric iron, has been shown to inhibit the growth of multiple strains of MAP in vitro and to significantly lower the MAP tissue burden of treated calves that were experimentally infected.[69,70] Gallium, if used as a feed additive in milk replacer, could represent an additional tool in the prevention of infection.

Monensin, an ionophore, was shown to reduce the number of MAP organisms in the tissues of calves experimentally infected and reduce MAP fecal shedding in naturally infected cattle and was associated with decreased odds of positive ELISA in animals raised in positive herds.[71–73] In the United States, monensin is approved for use in food-producing animals for the prevention of coccidiosis, and ameliorate feed efficiency, but not for the prevention or treatment of paratuberculosis. In Canada, monensin is also labeled for the reduction of MAP fecal shedding in mature cattle in high-risk herds, as a component of Johne disease control.

Manage Infected Cattle

Test and cull: Depending on the herd prevalence and the producer's goals (ie, eradiation or decreasing prevalence), culling may include all positive animals or may be targeting the most infectious cows. If the decision is made to cull only the most infectious cows, clear identification and possible segregation of the remaining positive cattle should be done. Clear identification will help in the management of the calving pen and colostrum administration. MAP-positive cattle that develop other production disorders, such as mastitis, lameness, or poor fertility, should be added to the cull list. The same test and cull strategies should be used with beef cattle. In addition, in dairy and beef herds whereby one or multiple bulls are used, annual testing should be conducted to ensure that bulls are MAP negative.

Improve Resistance

Vaccination: Vaccination in cattle has been used with mixed results. Vaccination has been shown to decrease MAP fecal shedding in infected animals, prevent progression of infected animals to clinical diseases, and, in conjunction with husbandry changes, can decrease the incidence of infection in herds.[74] However, vaccination does not fully prevent infection and is available only on a limited basis in cattle in the United States.[75] Because Johne disease vaccines may interfere with diagnostic testing for bovine tuberculosis,[76] the use of the vaccine is regulated and purchase and administration are limited to state-approved veterinarians. Emphasis should be placed on the fact that, in cattle, vaccination does not replace good husbandry and that its use should be reserved to herds with very high prevalence.

Genetic resistance: As stated earlier, more data are emerging showing some degree of host genetic susceptibility to MAP infection in cattle.[31] Using genetic testing as a tool to select animals that are more resistant to MAP infection may become the standard approach to Johne disease control in a near future.

SUMMARY

Since first reported in the late 1800s, JD remains one of the most important diseases of cattle worldwide. In cattle, the disease is debilitating and is characterized by weight loss and chronic diarrhea in the later stages of infection. However, cattle in the subclinical stages of the disease often show decreased milk production and are at a higher risk for the development of other common production diseases, such as mastitis. Infections with MAP are difficult to control because of the long incubation periods (1–7 years), the absence of clinical signs until advanced stages of the disease, and the lack of completely reliable diagnostic methods in the preclinical stages of the disease. It is general knowledge that most calves become infected very early in life. Therefore, control programs are based on preventing transmission from adult cattle shedding the MAP organisms in feces to young replacement stock on the farm. Control programs specifically focus on calving-pen management, milk- and colostrum-feeding practices, and rearing of young stock.

REFERENCES

1. Coussens PM. Mycobacterium paratuberculosis and the bovine immune system. Anim Health Res Rev 2001;2(2):141–61.
2. Whittington RJ, Marshall DJ, Nicholls PJ, et al. Survival and dormancy of *Mycobacterium avium* subsp. *paratuberculosis* in the environment. Appl Environ Microbiol 2004;70(5):2989–3004.
3. Grant IR, Hitchings EI, McCartney A, et al. Effect of commercial-scale high-temperature, short-time pasteurization on the viability of *Mycobacterium avium* subsp. *paratuberculosis* in naturally infected cow's milk. Appl Environ Microbiol 2002;68(2):602–7.

4. Godden S, McMartin S, Feirtag J, et al. Heat-treatment of bovine colostrum. II: effects of heating duration on pathogen viability and immunoglobulin G. J Dairy Sci 2006;89:3476–83.

5. Van Metre DC, Tennant BC, Whitlock RH. Infectious diseases of the gastrointestinal tract. In: Divers TJ, Peek SF, editors. Rebhun's diseases of dairy cattle. 2nd edition. St-Louis (MO): Elsevier; 2008. p. 279–83.

6. Lombard JE. Epidemiology and economics of paratuberculosis. Vet Clin North Am Food Anim Pract 2011;27(3):525–35.

7. USDA. Johne's disease on US dairies, 1991-2007. Fort Collins (CO): USDA-APHIS-VS, CEAH, National Animal Health Monitoring System; 2008. N521.0408.

8. USDA. What do I need to know about Johne's disease in beef cattle? Fort Collins (CO): USDA-APHIS-VS, CEAH, National Health Monitoring System; 1999. N309–N899.

9. USDA. Johne's disease on US dairy operations, 2002. Fort Collins (CO): USDA-APHOIS-VS, CEAH, Natl Anim Health Monit Syst; 2005. N427–N420205.

10. Whitlock RH. Johne's disease. In: Smith BP, editor. Large animal internal medicine. 4th edition. St Louis (MO): Elsevier; 2009. p. 881–7.

11. Aly SS, Thurmond MC. Evaluation of *Mycobacterium avium* subsp *paratuberculosis* infection of dairy cows attributable to infection status of the dam. J Am Vet Med Assoc 2005;227(3):450–4.

12. Whittington RJ, Windsor PA. *In utero* infection of cattle with *Mycobacterium avium* subsp. *paratuberculosis*: a critical review and meta-analysis. Vet J 2009;179(1):60–9.

13. Rhode RF, Shulaw WP. Isolation of *Mycobacterium paratuberculosis* from the uterine flush fluids of cows with clinical paratuberculosis. J Am Vet Med Assoc 1990;197:1482–3.

14. Kruip TA, Muskens J, van Roermund HJ, et al. Lack of association of *Mycobacterium avium* subsp. *paratuberculosis* with oocytes and embryos from moderate shedders of the pathogen. Theriogenology 2003;59(7):1651–60.

15. Ayele WY, Bartos M, Svastova P, et al. Distribution of Mycobacterium avium subsp. paratuberculosis in organs of naturally infected bull-calves and breeding bulls. Vet Microbiol 2004;103(3–4):209–17.

16. NRC (National Research Council). Diagnosis and control of Johne's disease. Washington, DC: National Academies Press; 2003.

17. Sweeney RW, Whitlock RH, Rosenberger AE. *Mycobacterium paratuberculosis* cultured from milk and supramammary lymph nodes of infected asymptomatic cattle. J Clin Microbiol 1992;30:166–71.

18. Streeter RN, Hoffsis GF, Bech-Nielsen S, et al. Isolation of *Mycobacterium paratuberculosis* from colostrum and milk of subclinically infected cows. Am J Vet Res 1995;56:1322–4.

19. Nielsen SS, Bjerre H, Toft N. Colostrum and milk as risk factors for infection with Mycobacterium avium subspecies paratuberculosis in dairy cattle. J Dairy Sci 2008;91(12):4610–5.

20. Chiodini RJ, Hermon-Taylor J. The thermal resistance of *Mycobacterium paratuberculosis* in raw milk under conditions simulating pasteurization. J Vet Diagn Invest 1993;5(4):629–31.

21. Taylor AW. Experimental Johne's disease in cattle. J Comp Path 1953;63:355–67.

22. Larsen AB, Merkal RS, Cutlip RC. Age of cattle as related to resistance to infection with Mycobacterium paratuberculosis. Am J Vet Res 1975;36:255–7.

23. Windsor PA, Whittington RJ. Evidence for age susceptibility of cattle to Johne's disease. Vet J 2010;184(1):37–44.

24. Sweeney RW. Pathogenesis of paratuberculosis. Vet Clin Food Anim 2011;27(3): 537–46.
25. Rossiter CA, Burhans W. Farm specific approach to paratuberculosis (Johne's disease) control. Vet Clin Food Anim 1996;12(x):383–415.
26. Fecteau ME, Whitlock RH, Buergelt CD, et al. Exposure of young dairy cattle to *Mycobacterium avium* subsp. *paratuberculosis* (MAP) through intensive grazing of contaminated pastures in a herd positive for Johne's disease. Can Vet J 2010; 51:198–200.
27. Chiodini RJ, van Kruiningen HJ, Merkal RS. Ruminant paratuberculosis (Johne's disease): the current status and future prospect. Cornell Vet 1984;74:218–62.
28. Roussel AJ, Libal MC, Whitlock RH, et al. Prevalence and risk factors for paratuberculosis in purebred beef cattle. J Am Vet Med Assoc 2005;226:773–6.
29. Elzo MA, Rae DO, Lanhart SE, et al. Factors associated with ELISA scores for paratuberculosis in an Angus-Brahman multibreed herd of beef cattle. J Anim Sci 2006;84(1):41–8.
30. Osterstock JB, Fosgate GT, Cohen ND, et al. Familial and herd-level associations with paratuberculosis enzyme-linked immunosorbent assay status in beef cattle. J Anim Sci 2008;86(8):1977–83.
31. Kirkpatrick BW. Genetics of host susceptibility to paratuberculosis. In: Behr MA, Collins DM, editors. Paratuberculosis: organism, disease, control. Oxofordshire, United Kingdom: CABI International; 2010. p. 50–9.
32. Kiser JN, White SN, Johnson KA, et al. Identification of loci associated with susceptibility to *Mycobacterium avium* subsp. *paratuberculosis* infection in cattle. J Anim Sci 2017;95(3):1080–91.
33. Hugot JP. CARD15/NOD2 mutations in Crohn's disease. Ann New York Acad Sci 2006;1072:9–18.
34. Radford-Smith G, Pandeya N. Association between NOD2/CARD15 genotype and phenotype in Crohn's disease-are we there yet? World J Gastroenterol 2006;12:7097–103.
35. Pinedo PJ, Buergelt CD, Donovan GA, et al. Association between CARD15/NOD2 gene polymorphisms and paratuberculosis infection in cattle. Vet Microbiol 2009; 134(3–40):346–52.
36. Ruiz-Larranaga O, Garrido JM, Iriondo M, et al. Genetic association between bovine NOD2 polymorphisms and infection by *Mycobacterium avium* subsp. *paratuberculosis* in Holstein-Friesian cattle. Anim Genet 2010;41(6):652–5.
37. Mucha R, Bhide MR, Chakurkar EB, et al. Toll-like receptor TLR1, TLR2, and TLR4 gene mutations and natural resistance to *Mycobacterium avium* subsp. *paratuberculosis* infection in cattle. Vet Immunol Immunopathol 2009;128(4):381–8.
38. Koets A, Santema W, Mertens H, et al. Susceptibility to paratuberculosis infection in cattle is associated with single nucleotide polymorphisms in Toll-like receptor 2 which modulate immune responses against *Mycobacterium avium* subspecies *paratuberculosis*. Prev Vet Med 2010;93(4):305–15.
39. Verschoor CP, Pant SD, You Q, et al. Polymorphisms in the gene encoding bovine interleukin-10 receptor alpha are associated with Mycobacterium avium spp. paratuberculosis infection status. BMC Genet 2010;11:23.
40. Ruiz-Larranaga O, Garrido JM, Manzano C, et al. Identification of single nucleotide polymorphisms in the bovine solute carrier family and 11 member 1 (SLC11A1) gene and their association with infection by Mycobacterium avium subspecies paratuberculosis. J Dairy Sci 2010;93(4):1713–21.
41. Gilmour NJ, Nisbet DI, Brotherston JG. Experimental oral infection of calves with *Mycobacterium johnei*. J Comp Pathol 1965;75(3):281–6.

42. Jørgensen JB. An improved medium for culture of *Mycobacterium paratuberculosis* from bovine faeces. Acta Vet Scand 1982;23(3):325–35.
43. Whittington RJ, Fell S, Walker D, et al. Use of pooled fecal culture for sensitive and economic detection of *Mycobacterium avium* subsp *paratuberculosis* infection in flocks of sheep. J Clin Microbiol 2000;38:2550–6.
44. Sweeney RW, Uzonna J, Whitlock RH, et al. Tissue predilection sites and effect of dose on *Mycobacterium avium* subs. *paratuberculosis* organism recovery in a short-term bovine experimental oral infection model. Res Vet Sci 2006;80:253–9.
45. Momotani E, Whipple DL, Thiermann AB, et al. Role of M cells and macrophages in the entrance of *Mycobacterium paratuberculosis* into domes of ileal Peyer's patches in calves. Vet Pathol 1988;25(2):131–7.
46. Wu CW, Livesey M, Schmoller SK, et al. Invasion and persistence of *Mycobacterium avium* subsp. *paratuberculosis* during early stages of Johne's disease in calves. Infect Immun 2007;75(5):2110–9.
47. Hostetter J, Steadham E, Haynes J, et al. Phagosomal maturation and intracellular survival of *Mycobacterium avium* subspecies *paratuberculosis* in J774 cells. Comp Immunol Microbiol Infect Dis 2003;26(4):269–83.
48. Clarke CJ. The pathology and pathogenesis of paratuberculosis in ruminants and other species. J Comp Pathol 1997;116(3):217–61.
49. Stabel JR, Palmer MV, Harris B, et al. Pathogenesis of *Mycobacterium avium* subsp. *paratuberculosis* in neonatal calves after oral or intraperitoneal experimental infection. Vet Microbiol 2009;136(3–4):306–13.
50. Bassey EO, Collins MT. Study of T-lymphocyte subsets of healthy and *Mycobacterium avium* subsp. *paratuberculosis*-infected cattle. Infect Immun 1997;65(11):4869–72.
51. Sweeney RW, Whitlock RH, Rosenberg AE. *Mycobacterium paratuberculosis* isolated form fetuses of infected cows not manifesting signs of the disease. Am J Vet Res 1992;53:477–80.
52. Benedictus G, Dijkhuizen AA, Stelwagen J. Economic losses due to paratuberculosis in dairy cattle. Vet Rec 1987;121(7):142–6.
53. Lombard JE, Garry FB, McCluskey BJ, et al. Risk removal and effects on milk production associated with paratuberculosis status in dairy cows. J Am Vet Med Assoc 2005;227(12):1975–81.
54. Gonda MG, Chang YM, Shook GE, et al. Effect of Mycobacterium paratuberculosis infection on production, reproduction, and health traits in US Holstein. Prev Vet Med 2007;80(2–3):103–9.
55. Sweeney RW. Paratuberculosis (Johne's disease). In: Smith BP, editor. Large animal internal medicine. 5th edition. St Louis (MO): Elsevier; 2015. p. 834–7.
56. Sweeney RW, Whitlock RH, McAdams S, et al. Longitudinal study of ELISA seroreactivity to Mycobacterium avium subsp. paratuberculosis in infected cattle and culture-negative herd mates. J Vet Diagn Invest 2006;18:2–6.
57. Collins MT, Wells SJ, Petrini KR, et al. Evaluation of five antibody detection tests for bovine paratuberculosis. Clin Diagn Lab Immunol 2005;12:685–92.
58. Collins MT, Gardner IA, Garry FB, et al. Consensus recommendations on diagnostic testing for the detection of paratuberculosis in cattle in the United States. J Am Vet Med Assoc 2006;299:1912–9.
59. Collins MT. Interpretation of a commercial bovine paratuberculosis enzyme-linked immunosorbent assay by using likelihood ratios. Clin Diagn Lab Immunol 2002;9:1367–71.
60. Collins MT. Diagnosis of paratuberculosis. Vet Clin Food Anim 2011;27:581–91.

61. Aly SS, Mangold BL, Whitlock RH, et al. Correlation between Herrold's egg yolk medium culture and real-time quantitative polymerase chain reaction results for *Mycobacterium avium* subspecies *paratuberculosis* in pooled fecal and environmental samples. J Vet Diagn Invest 2010;22:677–83.

62. Sweeney RW, Whitlock RH, Hamir AN, et al. Isolation of *Mycobacterium paratuberculosis* after oral inoculation in infected cattle. Am J Vet Res 1992;53:1312–4.

63. Sweeney RW, Collins MT, Koets AP, et al. Paratuberculosis (Johne's disease) in cattle and other susceptible species. J Vet Intern Med 2012;26:1239–50.

64. Raizman EA, Wells SJ, Godden SM, et al. The distribution of Mycobacterium avium ssp. paratuberculosis in the environment surrounding Minnesota dairy farms,. J Dairy Sci 2004;87:2959–66.

65. Berghaus RD, Farver TB, Anderson RJ, et al. Environmental sampling for detection of *Mycobacterium avium* ssp. *paratuberculosis* on large California dairies. J Dairy Sci 2006;89:963–70.

66. Lombard JE, Wagner BA, Smith RL, et al. Evaluation of environmental sampling and culture to determine *Mycobacterium avium* subspecies *paratuberculosis* distribution and herd infection status on US dairy operations. J Dairy Sci 2006;89: 4163–71.

67. Wells SJ, Godden SM, Lindeman CJ, et al. Evaluation of bacteriologic culture of individual and pooled fecal samples for detection of *Mycobacterium paratuberculosis* in dairy cattle herds. J Am Vet Med Assoc 2003;223:1022–5.

68. van Schaik G, Stehman SM, Schukken YH, et al. Pooled fecal culture sampling for *Mycobacterium avium* subsp. *paratuberculosis* at different herd sizes and prevalence. J Vet Diagn Invest 2003;15:233241.

69. Fecteau ME, Fyock TL, McAdams SC, et al. Evaluation of the in vitro activity of gallium nitrate against *Mycobacterium avium* subsp. *paratuberculosis*. Am J Vet Res 2011;72:1243–6.

70. Fecteau ME, Whitlock RW, Fyock TL, et al. Antimicrobial activity of gallium nitrate against *Mycobacterium avium* subsp. *paratuberculosis* in neonatal calves. J Vet Intern Med 2011;25:1152–5.

71. Whitlock RW, Sweeney RW, Fyock TL, et al. Johne's disease: the effects of feeding monensin to reduce the bioburden of Mycobacterium avium subsp. paratuberculosis in neonatal calves. In: Proceedings of the Am Assoc Bov Pract. Salt Lake City (UT); 2005. 191–2.

72. Hendrick SH, Kelton DF, Leslie KE, et al. Efficacy of monensin sodium for the reduction of fecal shedding of Mycobacterium avium subsp. paratuberculosis in infected dairy cattle. Prev Vet Med 2006;75:206–20.

73. Hendrick SH, Duffield TF, Leslie KE, et al. Monensin might protect Ontario, Canada dairy cows from paratuberculosis milk-ELISA positivity. Prev Vet Med 2006; 76:237–48.

74. Kalis CH, Hesselink JW, Karkema HW, et al. Use of long-term vaccination with a killed vaccine to prevent fecal shedding of *Mycobacterium avium* subsp. *paratuberculosis* in dairy herds. Am J Vet Res 2001;62:270–4.

75. Sweeney RW, Whitlock RW, Bowesock TL, et al. Effect of subcutaneous administration of a killed *Mycobacterium avium* subsp. *paratuberculosis* vaccine on colonization of tissues following oral exposure to the organism in calves. Am J Vet Res 2009;70:493–7.

76. Santema W, Rutten V, Koets A. Bovine paratuberculosis: recent advances in vaccine development. Vet Q 2011;31:183–91.

Moving?

Make sure your subscription moves with you!

To notify us of your new address, find your **Clinics Account Number** (located on your mailing label above your name), and contact customer service at:

Email: journalscustomerservice-usa@elsevier.com

800-654-2452 (subscribers in the U.S. & Canada)
314-447-8871 (subscribers outside of the U.S. & Canada)

Fax number: 314-447-8029

Elsevier Health Sciences Division
Subscription Customer Service
3251 Riverport Lane
Maryland Heights, MO 63043

*To ensure uninterrupted delivery of your subscription, please notify us at least 4 weeks in advance of move.

ELSEVIER

Printed and bound by CPI Group (UK) Ltd, Croydon, CR0 4YY

03/10/2024

01040388-0002